Written to Answer the Needs of First-Time Parents...
The Comprehensive Reference for All of Your Questions About:

Nutrition—how to get the most from the food you eat
Weight Gain, Weight Loss—how much is too much, too little?
Month-to-Month Developments—in you, your baby and the father
Remedies for Common Discomforts—backache, impatient bladder,
 insomnia, and more
Sonograms—is it worth the picture?
Birth Defects and Genetic Counseling
Advice for Expectant Fathers
Maternity Leave and Legal Rights
Single Mothers
The Pregnancy Beauty Book—complexion, hair, grooming
Miscarriage—dispelling the myths
Pediatrician or Family Physician?
Electronic Fetal Monitors—pros and cons
Caesarean—what every expectant mother should know
Infant CPR—an indispensable chapter on emergency and first aid
Sex—your most intimate questions answered
Stimulating Your Baby to Grow and Learn
Child-Proofing Your Entire Home—plus many other safety
 precautions

The Maternity Sourcebook

230 Basic Decisions
for Pregnancy, Birth and Baby Care

WENDY and MATTHEW LESKO

WARNER BOOKS

A Warner Communications Company

Copyright © 1984 by Wendy S. Lesko and Matthew Lesko
Warner Books, Inc., 666 Fifth Avenue, New York, NY 10103

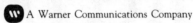 A Warner Communications Company

Printed in the United States of America

First Warner Books Printing: May 1984

10 9 8 7 6 5 4 3 2

Designed by Giorgetta Bell McRee

Library of Congress Cataloging in Publication Data

Lesko, Wendy.
  The maternity sourcebook.

  Includes bibliographies and index.
  1. Pregnancy. 2. Childbirth 3. Infants—Care
and hygiene. I. Lesko, Matthew. II. Title.
RG525.L46 1984   618.2   83-23380
ISBN 0-446-38375-9 (U.S.A.)
     0-446-38376-7 (Canada)

Contents

Introduction

We began writing this book several months before Morgan, our first child, was born. We had read dozens of books written for expectant parents but found fundamental problems with all of them. Our chief complaint was that they tended to offer only one point of view—either the "Doctor knows best" approach or an attitude of distrust regarding the medical profession and obstetrical technology. To make informed decisions, we wanted to know the facts, the pros and cons, and also be familiar with opposing viewpoints so as to make up our own minds about what was best for us.

We found, for example, that when we asked five obstetricians a question like "How long can a mother-to-be play tennis?" we received five completely different responses. Certainly when it comes to exercise during pregnancy as well as many other decisions, it boils down to one doctor's opinion against another's, particularly in those cases where there isn't enough conclusive scientific evidence, or existing research is contradictory. Not only are there few black-and-white answers, but given the endless variety of family, living and work arrangements nowadays, more often than not there are no "right" choices. Furthermore, many opportunities for the exchange of information and knowledge passed down through generations have disappeared with the decline of the extended family.

In this book, as a couple, we approach the 200-plus decisions which are encountered during the maternity cycle and the first year of life. We asked the obvious, sometimes naive, questions that anyone pregnant for the first time might wonder or worry about. Neither of us is an advocate of a particular childbirth philosophy, for example, or a single approach in disciplining a toddler.

Our principal objective throughout *The Maternity Sourcebook* is to give you enough information so that you have sufficient knowledge to know what questions to explore with an obstetrician, nurse-midwife, childbirth instructor, hospital delivery-room nurse, anesthesiologist, pediatrician, etc. Some medical terms are intentionally included along with definitions and pronounciations so you won't be intimidated by the jargon and won't feel left out of discussions with health professionals, especially during labor, when you may be confronted with making one decision right after another.

Besides being parents, both of us have spent a good deal of our professional lives tracking down information—Wendy, a reporter covering the U.S. Congress, a broadcaster for many years and currently the host of a nationally syndicated radio program for consumers; Matthew, founder of four information companies and author of several major reference books, including *Information USA*, which pinpoints the countless resources available from the federal government. In fact, the Library of Congress' National Referral Center and the government-sponsored National Health Information Clearinghouse provided us with computer printouts which helped us identify scores of organizations, federal agencies and medical schools involved with perinatal and infant research.

Experts at the National Institute of Child Health and Human Development (part of N.I.H.), the American College of Obstetricians and Gynecologists, and the American Academy of Pediatrics, along with individual researchers, mothers, nurse-midwives, obstetricians, pediatricians, psychologists and women contemplating pregnancy, were interviewed. Many of these same people checked the content and medical accuracy of practically every page of the manuscript.

It is our hope that this single volume will be comprehensive enough so you won't have to pore through half a dozen other books in search of pertinent information. However, organizations, clearinghouses, medical journals, newsletters, books and magazines which can provide you with more in-depth material are noted in all twelve chapters. Additional information sources along with a systematic approach for doing research on your own are included in the Appendix.

By all means, explore your options. Remain flexible but trust your own instincts. Before you know it, you, too, will be saying... "Having a child is one thing in life that actually turned out to be *better* than we thought it would ever be!"

Wendy and Matthew Lesko

Washington, D.C.
October 1983

Acknowledgments

Our special thanks to Marji Bayers for her enormous contribution to research and writing as well as her dedication to the objectives of this book, and to Rafe Sagalyn, our literary agent, whose idea it was in the first place.

This kind of book is so dependent on information and ideas from such a multitude of sources that it is impossible to express our appreciation individually to all those whose help was indispensable. We do want to single out a few of you who shared with us your expertise and philosophy and then volunteered much time reviewing portions of the manuscript: Charlotte Catz, M.D.; Donald McNellis, M.D.; Michaela Richardson; Brent Jaquet; Duane Alexander, M.D.; Thortsen Fjellstedt, Ph.D.; Gary Hodgen, Ph.D.; Dolores Bryla at the National Institute of Child Health and Human Development; Linda Hewes, CNM; Mort Lebow and Laurie Hall at the American College of Obstetricians and Gynecologists; Elaine Bratic and members of the Healthy Mothers, Healthy Babies coalition; Sally Tom, CNM with the American College of Nurse-Midwives; Ricky Grad, R.N. of the Alliance for Perinatal Research; Jean Lockhart, M.D.; Josephine Schuda and Joy Sotolongo of the American Academy of Pediatrics; Elaine Lawless of the National Child Passenger Safety Association; Joanne Dunne and Linda Todd with the International Childbirth Education Association; Judy Herzfeld, Ph.D., with Harvard Medical School; Ginny Crandall, CNM; Keith Johnson at the U.S. Pharmacopoeia; Dana Raphael, Ph.D., of the Human Lactation Center; Paula Pachon of the National SIDS Clearinghouse; Lucy Scott, Ph.D., of Parenthood After Thirty; Maryan McNaughton; Elayne Clift with Women in Health Roundtable.

PART I

YOUR PREGNANCY

①
Health Questions

READ THIS RIGHT AWAY

You may feel you have loads of time—nine months—to learn all you want to know about pregnancy, and, for the most part, that's true. But here are a few suggestions and some important facts you should know right away, because being unaware of them can seriously affect you and your baby in these early weeks of development.

It is so easy to get swallowed up by every "beware" and "don't." Just remember that only a tiny number of babies born here in the United States—between 2 and 3 percent—have birth defects. So we suggest, don't be too worried, and enjoy this time as much as possible.

Dollars and Cents

• *Insurance coverage.* Double-check to find out the payment schedule for your "pregnancy package," including lab tests. If you can, don't pay for all your prenatal care at once, just in case you decide later to switch doctors, as you might have trouble getting a refund.

• *Childbirth-education groups.* Many offer a free "early-pregnancy class" for expectant parents, which provides a good opportunity to check out whether you like the organization's philosophy before signing up for a six- or eight-week course.

• *IRS deductions.* Keep receipts and canceled checks for such items as prenatal vitamins if you plan to itemize your medical deductions. Also keep a record of mileage to and from the doctor's office or birth center. Check with the local IRS office or tax preparer to find out

3

what deductions are allowed in your particular case (that is, childbirth classes, books on pregnancy, special pregnancy-exercise classes).

• *Contact lenses.* Don't buy new lenses, especially hard contacts, since they probably won't fit after your baby is born, because your corneas will revert to their prepregnancy shape. Right now they may be a different size, owing to fluid retention.

• *Yard sales.* Particularly during the summer and early fall, they are a good place to buy nursery equipment and even baby clothes. These are generally in good condition, and buying them secondhand can save you considerable money.

• *Previous cesarean birth.* Given the official guidelines favoring an attempted vaginal birth after cesarean (VBAC), make sure your obstetrician is willing to give VBAC a try if you are keen on the idea. Your doctor's bill will be less, and so will your coinsurance payments, if you have a VBAC.

Medical Alert

• *Medications.* The use of drugs, including aspirin and other over-the-counter remedies, should be suspended unless you and your physician or midwife decide it is absolutely necessary to continue treatment throughout pregnancy.

• *IUD still in place.* If you are pregnant with an intrauterine device still in place you run a much greater risk of miscarriage. It's a simple procedure to remove it and eliminate the risk, as soon as you know you are pregnant.

• *Diabetes.* If you are a diabetic, your diet and insulin balance are vitally important to your baby's health, especially during the first two months.

• *Dental care.* Besides needing more calcium, you may have softer gums, more plaque buildup and perhaps more cavities. Get your teeth cleaned, and remember to brush and floss regularly. Avoid all major dental work or, if it is unavoidable, postpone it until the second trimester, and do not use gas anesthesia.

• *Previous ectopic pregnancy.* You stand a greater chance than other women of having the fertilized egg again implant itself outside your uterus. Watch out for any warning signs and notify your doctor immediately.

• *Previous abortion.* One or two elective abortions will not alter the likelihood of having a normal pregnancy or healthy child; however, not enough research has been done to learn how pregnancy outcome is affected if you have had more than two abortions.

• *DES exposure.* If you are one of two million women whose mothers took the drug diethylstilbestrol during their pregnancies, you have a slightly higher chance of miscarriage, preterm birth and ectopic pregnancy. Make sure your doctor or midwife is aware of your exposure to DES.

● *Vaccines.* The effects of vaccines on your unborn baby are not yet known, but particularly worrisome are "live" vaccines such as smallpox, rubella (German measles) and yellow fever. Only "killed" vaccines such as flu, rabies, tetanus, cholera and diptheria should be prescribed by a physician who knows you are expecting.

● *Diathermy.* If you are undergoing medical treatment by diathermy (heat), warn your therapist not to use excessively high temperatures.

Food and Drink

● *Eating for two.* The old wives' tale that the less you eat, the smaller the baby and the easier the delivery isn't true. Another myth is that after you gain eight pounds for your baby, the rest is fat. However, eating for two doesn't mean you need to consume twice as much food now that you're pregnant.

● *Dieting.* Don't skip meals or take water pills or diuretics. Your baby needs a constant stream of nutrients every day.

● *Raw meat.* Toxoplasmosis, a parasitic disease, is sometimes found in raw meat. Avoid steak tartare and eat only thoroughly cooked meat; if you handle it raw, wash your hands carefully afterward. The prenatal test called TORCH can determine if you already carry an immunity to the disease.

● *Booze.* Babies born to mothers who drink excessive amounts of beer, wine or hard liquor are likely to have some mental and physical defects. Some studies suggest that even small amounts of alcchol can cause damage, particularly during the first trimester.

● *Cigarettes.* Since smoking slows your circulation, it is also believed to inhibit the amount of nutrients and oxygen that pass through the placenta, possibly hindering your baby from growing and developing normally.

Your Surroundings

● *Occupational environment.* Evaluate your workplace, whether it is an office or a factory, to make sure you aren't exposed to such known toxins as heavy metals and gas anesthetics. A temporary change in job responsibilities may be the safest route.

● *Household pesticides or insect "bombs."* If you must spray, cover and put away all food, don't spray in closets and try to stay out of the house for 24 hours afterward.

● *Paint, paint thinner, or stripper.* Stay away from them or anything that gives off fumes.

● *Flea-dipping.* Postpone doing this to your cat or dog until after pregnancy.

• *Hair sprays.* The effects of these and other aerosols are still unknown, so be cautious.

• *Cats and litter boxes.* Cat feces can carry toxoplasmosis (also found in raw meat), a disease that can impair your baby's brain development. A veterinarian can do a simple test to see if your cat carries this parasitic infection. Try to stay away from litter boxes or anything else that may be contaminated by fecal matter. Kittens are more likely to be carriers than older cats.

• *Infectious diseases.* Stay away from anyone who has a fever or infection. See your doctor or midwife immediately if you have been exposed to rubella (German measles).

Miscellaneous Precautions

• *Buckle-up.* Medical research proves that in an automobile crash the most serious risk to your baby is that *you* will be injured. The American Academy of Pediatrics and the American College of Obstetricians and Gynecologists advise attaching your seat restraint by first sitting tall and placing the lap belt as low as possible on your hips—bikini fashion—under the baby. Wear the shoulder harness, too, since it gives you and your passenger important added protection.

• *X rays.* Because radiation has its greatest impact on growing cells, if you are X-rayed without adequate safeguards such as a lead apron to shield your abdomen, your baby runs a risk of birth defects or, possibly, childhood leukemia. No birth defects have been found to result from dosages over 10 rads, but leukemia has developed in babies exposed to lower levels. X rays to your stomach, abdomen, lower back, kidneys, hips and pelvis are particularly dangerous. Dental and chest X rays are not so worrisome, provided a skilled technician or radiologist runs the test. Still, the U.S. Food and Drug Administration in its March 1979 report, *FDA Consumer*, states that "no threshold level of exposure is completely safe." Ask if an ultrasound scan (sonogram) can be used instead. A sonogram emits sound radiation, not light, making it a far safer procedure.

• *Hot tubs and saunas.* High core body heat or "hyperthermia" is known to cause central-nervous-system disorders and other anomalies. The danger level of heat or "fever" has not yet been determined, but a University of Washington study published in the *Canadian Medical Association Journal* in July 1981 concludes that expectant mothers should limit their time in hot tubs (no more than 15 minutes at 39°C) and saunas (less than 10 minutes at 81.4°C), even when interrupted by short cooling-off periods.

• *Some sexual acts.* Blowing into the vagina is dangerous during pregnancy, since it can actually force air bubbles into your bloodstream, leading to embolism and stroke.

• *Douching.* Hand bulb syringes should not be used during pregnancy, because of the danger of air embolisms. Consult your physician or midwife for guidelines on douching.

● *Vitamin junkies.* Limit your extra vitamins to the ones prescribed in consultation with your obstetric caretaker. Megadoses of vitamin A and vitamin D are known to cause mental retardation.

Common Misconceptions

● The major support organ, the placenta, does not act as a barrier but is more like a sieve. Oxygen, nutrients and, unfortunately, some viruses and toxins are able to pass through to your baby.

● Raising your arms will not cause the umbilical cord to wrap around the baby's neck. Though the cord is wrapped around the baby's neck in approximately 25 percent of all births, it has absolutely nothing to do with the mother. The muscles involved when you reach for something on a high shelf work independently of your passenger, since it lives in its own protective, fluid-filled sac inside your uterus.

● Your baby stands no chance of drowning if you bathe or swim. Since the fetus is floating free in liquid, there is no possibility of its drowning even if water could enter the uterus. "Flooding" is next to impossible, owing to the hard mucous plug lodged in the cervix, sealing off the uterus from the vagina.

OLDER FIRST-TIME MOTHERS

Age 30 used to be the cut-off point separating "low-risk" younger women and "high-risk" expectant mothers. Now most obstetricians say 35, while others hold that real concern is unnecessary until age 40. Women in their thirties and forties do inherit certain statistical risks, such as producing a baby with Down's syndrome, although the chance of that happening is still small. Certainly the higher overall incidence of health problems, including hypertension, diabetes and heart disease, comes with the aging process, and if you enter pregnancy with any one of these conditions—regardless of age—your risks are undeniably greater. But today's emphasis on good physical fitness and medical advances in all areas are responsible for narrowing the gap between biological and chronological age. Many experts believe social and economic factors greatly influence the absolute levels of risk at any age.

Total Number of 1981 Births	
30–34 years	581,454
35–39 years	146,056
40–44 years	23,326
45–49 years	1,190

(Source: National Center for Health Statistics)

Selma Taffel of the government's National Center for Health Statistics claims, "Although women in their thirties face a higher risk of bearing infants with certain congenital anomalies than younger women do, the data on birth weight and prenatal care tend to suggest that delayed childbearing, because it is associated principally with well-educated women, carries *fewer* health risks now than perhaps was true a decade or more ago." While almost everyone agrees that older women stand a better chance now than ever before of having healthy babies with no major problems, many obstetricians view sonograms, electronic fetal monitors and other medical advances as chiefly responsible. Of course not every complication can be prevented or controlled. As Dr. Roger Freeman, author of *Safe Delivery*, says, "These days if a woman eats right and exercises and things don't come out right she has lots of guilt—years back it was God's fault."

Don't get thrown by the medical term "elderly primigravida." The expression simply refers to a woman in her thirties or forties who is pregnant for the first time. In the minds of many physicians, it does not necessarily imply a high-risk pregnancy. Pamela Davis and Kathy Weingarten, authors of *Sooner or Later: The Timing of Parenthood in Adult Lives*, maintain that "there is no single dramatic moment at which the risk of pregnancy and childbirth suddenly escalate. Rather, the increments in risk are gradual." Misleading statistics are partly to blame for the muddy picture of just when and how age affects pregnancy. For one thing, most studies on risk and maternal age tend to work in increments of five years because it is easier, not because those cutoff lines are meaningful. In comparing the age groups 30 to 34 and 35 to 39, for example, the average risk for each group is affected by the pregnancies of the 30- and 39-year-olds. So, although the risks for a woman of 35 are not significantly greater than those for a 34-year-old, the statistics from their respective groups show a marked increase. Take, for instance, the estimated incidence of Down's syndrome, which gradually rises with advancing maternal age.

Mother's Age	Down's Syndrome Estimated Incidence*
30	1 in 830–1110
31	1 in 770–1110
32	1 in 670–910
33	1 in 530–710
34	1 in 420–530
35	1 in 260–400
36	1 in 200–310
37	1 in 160–240
38	1 in 120–190
39	1 in 95–150
40	1 in 73–120
41	1 in 56–93
42	1 in 43–72
43	1 in 33–57
44	1 in 25–44
45	1 in 19–35
46	1 in 15–27
47	1 in 11–21
48	1 in 9–17
49	1 in 7–13

*These rates, published in 1981, do not take into account other predisposing risk factors aside from maternal age.

(Source: Birth Defects Institute, New York State Department of Health)

Many theories attempt to explain why chromosomal aberrations occur more frequently in older women. With regard to paternal age, there is suggestive but still not conclusive evidence that fathers over age 50, perhaps 55, may have a slight effect on the incidence of Down's syndrome (see "Birth Defects and Genetic Counseling," p. 76, and "Amniocentesis: Risky or Not?" p. 82).

The gradual rise in age-related risks is best visualized in a J-shaped curve. Teenagers and women over 40 figure at the top of both sides of the "J," while along the bottom lie the 20- to 29-year-old mothers, with the line then climbing sharply as women age. Unlike Down's syndrome, which unequivocally climbs year by year, other risks are not as clear-cut; and in fact, many pregnancy complications are in no way affected by advancing maternal age.

DIRECTLY RELATED TO AGE	INDIRECTLY RELATED	UNRELATED TO AGE
Miscarriage. Likelihood increases with age be-	*Toxemia* (placenta may cease to function). In-	*Ectopic Pregnancy* (egg implanted outside

DIRECTLY RELATED TO AGE	INDIRECTLY RELATED	UNRELATED TO AGE
cause of higher rate of birth defects; uterus may have less room to grow due to fibrous benign tumors, primarily in women over 40	cidence higher among first-time mothers, especially teenagers, although, since high blood pressure is one of the symptoms, toxemia may be indirectly linked to advancing age	womb). Not associated with age but not uncommon among older women with histories of tubal or ectopic pregnancies who used fertility drugs
Genetic Defects. Incidence of chromosomal abnormalities such as Down's syndrome rises with age	*Premature Delivery.* Mothers age, 30–34 are least likely to give birth to low-weight infants (incidence of low birth weight is closely linked with preterm delivery), while mothers in their forties are more likely to bear smaller babies	*Placenta Problems.* Not as common in first-time mothers and non-smokers
Twins. Multiple births tend to increase with advancing age, generally peaking among women 35 to 39, then declining		*Long Labor.* Length of labor is not related to mother's age but depends primarily on whether or not this is first child
Cesarean Delivery. Rate increases with age, particularly for first-time mothers 35 and over	*Labor Disorders.* Some theorize that among older women contractions may not be as effective because of less efficient muscular lining of uterus	*Postdelivery Hemorrhage or Infection.* Related to birth environment and other factors, not to age

Most obstetricians, tending not to take any chances, treat women in the age bracket 35 to 45 with kid gloves. Part of the reason is that it is impossible to predict how your body will handle the physical demands of pregnancy and especially childbirth, because you have an "untested pelvis." Of course, this holds true for every first-time mother regardless of age, but the uncertainty becomes more relevant in those so-called premium pregnancies, where this is a woman's only or last chance to have a child. The cesarean (C-section) rates for women over 30 are higher than for other age groups, and according to the National Center for Health Statistics, in 1981 the rates "were highest in the Northeast at 20% among older women, among married women, and in proprietary [private] hospitals." Where some physicians will order every diagnostic test and be more inclined to perform a cesarean, other obstetricians take no special precautions so long as there are no signs of potential complications.

Much of the way you are treated depends on the "customary

practice in that community setting," according to Dr. Joan Mulligan, professor at the University of Wisconsin's Medical School. If an obstetrician deviates from the way "older" women are traditionally managed in that community, he or she runs a greater chance of being charged with malpractice if anything goes wrong. A lawsuit for failure to perform a cesarean is by no means uncommon, which explains why surgery is often done at the least sign of "trouble"; yet not all hospitals have a dramatically higher cesarean rate among first-time mothers over 35.

Special Considerations

The following advance preparations contribute to your degree of control and participation in your medical care as well as to your morale throughout pregnancy and childbirth.

(1) *Health-care team.* If you are thinking in terms of this being your only chance to have a baby, you should not have much trouble finding an obstetrician specializing in so-called premium pregnancies, who probably will be more interventionist (continuous electronic monitoring during labor; more likely to do a C-section). However, if you are healthy and don't want to be treated automatically as a high-risk pregnancy, most likely you will have to scout around. Inquire about your hospital's policy on allowing the patient and doctor to decide, for instance, on the use of fetal monitors. Should you choose a certified nurse-midwife and perhaps an out-of-hospital birth center, check on the credentials and experience of the backup physician.

(2) *Genetic counseling and amniocentesis.* Don't go to see a genetic counselor without first finding out about his/her qualifications and fees, which often are not covered by insurance. More important, if you decide to have amniocentesis, check out the reputation of both the doctor doing it as well as the lab responsible for analyzing the cells. (see "Birth Defects and Genetic Counseling," p. 76, and "Amniocentesis: Risky or Not?" p. 82).

(3) *Nutrition and fitness.* Don't diet now, even if you are overweight; monitor your weight instead, so that it increases gradually. Although physical fitness cannot stop the aging process, it can help boost your stamina to handle the added demands of pregnancy and childbirth. Just don't overdo it. Should problems develop, "pelvic rest," meaning no exercise, and possibly bed rest, may be the best course.

(4) *Childbirth classes.* Besides selecting a program that coincides with your philosophy, you may want to see which instructors tend to attract an older crowd if you think you might feel self-conscious about being the "grandparent" in the class (see p. 106).

(5) *Prevention of premature delivery.* If you have had previous preterm labor, get your doctor or midwife to teach you how to detect the subtle symptoms of early labor (see "Premature Labor: Catching It in Time," p. 167).

(6) *Cesarean preparation.* Since you stand a greater chance of having a C-section, read up on it (see "Cesarean: What Every Expectant Mother Should Know," p. 260). Talk with your doctor about medications, the type of incision to be made, whether the father is allowed in the operating room, the hospital's policy on being with the baby after delivery, etc. Parents who have a better notion of what to expect and have made their preferences known ahead of time tend to be more satisfied than those who focus only on a vaginal delivery and unexpectedly end up with a cesarean.

(7) *Switch doctors.* If you see an obstetrician who specializes in high-risk pregnancies but your pregnancy turns out to be an ordinary one, find out if he or she intends to be with you during labor or pass you on to another obstetrician. Of course, if you are dissatisfied or uneasy with your physician, shop around for someone else (see p. 94).

(8) *Child Care.* If you intend to return to work, don't wait until your baby is born to make arrangements (see "Day Care, Live-Ins and Babysitters," p. 334).

There is no doubt that you will handle pregnancy differently now—both emotionally and physically—than if you were in your early twenties, but unless you have health problems, don't waste energy worrying. Dr. Lucy Scott, of the Parenthood After Thirty project, says: "Yes, there are risks. Don't expect a total guarantee that you will have a trouble-free birth and healthy baby but if you are in good physical health, if you take advantage of preconception counseling, early, high-quality prenatal care, amniocentesis and the latest obstetrical technology, your overall risks are about the same as they were for women in all age groups in the 1960s."

Information Sources

ADDITIONAL READING

Having a Baby After 30, by Elisabeth Bing and Libby Colman (New York: Bantam, 1975). Full of personal experiences of parents over 30.

It's Not Too Late for a Baby: For Women and Men Over 35, by Sylvia Rubin (Englewood Clifts, N.J.: Prentice-Hall, 1980). Comments and advice about pregnancy for older women.

Parents After Thirty, by Murray Kappelman and Paul Ackerman (New York: Wideview Books, 1981). Handbook on making the right decision, guidelines for prenatal care.

Pregnancy After 35, by Carole McCauley (New York: Pocket Books, 1976). Genetics, nutrition and emotional stress are among topics discussed.

The Pregnancy After 30 Workbook, by Gail Brewer (Emmaus, PA.: Rodale Press, 1978). Discusses risks, nutrition, breast-feeding and parenting.

Sooner or Later: The Timing of Parenthood in Adult Lives, by Pamela Davis and Kathy Weingarten (New York: W.W. Norton, 1982). Interviews with both women who decided to have a family and those who did not.

Women Can Wait: The Pleasures of Motherhood After 30, by Terry Schultz (New York: Doubleday, 1979). Full of interviews discussing the issues involved in delayed childbearing.

ORGANIZATIONS

March of Dimes
1275 Mamaroneck Ave.
White Plains, NY 10605
International Directory of Genetic Services, which lists genetic-counseling centers throughout the world and the services offered at each center; other information also available.

Parenthood After Thirty
451 Vermont
Berkeley, CA 94707
This clearinghouse provides training, consultation, workshops and resources for professionals and those individuals making choices about parenthood.

YOUR BABY'S LIFE-SUPPORT SYSTEM

From the moment of conception until birth, special organs and chemicals assemble to form the complex apparatus that nurtures and sustains your baby's life.

Corpus Luteum. Each month your body prepares for a possible pregnancy. After ovulation a hormone-producing structure forms at the exact spot in your ovary where the mature egg is cast forth, sometimes producing a nagging, cramplike pain. During the first three months of pregnancy this compact mass of tissue is responsible for secreting plenty of estrogen and progesterone, hormones essential for making your uterus receptive to the fertilized egg. Another hormone, known as chorionic gonadotropin, is produced by specialized cells of the embryo to stimulate the corpus luteum so that it does not deteriorate until the placenta becomes self-supporting and can take over the manufacture of hormones as well as the primary responsibility for fetal growth.

Placenta. Literally meaning a large, flat cake, the placenta is the principal link between you and your baby, with a life-span only the length of gestation. It takes about three months to construct this major organ, which serves as the fetus's lungs, stomach, intestines and kidneys. In addition to nurturing, the placenta also acts as a partial barrier between the different genetic constitutions of mother and child. The other main mission of this organ, which weighs between one and three pounds at birth, is to function as a gland, producing progesterone and other hormones and enzymes essential for maintaining pregnancy.

Amniotic Sac, or "Bag of Water." This transparent capsule cushions and protects the developing fetus. It keeps the baby at an even temperature and allows the fetus to move with ease in utero; some speculate that babies even experience weightlessness. The fluid, composed of 98 percent water, traces of protein, sugar, calcium, vitamins and digestive enzymes, is constantly replenished. Throughout life in the womb, your baby drinks and inhales it. At the end of nine months, the total amount of amniotic fluid is roughly one quart.

Uterus, or Womb. Weighing only two ounces prior to pregnancy, this unique muscular organ now expands to house the fetus and its entire support system. The uterine cavity is lined with a membrane (endometrium) containing hundreds of glands. It is this lining that fills with blood and tissue during each menstrual cycle to prepare for the possible arrival of a fertilized egg. When, after one month, the ovum does finally appear it has a home all ready and waiting. The layer outside this membrane is formed of the muscles that will be used for labor contractions. At full term the enlarged uterus will weigh two pounds.

Umbilical Cord. This lifeline links the fetus with the placenta and ranges from 12 to 36 inches in length when complete at 20 weeks. One vein in the cord carries oxygen and food from the placenta to the baby. Blood from the fetus flows through two umbilical arteries to the placenta, where it gives up carbon dioxide and other fetal waste products. The umbilical cord forms by the end of the first month.

Hormones. Hormones get credit for making many things happen during pregnancy. What actually brings on labor remains a mystery, although the delicate interplay of several key hormones described below is known to be partly responsible.

- **Estrogens:**   Prepare mucous-membrane
                                   lining of the womb for the
                                   fertilized egg
                                   Ready breast cells and glands
                                   for milk production

- **Progesterone**   Thicken lining of womb so
  and other progestogens: fertilized egg can nest, or "im-
                                   plant," itself
                                   Calm muscles of uterus so
                                   they don't contract, expelling
                                   the baby prematurely
                                   Relax smooth muscles such as
                                   those in the intestines
                                   Stimulate breast growth
                                   Provide growth hormone for
                                   fetus

- **Oxytocins:**   Cause uterine contractions
                                   Maintain rhythmic contrac-
                                   tions with the help of prosta-
                                   glandins
                                   Release milk from breast

- **Prostaglandins:**   Help regulate uterine blood
                                   flow
                                   May be responsible for release
                                   of oxytocin, thus playing a
                                   role in initiating labor

Adding components of the support system all together, you can understand how many prenatal specialists recommend a weight gain of roughly 25 pounds:

Baby	7.5 lbs. (average)
Placenta	2.0 lbs.
Amniotic Fluid	2.0 lbs.
Uterus	2.0 lbs.
Increased Blood Flow	4.0 lbs.
Fat and Water	6.0 lbs.
Enlarged Breasts	1.0 lb.
Total Weight Gain	24.5 lbs.

Your weight gain should be modest until you pass the halfway point, largely because your new pregnancy equipment is still incomplete. By the twentieth week, though, the entire apparatus is operational and will remain in high gear until birth (see "Nutrition and Essential Extra Pounds," p. 26).

Estimated Timetable For Support System

First Week
- *Day 1* Moment of conception: the corpus luteum already is working to secrete the growth hormones to provide environment necessary for fertilized egg
- *Day 5* Cell division causes formation of hollow ball within which an embryonic mass grows. Innermost cells will become digestive system, lungs and rest of respiratory tract, except nose; middle cells will form muscles, bones, connective tissue, circulatory system and reproductive organs; central nervous system, skin, eyes and ears will evolve from outermost cells
- *Day 7* This tiny mass burrows into the lining of your uterus. Immediately after "implantation," the embryo is *especially* sensitive to drugs, ionizing radiation and other environmental substances

Second Week
- *Day 14* Mother's blood flow is hooked up to the placenta site

Third and Fourth Weeks
- *Day 21* Yolk sac, soon to become amniotic sac, or "bag of water," develops just below tiny embryo

Fifth Week
- Placenta begins to take more definite shape

Sixth Week
- Chorionic gonadotropin, the hormone that continues to stimulate the corpus luteum, reaches a sufficiently high level at this time for it to be detected in a urine or blood test, thus confirming your pregnancy

Twelfth Week
- Placenta in operation and corpus luteum goes out of business

Twentieth Week
- Placenta and umbilical cord fully functioning

MONTH-BY-MONTH DEVELOPMENTS

Here are some physical and emotional changes you might experience during the next nine months. Some of us are lethargic and nauseated, while others never feel under the weather. Besides leafing through the previous section, "Your Baby's Life-Support System," to understand what actually triggers these metabolic and mental changes, refer to pp. 47 and 57.

Remember, every pregnancy is unique. In contrast, the miraculous pattern of growth of your unborn child rarely deviates from the timetable outlined below.

MOTHER

You cannot overestimate the changes that occur during these first three months. The demands are great as your body gears up to create and support another life. It takes time for your metabolism to adjust to the stepped-up production of certain hormones. Fatigue, nausea and mood swings are common, but usually they subside after about 12 weeks.

Physical

Sleepiness, mood swings, even food cravings and aversions are triggered in part by increased levels of estrogen and progesterone

Distribution of blood is temporarily out of kilter, because of progesterone relaxing muscular wall of blood vessels, causing dizziness or light-headedness

Sluggish gastrointestinal tract is due to higher amounts of progesterone, sometimes bringing on nausea

Breast changes and activated milk-duct apparatus are due to elevated level of chorionic gonadotropin, the hormone detected in pregnancy tests

Urinary tract muscles are relaxed, owing to higher amounts of progesterone, causing frequent urination

Almost every organ undergoes some sort of change, beginning now and continuing throughout pregnancy

Weight gain: about 1 lb./month

Common Emotions

Joy and excitement
Ambivalence about being pregnant

BABY

The transformation of fertilized egg to a miniature human being occurs within these three short months. The developing offspring is remarkably sensitive to X rays, drugs and other potentially toxic agents during this critical period, when the nervous system and all major organs are formed and physical refinements such as toenails and taste buds begin.

First Month

Embryonic mass implanted in lining of uterus by first week

Fetal placenta starts to form

Brain, lungs and digestive tract develop

Neural tube, the future nervous system, is created

Heart begins to beat, probably by third week

Ears, eyes and nose begin to form

Whole embryo (meaning "to swell") is developed by fourth week

Second Month

Embryo is about 1 in. long, weighs approximately ⅓ oz.

Human face appears

Spinal column is formed

Intestines and internal organs are present

Brain has divided into three parts

Hands, fingers, knees, ankles and toes begin to take shape

Embryo resembles tiny human being with its features and organs created

Bones begin to develop

MOTHER	**BABY**

YOUR FIRST TRIMESTER
   Common Emotions (cont.)
Anxiety about miscarriage and whether your baby is normal

Testiness and irritability, possible crying spells

FIRST THREE MONTHS IN THE WOMB

Third Month

Now called "fetus" (meaning offspring)

Fetus is 3 in. long, weighs about 1 oz.

Sex can now be identified

Mouth opens and closes

Baby swallows amniotic fluid

Kidneys function

Fingernails and signs of toenails are present

Moves arms and hands and kicks legs, although not felt by mother

---

YOUR SECOND TRIMESTER

You have just passed a physiological landmark. The baby's support system, including the placenta, is ready to work around the clock. Your body doesn't have to work so hard during the second trimester, and even your emotions have grown accustomed to the hormones that are partly responsible for changing moods. For the time being there is less bladder pressure and little nausea, and you are not so tired.

Physical

Center of gravity shifts forward to compensate for curvature of lower back

Fat is stored during first two trimesters that will serve as needed calories for growth spurt at end of pregnancy

Colostrum, the forerunner of milk, may seep through nipples

THE MIDDLE MONTHS
IN THE WOMB

The fetus is gaining weight and growing taller each day. Major brain development is rapid from the fourth month until 1½ years after birth. The brain begins to orchestrate functions of the organs and to stimulate fetal movement. The intake of calcium is important during this trimester for the construction of 222 bones.

Fourth Month

Fetus is 8–10 in. long, weighs 6 oz.

Joints are evident

Muscles can actually contract

Slow eye movements

Baby may begin to recognize your voice as early as twenty-sixth week, some theorize

Bones begin to change from cartilage to real bone

YOUR SECOND TRIMESTER
Physical (cont.)

Eyes, specifically pupils, change shape due to fluid retention and hormones

Vaginal secretion becomes heavier because of hormonal changes

Oxygen intake is increased by 20–30 percent over prepregnancy level

Uterus grows from the size of a fist to that of a small melon by 14 weeks

Blood pressure returns to normal as body produces more blood

Weight gain: 3–4 lbs./month

Common Emotions

Period of normalcy; more relaxed

Comfortable with idea of motherhood

Heightened sexuality

Growing concern about appearance and weight gain

Increasing attachment as baby moves and kicks

THE MIDDLE MONTHS
IN THE WOMB

Fifth Month

Fetus is 12 in. long, weighs about 1 lb.

Fetal placenta and umbilical cord fully operational

Heartbeat easily heard

Baby's movement felt by mother

Fingernails grow

Sixth Month

Fetus is 14 in. long, weighs 1.5 lbs.

Eye movements are rapid

Eyebrows and eyelashes grow

Skin is wrinkled and red

Baby may suck thumb

YOUR THIRD TRIMESTER

The homestretch may seem to take much longer than three months, particularly if you pass your due date. It's not uncommon to feel like a beached whale and have last-minute thoughts of panic and indecision about motherhood, especially when you cannot find a comfortable position at night.

Physical

Blood volume increases 30–40 percent, approximately 2 pints; increase

LAST THREE MONTHS
IN THE WOMB

This is the final growth spurt when the fetus gains 0.5–1 lb. a week. If your baby is born in the seventh month, it has about a 50 percent chance of survival. Survival rate jumps to about 90 percent if born at 34 weeks. Your baby acquires the last bit of equipment before birth: antibodies and protective coating of skin.

Seventh Month

Fetus is 15 in. long, weighs about 2–2.5 lbs.

YOUR THIRD TRIMESTER
Physical (cont.)

in hemoglobin mass often requires iron supplements

Volume of amniotic fluid approaches one quart

Pelvis joints soften and become wobbly partly because of increased production of the hormone relaxin

Uterus "practices" painless contractions

Metabolism speeds up near birth

Heart adapts to additional work load, actually enlarges and picks up 10 beats per minute

Weight gain: 3–4 lbs./month

Common Emotions

Proud, yet resentful of discomfort

Depressed about figure and impatient with pregnancy

Increased dependence on mate, family and/or friends

Last-minute identity crisis; concern about how your life-style will alter

Nervous about labor; anxious about unexpected events that might occur during childbirth; concern over whether your baby will be healthy and normal

"Nesting" instinct to get everything ready

LAST THREE MONTHS
IN THE WOMB

Seventh Month (cont.)

Moves frequently, stretches and kicks

Skin smoother as fat forms underneath

Protective blanket of downy hair and cheesy substance called "vernix" cover body

Eighth Month

Fetus is 16.5 in. long, weighs 4 lbs.

Eyes are formed and open

Baby usually will get in position and will stay that way until birth

This month or next baby will usually "drop" lower into pelvis

More hair on head

Ninth Month

Fetus is 20 in. long, weighs 7.5 lbs.

Brain cells develop most rapidly during this final month

Downy hair disappears, but protective coating remains

Inner ear is formed

Antibodies develop to battle whatever disease(s) you have had or have been immunized against

Head measures same circumference as shoulders

Information Sources

ADDITIONAL READING

A Child Is Born, by Lennart Nilsson *et al.* (New York: Dell, 1979). Remarkable photographs of the fetus in utero.

The First Nine Months of Life, by Geraldine Lux Flanagan (New York: Simon & Schuster, 1962). Photographs of the developing fetus.

The Secret Life of the Unborn Child, by Thomas Verny (New York: Summit, 1981). Provocative concept that everything an expectant mother thinks and feels is transmitted to her unborn child and helps shape his or her personality.

DUE DATE: KEEP IT A SECRET

A date nine months away suddenly takes on great significance once pregnancy is confirmed. It's natural to pin your hopes on your "due date" and forget that it is only the *estimated* day of delivery (EDD). Think about resisting the temptation to announce exactly when the baby is expected. It may seem unimportant now, but during the final month, when well-meaning friends and relatives keep bugging you with the question, "Any news?" you may wish you had kept it a secret.

That only one baby in ten arrives on the exact due date is an oft-quoted figure, but a *Parents* magazine 1982 poll of 64,000 mothers found a surprising 19 percent delivered on their EDD. Even with this discrepancy, that leaves more than 40 percent of all babies born after their due date.

Nothing is magical about figuring out the projected birth date. The formula is pegged to a known date, the onset of the last menstrual period, since it was then that your womb actually began to prepare itself to receive and nurture the fertilized egg. Instead of counting the required 280 days or 40 weeks from the first day of your last period, simply count backward three calendar months and add seven days to get the due date.

Even though due dates are straightforward calculations, it's easy for them to be off, for several reasons:

- wrong day for beginning of last period
- erratic menstrual cycle
- ovulation may occur earlier or later than the usual fourteenth day after the onset of menstruation

The foregoing method is geared to a 28-day cycle, so if you menstruate at longer intervals, a few more days should be added to your EDD.

Sophisticated high technology, specifically sonograms (ultrasound scans), can take a lot of the guesswork out of predicting the due date, especially if you are unclear about when your last period started. An ultrasound scan can determine the gestational age by measuring the baby's crown and rump during the first trimester. Some experts caution, however, that sonograms done during the last trimester are not accurate as to EDD because of variations in fetal growth rates. (See "Sonogram: Is It Worth the Picture?" p. 73).

Rather than pinpoint a specific day, since delivery frequently comes two weeks before or after the due date, some doctors and midwives simply say that labor probably will begin sometime between the thirty-eighth and forty-second week. Not only are you less likely to be discouraged if nothing happens on the projected birth date, but it is much easier to be vague when you are hounded by friends and relatives about when the baby is expected. In the words of a pamphlet published by the American College of Obstetricians and Gynecologists: "Even at this stage, infants keep their parents guessing. Get used to it; they go on doing it all their lives."

PRENATAL CHECKUPS: OPTIMIZING YOUR VISITS WITH YOUR DOCTOR

From the time you discover you are pregnant until labor begins, you will visit your doctor or midwife approximately 12 times: once every month until the twenty-eighth week, then every other week and finally, during the last month, weekly. These prenatal checkups not only monitor you and your baby's progress during gestation but provide an opportunity to build a relationship of understanding and mutual trust between you and your medical adviser. Each appointment will follow a predictable pattern.

CHECKPOINTS	METHOD
Weight gain	Stand on scales fully clothed. Weight gain should be gradual.
Blood pressure	A cloth band is wrapped around the upper arm and inflated; a stethoscope is placed on the artery in the arm to monitor blood pressure.
Signs of pregnancy-related illnesses (toxemia, diabetes)	With a dipstick, your urine specimen is checked for the presence of protein and sugar.
Growth rate of uterus and fetus	Fundal height (fundus refers to top of uterus) is calculated in centimeters, using tape measure between pelvic bone and uppermost section of uterus. At 5

CHECKPOINTS	METHOD
	months, the fundus is usually at the navel.
Fetal well-being	A fetoscope (similar to stethoscope) placed on your abdomen can pick up the baby's heartbeat at 20 weeks; a doptone ultrasound device can do this at 12 weeks so you can hear it. Baby's position is checked externally, by feeling location of head, limbs and buttocks.

Your initial appointment will include a review of your medical history and the father's and a thorough physical exam. If hereditary diseases run in your family or if you will be age 35 or older at the projected date of delivery, amniocentesis may be recommended (see "Amniocentesis: Risky or Not?" p. 82). If you are uncertain of when you last started to menstruate, an ultrasound scan may be suggested to pin down the baby's age in utero (see "Sonogram: Is It Worth the Picture?" p. 73). Several tests will be performed at the first prenatal checkup, including some blood tests. A blood sample can reveal a surprising amount of information about your general health:

• *Blood type.* You are either type A, B, AB or O, and you may or may not have what's termed an Rh factor. If you are diagnosed as Rh negative, you are missing a substance most people have in their red blood cells. If the father is Rh positive, the fetus will be positive and your own body may begin to produce antibodies to fight off the baby's Rh factor. This is called "Rh sensitivity," and you will have to be watched more closely throughout the nine months, so that countermeasures can be taken for control (see "Anemia, Herpes, Toxemia and Other Complicating Factors," p. 170).
• *Complete blood count* (CBC). This test counts the number of red and white blood cells in your body and measures the amount of oxygen-carrying hemoglobin as well as the total volume of cells and plasma. Low red blood count and/or low hemoglobin may mean you are anemic and need iron.
• *Serology test.* There are a number of different ones, but they all indicate if you have syphilis or Herpes Simplex Virus Type 2.
• *Rubella titre.* A test to find out if you have been exposed to rubella (German measles); if you have been, you are probably immune; if not, you should be careful to avoid exposure; rubella during the first three months of pregnancy can have serious effects on the developing fetus.
• *Toxoplasmosis* (Cat fever). Optional blood test is run to see if you've been exposed to this parasitic disease, which is contracted from a cat

that is a carrier or by eating raw meat. If you've been exposed, you may now be immune. The antibodies will show up in your blood, as they do in the case of rubella.

Often a multivitamin is prescribed routinely, along with an iron supplement. You may want to ask your doctor or midwife precisely why supplements are suggested, particularly if the results of your blood test are not yet known (see "Nutrition and Essential Extra Pounds," p. 26).

It is not uncommon for expectant mothers to develop high blood pressure, urinary tract infections and other problems during pregnancy. An explanation of these and other conditions, along with a review of different approaches to treatment, is found in "Anemia, Herpes, Toxemia and Other Complicating Factors," p. 170. You should not hesitate to call your health adviser between scheduled checkups if you experience any of the following symptoms:

- vaginal bleeding or spotting
- continuous abdominal pain
- severe nausea or vomiting
- fainting spells
- blurred vision
- persistent headaches
- sudden swelling
- chills, fever or rash
- sudden weight gain
- unusual vaginal discharge
- burning when you urinate
- decreased fetal activity (if you notice a marked reduction in movements during those periods of the day or night when your baby is normally active).

Internal exams, like many aspects of prenatal care, vary from practitioner to practitioner; such an exam will be done either at the start of the ninth month or at 39 or 40 weeks, although some preliminary research suggests pelvic exams before the fortieth week may rupture the membranes (break your bag of water) and trigger labor. By the ninth month your baby's weight can be estimated fairly accurately by experienced hands, and many doctors and midwives want to recheck your pelvic dimensions to judge whether the birth canal seems roomy enough. An internal exam also helps to determine signs of readiness for labor.

- *Consistency.* change of cervix from firm to soft
- *Dilation.* widening of cervix, which gradually opens to about 4½ inches (10 centimeters) just before baby's head emerges

- *Effacement.* thinning out of cervix as it is drawn up to become part of the lower section of uterus
- *Station.* descent of baby's head
- *Position.* forward movement of cervix as labor progresses, in contrast to its far-back, difficult-to-reach position.

Even if your baby has "dropped" down in your pelvis and you are perhaps two centimeters dilated and 20 percent effaced, remember that contractions may not begin for several days, and possibly longer. On the other hand, though there may be no signs of approaching labor at the office visit, these conditions can develop overnight (see "Signs of Labor: True or False?" p. 213).

Don't be too discouraged if your due date passes and there is no sign that labor is imminent. At 41 or 42 weeks, depending on your medical adviser's judgment, several tests may be run to check the strength of the placenta and your baby's health. These screening techniques, which are quite safe, accurate and painless, are described in "Postdue...If You're Late," p. 210).

How to Optimize Your Office Visits

At first you are apt to feel there is never enough time to ask about all that's on your mind, but after the third or fourth appointment, most likely you will be more relaxed about being pregnant and have fewer concerns. Your list of questions will probably grow long again during the final trimester, when you begin to focus on labor and delivery—that is, to ask questions about the use of electronic fetal monitors, birth equipment and so on (see "Final Countdown Checklist," p. 193).

Although a dozen checkups may seem like a lot of time spent with your medical adviser, it amounts only to about five hours over the course of nine months. Here are some suggestions on how to promote good dialogue, avoid getting stock answers and avoid being intimidated.

(1) Jot down questions before each appointment and list them in order of importance, since you may not get through them all.
(2) Consult the relevant section in this book and read up on the issue beforehand, so you will be in a better position to know what questions to ask and ensure that it is a two-way conversation. *
(3) Choose a nonthreatening approach when phrasing your questions and don't be too set in your own ways or rigid about a particular point of view.
(4) Try to ask specific questions and mention information sources or

---

*You may also want to browse through the Appendix, specifically "Research on Your Own" (p. 451).

scientific studies that will let your doctor know you are informed and serious.

(5) Discuss all options; beware if only one opinion or treatment is offered.

(6) Take your husband or "labor coach" along, particularly when you plan to talk with your physician about specific procedures such as prepping, positions during labor, Leboyer delivery.

Sometimes expectant parents demand black-and-white answers, forgetting that medicine consists of educated guesses. That is why full-fledged dialogue is so important throughout your pregnancy. Nowadays most doctors expect lots of questions, but if your physician seems impatient or makes you feel ill at ease, consider shopping around for someone else (see "Switching Doctors," p. 94).

NUTRITION AND ESSENTIAL EXTRA POUNDS

Nutrition

Life begins as one cell, which multiplies itself several billion times before birth. This miraculous growth process requires energy—about 2300 calories daily. The old-fashioned notion that expectant mothers must eat for two should not be taken literally, but an extra 200 to 350 calories and increased amounts of almost all nutrients are necessary every day. For many years the baby in utero was considered relatively protected from specific nutritional deficiencies, taking whatever it needed from the mother's body. Although certain nutrients such as calcium seem to go to the baby regardless of the mother's needs, clearly the developing child is not an actual parasite. Nor is it immune to excessive amounts of certain vitamins (for instance, too much or too little vitamin A can cause birth defects).

The interplay between protein, carbohydrates, fats, vitamins and minerals—the basic components of food—demonstrates why it is so important to eat a wide variety of dairy products, meats, grains, fruits and vegetables. Ample amounts of protein, especially high-quality protein, are necessary for amino acids, which represent the essential building blocks of all new tissues, and for growth. Adequate amounts of carbohydrates are crucial for fuel; otherwise protein will be used for energy instead of construction, which may result in fewer cells in every organ including the baby's brain. Fats, which also transport certain vitamins and help the body process them, are another concentrated source of energy. Vitamins such as ascorbic acid help metabolize protein and also are needed for the absorption of iron and other minerals.

It appears that a steady stream of approximately 50 nutrients, including water, is equally important every day of the maternity cycle. Brain development begins early, with each region having its own rate of growth, although it is believed that there are definite growth spurts, at which time the brain is particularly vulnerable to nutritional insults. This is one reason poor eating habits and dieting—even a 24-hour fast—may have serious consequences.

The Recommended Dietary Allowances (RDA) issued by the Food and Nutrition Board of the National Academy of Science in 1974 are regarded as the safest bet, at least until more is known about the numerous interactions with regard to nutrition, the developing individual's genes, drugs and environmental components. These RDA should be viewed as guidelines that need some adjustment; for instance, if you are physically active, most likely you and your baby will need more than 2300 calories a day.

RECOMMENDED DIETARY ALLOWANCES	NONPREGNANT	PREGNANT
Energy	2000 cal	2300 cal
Protein	44 g	74 g
Vitamin A	800 mg	1000 mg
Vitamin D	5 mcg	10 mcg
Vitamin E	8 mg	10 mg
Vitamin C	60 mg	80 mg
Folic Acid	400 mg	800 mg
Niacin	13 mg	15 mg
Riboflavin	1.2 mg	1.5 mg
Thiamine	1 mg	1.4 mg
Vitamin B_6	2 mg	2.6 mg
Vitamin B_{12}	3 mcg	4 mcg
Calcium	800 mg	1200 mg
Phosphorus	800 mg	1200 mg
Iodine	150 mcg	175 mcg
Iron*	18 mg	48 mg
Magnesium	300 mg	450 mg
Zinc	15 mg	20 mg

*Daily supplementation often recommended
Iron   30–60 mg

Particular attention should be given to the increased requirements for the following nutrients:

NUTRIENT	GOOD SOURCES	KEY FUNCTIONS
Protein	milk, cheese, eggs, meat, fish, poultry, dried legumes (peas, beans, lentils), cereals, nuts, bread, peanut butter	Protein builds all tissues, constitutes part of the structure of every cell, creates hemoglobin for blood and forms antibodies to fight infection
Calcium	milk and dairy products, egg yolk, broccoli, greens, sardines and salmon with bones	Calcium builds teeth and bones; plays a leading role in the contraction and relaxation of muscles, including the heart
Iron	liver, red meat, dried fruits, egg yolk, dark-green leafy vegetables, whole grain and enriched bread and cereals	Iron is present in all body cells and is one of the constituents of hemoglobin, which carries oxygen to the tissues by blood circulation
Folic Acid	liver, kidney, brewer's yeast, mushrooms, asparagus, broccoli, lima beans, spinach, orange juice, lemons, bananas, strawberries, cantaloupe	Folic acid is needed for assimilation of protein in the body and for regeneration of blood cells
Vitamin B_6	wheat germ, meat, liver, corn, soybeans, whole-grain cereals, peanuts	Vitamin B_6 aids in the formation of hemoglobin and helps body use protein, carbohydrates and fat
Vitamin B_{12}	milk, eggs, cheese, liver, muscle meats, kidney	Vitamin B_{12} is essential for forming red blood cells; helps in forming all cells in the body and functioning of nervous system
Vitamin A	whole or fortified milk, butter, fortified margarine, eggs, liver, tomatoes, cantaloupe, dark green vegetables, yellow-fleshed vegetables and fruit	Vitamin A promotes skeletal growth and tooth structure; also forms skin and mucous membranes that increase resistance to disease

NUTRIENT	GOOD SOURCES	KEY FUNCTIONS
Vitamin C	citrus fruits and juices, most berries, tomatoes, cabbage, mango, broccoli, cauliflower, spinach, green pepper	Vitamin C forms collagen, a protein that "glues" cells together; also needed for the absorption of iron, some proteins and folic acid
Vitamin D	eggs, fortified milk, butter, fortified margarine, fish-liver oils	Vitamin D promotes normal bone and tooth development; helps absorb calcium and phosphorus

Fortunately, you don't have to be a trained nutritionist to plan meals for yourself and your baby. The "Basic Four" provide the framework for a balanced diet in accordance with the RDA. The four food groups—milk products, meats, vegetables and fruits, grains—can accommodate what's in season as well as one's individual tastes. The beauty of this system, says Elizabeth Whelan, in *Eating Right: Before, During and After Pregnancy*, is that "as long as you include all the recommended portions throughout the course of the day, it makes no difference how you put them together."

SAMPLE DAILY MENU

Food Group	Amount
Milk: for calcium, protein and riboflavin Whole milk, nonfat milk, evaporated milk, nonfat dry milk; cheddar and Monterey Jack cheeses (1½ oz = 1 cup milk); 1¾ cups ice cream = 1 cup milk	1 quart (4 cups)
Meat, fish, poultry, cheese, beans, peanut butter: for protein, iron, B vitamins one serving is: 2 to 3 oz. cooked meat, fish or fowl ½ cup cottage cheese 1 cup cooked dry beans or peas 4 tbs. peanut butter 2 to 3 oz. liver	2 servings
Egg or another small serving of meat	1 serving

Food Group	Amount
Dark green and deep yellow vegetables and fruits: for vitamins A and C	½ cup
Broccoli, greens, spinach, sweet potato, yams, yellow squash, pumpkin, carrots, cantaloupe, dried apricots	
Citrus fruits or other foods high in vitamin C	½ cup
Orange or juice, grapefruit or juice, greens, broccoli, green peppers, chili peppers, strawberries, cantaloupe	
Other fruits and vegetables	2 servings (1 cup)
White potato, cabbage, tomato, corn, green beans, green peas, apple, banana, prunes, raisins (and other vegetables, fruits or juices)	
Whole-grain or enriched bread and cereals: for B vitamins, carbohydrates and iron	5 servings
One serving is: 1 slice bread ½ cup macaroni or spaghetti 1 tortilla ¾ cup ready-to-eat cereal 1 bagel ½ cup rice, enriched or converted ½ cup grits	
Margarine, butter, salad dressing, dessert, additional servings of bread, fruit, meat, milk and other foods	As you wish, if you are not gaining too much weight

There are several other essential complements of the Basic Four plan:

Water and fluids   Approximately 6–8 glasses/day. You don't have to drink that much if you are getting fluids from other sources, such as iceberg lettuce. Fluids are as important as solid foods and are necessary for all chemical reactions to help regulate the elimination of wastes from your body.

Salt
"Salt to taste" is the prevailing view. The policy of restricting the amount of sodium has been reversed, to correct the misconception that too much salt contributes to edema (swelling) and toxemia (preeclampsia). Adequate sodium is essential for keeping the blood circulating, which, in turn is necessary for maintaining an adequate blood flow through the kidneys and placenta.

Iron supplements
Iron tablets often are recommended during pregnancy, because the average diet cannot satisfy the increased needs of both the mother and her baby. However, some physicians advise against taking supplements during the first trimester when embryonic development may possibly be affected. Tell your medical adviser if you have had an unusual reaction to iron medicine in the past. Take pills with water or juice rather than milk, which may interfere with the absorption of iron.

Multiple vitamins
Although increased amounts of vitamins and minerals are required during pregnancy, the need for routine supplementation remains controversial. Some argue that prenatal multivitamins are an unnecessary expense, while others see them as a form of insurance. Even advocates who automatically prescribe vitamin supplements confess that they are not a substitute for a well-balanced diet. Check to make sure you are getting the multivitamin pill that meets your particular needs; for instance, if you are a vegetarian, B complex probably is necessary. Vitamin therapy, which places great emphasis on supplements, is discussed next.

Many holistic health centers advocate reinforcing prenatal diets with vitamin and mineral supplements. During pregnancy "supplement testing" is often performed every four to six weeks; a common method is muscle testing to determine the condition of various organs and their needs for special nutrients; for example, the kidneys can be checked by feeling a corresponding pressure point in the leg. Therapists caution that the dosage and particular brand of vitamin and mineral supplements should be prescribed on an individual basis and modified throughout pregnancy. Explicit directions on taking supplements (before or with meals, for instance) should be given. A popular offshoot of vitamin therapy or applied kinesiology is the use of B-complex vitamins for nausea. If you eat right, supplements are an unnecessary expense, argue many nutritionists, and the established medical community warns that nutrition therapy should not be a substitute for a well-balanced diet.

Although the Basic Four is the standard diet recommended by most health professionals, there are alternatives, particularly if you avoid eating meat. Lacto-ovo vegetarians should have no difficulty getting adequate amounts of milk, cottage cheese and other dairy products that are protein-dense, though supplements may be advisable to ensure enough calcium, iron, folic acid and vitamins A, C, D and B complex. Vegans, who eat no animal products, have to be very careful to get 30 grams of protein daily. Soybeans and soy products also contain all essential amino acids, but since most vegetable proteins are still incomplete, complementary foods such as whole grains should be eaten with proteins, at the same meal. Vegans may need a calcium supplement and additional supplements of vitamin D, riboflavin and B_{12}. Most health professionals agree with Gail and Tom Brewer, authors of *What Every Pregnant Woman Should Know*, who flatly insist that an absolutely vegetarian or vegan diet "should be modified to include eggs and milk products . . . for the sake of her baby, the sensible mother will obtain all the high quality, complete protein she needs regardless of its source."

Soliciting Sound Advice

Nutrition is one subject that you should spend time discussing with your health adviser to make sure you are getting the proper balance of essential nutrients. Keep in mind, though, that most medical schools devote little time to diet.

Even if your physician does not routinely ask about your diet, you may want to take the initiative by recording your eating habits for his or her assessment. A 24-hour recall simply means that you write down everything you ate for the past 24 hours. If it's an unusual day and you ate tons of hors d'oeuvres at a cocktail party, keep track of what you eat for another 24 hours. Include snacks and your fluid intake. Other factors to bring up with your doctor are any fluctuations in your prepregnancy weight and your level of physical exercise. If your physician doesn't seem to appreciate your interest in nutrition, you may want to consider switching to another health adviser or ask for the name of a qualified nutritionist. By and large, midwives devote considerable time to diet, and a 24-hour food diary will sharpen the discussion during one of your short prenatal checkups.

Food for Thought

Some nutritional tips to keep in mind when shopping, cooking and eating:

● *Whole-grain products.* These are more nutritious than enriched ones. For instance, brown rice has nearly four times the protein and calcium value of white enriched rice, and about double the iron content.

● *High-quality or "complete" protein.* Some vegetables, grains and seeds are incomplete- or low-quality-protein foods that are either missing one or more of the essential amino acids or have incorrect proportions of them. By combining two complementary sources of protein, such as pasta with cheese or rice with lentils, you can increase the usable protein.

● *Lack of appetite.* During the first month or two, especially, this may be due to morning sickness. Drinking very hot or very cold liquids may help. Other suggestions are discussed in detail in "Common Discomforts and Some Remedies," p. 47.

● *Avoid raw meat.* It can carry toxoplasmosis, the parasitic infection responsible for certain birth defects, although you probably are immune and therefore so is your unborn child.

● *Megadoses of vitamins.* Too much of many vitamins can be dangerous to your baby. The evidence is strongest with respect to large doses of vitamin A. Don't pop any pills until you check with your health adviser.

● *Intolerance to milk.* This is not uncommon. Cheese is an excellent substitute (1.5 ounces of cheddar, Swiss or brick cheese, 6 ounces of Camembert or 3 ounces of blue cheese is equivalent to 8 ounces, or 1 cup, of whole milk). Homemade yogurt often is more digestible if you are intolerant of lactose. Calcium pills may be taken, but they do not adequately replace the important nutrients found in milk and its by-products.

● *Cigarettes and coffee.* These tend to suppress your appetite. Either cut down on or quit smoking, and limit your caffeine intake.

● *Alcohol.* Alcohol can interfere with the absorption of essential nutrients, possibly decrease the transport of amino acids across the placenta and reduce the supply of folic acid or zinc to the developing baby.

● *Expecting twins.* This means an increase in your caloric and protein intake above the recommended dietary guidelines for a singleton pregnancy.

Eating right every day during pregnancy is perhaps your biggest responsibility, and, luckily, it is the one decision during the next nine months over which you exercise complete control. Most of us know from experience that our bodies can tolerate some dietary carelessness without serious consequences, but casual neglect at any time now poses a definite risk. Actually, there are only a few basic guidelines to follow:

- Dietary variety but not in hit-or-miss style
- Three meals a day plus highly nutritional snacks
- No dieting and no diuretics
- Individualized Basic Four meal plan
- Iron and vitamin supplements if they are prescribed for you
- Salt intake not necessarily restricted
- Increased caloric intake if you're physically active
- Plenty of water each day
- Attention to food labels

Like many new mothers, you may discover, too, that by establishing a well-balanced diet during pregnancy you've permanently improved your own eating habits, and you'll be in a better position to feed your baby the right mix of foods when the time comes.

Essential Extra Pounds

Everyone seems to agree that pregnancy is not the time to diet, even if you are overweight. The consensus is that you should put on weight in a gradual and steady pattern. "The great emphasis on total weight gain is almost certainly misplaced," writes Dr. Roy Pitkin of the Committee on Nutrition, American College of Obstetricians and Gynecologists. "Of much greater importance is the pattern of accumulation." But advice about total weight gain fluctuates all over the scale. Some expectant mothers are still warned to stay within a 15–20 pound limit; more frequently, pregnant women are told to concentrate on eating the right foods rather than watching their weight. Yet this open-ended "eat plenty of the right foods" approach carries risks, as in the case of the petite mother-to-be who was told to gain 40 pounds, only to develop serious joint problems later.

No one really knows what is the optimal number of pounds, particularly if you are not "average," but slender or chubby, at the start of your pregnancy. Some research does suggest, however, an association between weight gain and pregnancy outcome and recommends that women of normal weight for their height before pregnancy gain between 24 and 30 pounds, that overweight women put on only 15 to 24 pounds and that underweight expectant mothers try to gain an average of 30 pounds. Some thought should also be given, of course, to your bone structure, height, metabolism and level of physical activity.

If you have been battling the needle on the scale for years, you may have some difficulty accepting the undisputed need to put on pounds, but remember that if you eat wisely, most of the added weight is in lean body (protein) tissue. The baby, placenta, amniotic fluid and growth of the uterus and breasts account for about 14 to 16 pounds. Another 10–12 pounds are from general growth of your body and storage of nutrient reserves. The rate of weight gain correlates with these physiological developments. Usually one-fifth of the total number of pounds is gained in the first trimester and two-fifths are gained in each of the other two trimesters.

After birth, some new mothers have to work at trimming off the final five to ten pounds, while for others weight just seems to disappear. Your eating habits, individual metabolism and degree of caloric expenditure will largely determine how quickly you return to your prepregnancy weight. Many health authorities claim women who breast-feed tend to get back into shape much sooner than those who do not. Even though mothers who nurse need to eat even more than they did while pregnant, to produce nearly a quart of milk a day, it is estimated that the energy expended on lactating burns off about 500 additional calories daily.

SAMPLE WEIGHT-LOSS SCHEDULE

Total weight gain at 40 weeks	26 lbs.
Weight lost during childbirth	
Baby	8 lbs.
Placenta	2 lbs.
Amniotic fluid	2 lbs.
Weight lost during first 2 weeks postpartum	
Maternal blood volume	4 lbs.
Uterus and breast tissue	4 lbs.
Extracellular fluid	4 lbs.
Weight lost after 3–6 months breast-feeding	
Maternal fat stores	2 lbs.
Total weight lost	26 lbs.

This is one time in your life when you should worry if you are *not* putting on pounds. Remember, during the last trimester your baby gains nearly an ounce a day. Charting your weight gain is one crude method of monitoring your baby's physiological development. Notify your doctor or midwife if you experience a sudden jump in weight or weight loss (don't worry if you notice a drop between 38 and 40 weeks; it's normal and may be caused by a reduction of certain hormones in preparation for labor). Simple tests can be run to check on the well-being of the placenta and your baby (see "Postdue ... If You're Late," p. 210).

It is only natural to get depressed about your ever-expanding middle, but miraculously, you will probably shrink back to size long before your baby is walking.

Information Sources

ADDITIONAL READING

Diet For a Small Planet, by Frances Moore Lappe (New York: Ballantine, 1971). If you have to watch your pocketbook or if you are a vegetarian, this is a comprehensive guide.

Eating Right: Before, During and After Pregnancy, by Elizabeth Whelan (New York: American Baby Books, 1982). This 70-page paperback outlines the Basic Four food groups.

The Farm Vegetarian Cookbook, edited by Louise Hagler (Summertown, TN.: The Book Publishing Co., 1978). This book is based on a soy diet—no meat, fish, poultry, eggs or animal dairy products; approximately 200 pages of recipes.

Nourishing Your Unborn Child: Nutrition and Natural Foods in Pregnancy, by Phyllis Williams (New York: Avon, 1975). A no-nonsense guide, written by a pediatrics nurse, that tells you what to eat, rather than just what to avoid, and supplies menus.

The Brewer Medical Diet for Normal and High-Risk Pregnancy, by Gail S. Brewer with Thomas Brewer, M.D. (New York: Simon & Schuster, 1983). Nutritional guidelines and worksheets to help you plan an individualized diet.

ORGANIZATIONS

American Dietetic Association
430 N. Michigan Ave.
Chicago, IL 60611
The Association provides referrals to registered dieticians.

Columbia University Institute of Human Nutrition
701 W. 168th St.
New York, NY 10032
A newsletter and literature are available.

Society for Nutrition Education
1736 Franklin St.
Oakland, CA 94612
This organization is concerned with the nutritional management of high-risk pregnancies.

REDUCING RISKS: DRINKING, SMOKING, DRUGS

While nothing can guarantee that your child will be healthy and normal, moderation in or complete avoidance of certain substances cannot hurt—and may, in fact, reduce the risk of birth defects. Heavy drinking is known to cause mental retardation and certain deformities. Extensive research proves cigarette smoking jeopardizes not only the child's health but also the mother's. Some animal studies, although controversial, implicate caffeine. And even though only a handful of over-the-counter and prescription drugs have been shown to cause abnormalities in or other problems for the developing fetus, the chance always exists that other drugs may do so too.

Alcohol: Warning to Social Drinkers

Heavy drinking is known to be harmful during pregnancy—at any time, for that matter—but the debate about total abstinence versus "social" drinking continues. That small amounts of alcohol could harm the fetus was suspected even in ancient times. Today tourists visiting the ruins of Carthage are still told of the laws forbidding a bride and groom from drinking on their wedding night in order to prevent the birth of an abnormal child.

Until recently, many physicians and midwives were not alarmed by moderate drinking during pregnancy. In July 1981, the Surgeon General of the United States warned all mothers-to-be (and even those considering pregnancy) not to drink—at all. However, many health professionals recommend that expectant mothers limit themselves to no more than two drinks a day.

WHAT'S IN A DRINK?

A 12-oz. can of beer, a 5-oz. glass of table wine and a mixed drink with 1.5 oz. of 80-proof alcohol all contain approximately the same amount of absolute alcohol.

The Surgeon General's 1981 report, based primarily on studies of 14,000 pregnant women and their newborn babies, specifically cautioned against drinking any alcohol during the first trimester—the early months—of pregnancy. The government also encouraged women to take notice of the alcoholic content in food and drugs (for instance, in liquored desserts, cough syrups). This warning has been recently extended through the third trimester. A 1982 study of monkeys and their fetuses conducted at the government's National Institutes of Health (NIH) found evidence of severe oxygen deficiency, possibly resulting in brain damage. Soon after giving five monkeys the equivalent of three to five drinks, blood vessels in the umbilical cords turned white, reducing normal circulation for about one hour. Photographs of the blanched cords, published in the November 1982 issue of *Science*, are startling. "Based on these experimental results obtained in laboratory primates," warn the NIH researchers, "we offer a prudent recommendation that pregnant women consider total abstinence from ethanol [alcohol] throughout pregnancy."

If this research on monkeys proves true for humans, the dangers of drinking while pregnant may be greater than ever realized. Few studies dispute the government findings. Out of 152 medical papers published in 1979 and 1980, only 2 concluded that it was safe for expectant mothers to drink moderate amounts of alcohol. It will be years before the preliminary data regarding the potential danger to offspring of light and moderate drinking are confirmed or rejected. For this reason, reaction by the medical community to the warnings issued by the Surgeon General is mixed.

Our random sampling of obstetricians around the country revealed that the majority are advising their patients to keep their drinking to a minimum. Along with the Surgeon General, hard-liners, like Dr. Dwight Cruykshank of the Medical College of Virginia, discourage expectant mothers from drinking not only during the first trimester but throughout their entire pregnancy, arguing that the baby's brain is the organ most affected by alcohol. Among the skeptics is the Executive Director of the American College of Obstetricians and Gynecologists, Dr. Warren H. Pearse, who says, "the Surgeon General's advisory is an overly conservative reaction... there's no need for an absolute prohibition." In fact, a glass of wine is often "prescribed" during the last month or two if an expectant mother cannot relax or is in false labor.

Evidence has been building for the past decade that women who drink very heavily—more than six drinks a day—run the risk of miscarriage, stillbirth or bearing a baby with fetal-alcohol syndrome. The principal features of this syndrome include central-nervous-system disorders, retarded growth, abnormal facial features such as folds on the inner part of the eyelids and skeletal defects.

Periodic binge drinking most likely is not a safe alternative. Mothers who are not chronic drinkers or alcoholics but occasionally consume a lot may also run the risk of bearing a baby with some fetal-alcohol-syndrome abnormalities. The government's National Institute of Alcohol Abuse and Alcoholism claims 178 studies demonstrate that average alcohol consumption may not be as important as high blood alcohol level at critical times during embryonic development.

Heavy drinking doesn't make sense at any time, and even moderate consumption of beer, wine or other liquors could mean you're taking a real chance. The effect of cumulative "starvation" of your baby's brain cells from just one or two drinks is unknown, but in light of the 1982 NIH study on monkeys, there is at least a theoretical link between repeated moderate drinking and mental retardation in the offspring.

Nonalcoholic concoctions may be the safest bet, so experiment with drinks such as iced tea with pineapple juice, cranberry juice with lime, orange eggnog, or tomato or orange juice.

Cigarettes: Kick the Habit

Not even the Tobacco Institute would advocate cigarette smoking for expectant mothers. "No Smoking—Fetal Growth in Progress," the slogan of the International Childbirth Education Association, sums up the prevailing view. The detrimental effects of tobacco were suspected in the late nineteenth century, based on women working in tobacco factories who had a high rate of miscarriage or lost their babies soon after birth. Research has been continuous since the 1920s, and even though alcohol, diet and other habits of pregnant smokers can disrupt the accuracy of scientific data, much of the evidence is damning and indisputable.

It is a fact that the placenta, the major component of your baby's support system, cannot filter out nicotine and many other chemical compounds contained in tobacco smoke. Nicotine constricts the blood vessels and reduces blood volume, which, in turn, decreases the supply of oxygen and food to your baby. An encouraging although controversial study suggests that the risks connected with smoking are *eliminated* if the mother quits before her fourth month of pregnancy.

The disturbing consequences of tobacco smoke, of course, are directly proportional to the number of cigarettes smoked. Heavy smokers stand about two times the chance of pregnancy complications and infant mortality than expectant mothers who smoke less than a pack a day do, although most studies conclude that light smokers still have a greater risk than nonsmokers of losing their baby or having a less healthy child. The dangers include the following:

- miscarriage
- fetal growth inhibited, causing underweight babies (5.5 pounds or less) who are more likely to develop health problems in early infancy than babies of average weight
- premature delivery prior to 38 weeks, particularly among women who smoke more than a pack a day

- premature separation of placenta from wall of uterus, which is a major threat to baby
- cesarean birth. This possibility based on findings that among smokers the placenta is more likely to be located over the cervix rather than high up in the uterus, a condition that usually necessitates abdominal delivery
- breast-milk production decreased among mothers who smoke more than 20 cigarettes daily
- sudden infant death syndrome (SIDS) seems to occur more frequently to babies born to mothers who smoke
- pneumonia and bronchitis are more common in infants less than one year of age if parents smoke
- maternal smoking may be linked to childhood asthma and painful middle-ear infections, which usually call for antibiotics.

Numerous suggestions aimed at pregnant smokers deserve your consideration; some of the more controversial recommendations should be discussed with your doctor or midwife:

(1) Switch to a brand of cigarettes you find distasteful and buy only packs, not cartons. Smoke only half of each cigarette, and put it down after each puff.
(2) Try to avoid alcohol, coffee and other beverages that you associate with cigarette smoking.
(3) Persuade friends and family members to avoid smoking around you during your pregnancy.
(4) Cut down gradually if "cold turkey" is too stressful.
(5) Prevent low birth weight, if you are unable to stop smoking, by increasing your dietary intake. Some researchers say that it is unlikely that this nutritional strategy could offset the negative effect of stunted fetal growth.
(6) Extra vitamin C? Some experts suggest an increase of ascorbic acid by about 40 percent, but leave it to the professional to decide, since megadoses of vitamin C are known to be dangerous to the baby in utero.
(7) If you are unable to quit, at least stop smoking for the last few days of pregnancy to ensure more oxygen is available to your baby during the critical time of delivery.

Marijuana and Other Recreational Drugs

What is known about the biological effects of marijuana is at about the same stage today as the evidence surrounding cigarettes was 40 years ago. Even less is known about cocaine, LSD and other hallucinogens. Research on pregnant women is practically nonexistent, and animal studies have produced inconclusive results. The government's

National Institute of Drug Abuse warns pregnant women to avoid drugs, on the ground that they pose an unnecessary risk to the fetus and the mother. An added concern with illegal street drugs is that they may have been adulterated with other chemicals.

Smoking marijuana once a week or less is believed to be harmless, but the same research concludes that in heavy marijuana smokers the drug interferes with white cell formation, reducing the body's ability to fight infection. In contrast to tobacco smoke, marijuana is suspected of being more destructive to the lung's defense against bacteria. This problem may be aggravated, since "grass" is usually inhaled deeply into the lungs and held there for as long as possible.

A Canadian study analyzing the babies of 291 women who smoked five to seven joints a week found no major differences between them and a control group of nonusers. Babies of mothers who smoked marijuana tended to become more easily startled, but there was no difference in birth weight or incidence of birth defects. However, animal studies have yielded more forbidding conclusions. A 1982 report by the National Academy of Sciences implicated Delta-9-THC, the major ingredient in marijuana, as responsible for birth defects when given in large doses to experimental animals; it did find that THC does not appear to break chromosomes, although possible genetic damage of the embryo has not been ruled out. Research showed that monkeys which were given marijuana for several years were four times as likely to lose their offspring either by miscarriage or by stillbirth. More recent still is a study of 1690 mothers and their newborns at the Boston University School of Medicine, discussed in the journal *Pediatrics*, which found babies of marijuana smokers were more likely to be born with characteristics similar to those of fetal-alcohol syndrome: weighing less, with smaller heads and abnormal features. As for nursing mothers, marijuana tends to reduce the level of prolactin, the hormone necessary for milk supply. The chemical that produces the marijuana high is concentrated in breast milk and shows up in nursing infants.

Even less is known about cocaine and other street drugs. Expectant mothers are more vulnerable to respiratory infections, and "snorting coke" only increases the likelihood. A 1970 study involving 148 pregnancies, regarding the effects of LSD on the developing fetus, found there was some indication of a relationship between "acid" and miscarriage, premature delivery and birth defects, though it was not clear-cut.

Caffeine: Is Trouble Brewing?

Since the 1940s caffeine has been suspected as dangerous to the developing fetus, but recently the risk has been discounted. Given the contradictory findings, during pregnancy you may want to watch your intake of coffee, tea, cola, chocolate candy bars, cough syrups and other foods and drugs containing this active ingredient. Some experts advise limiting caffeine consumption to two cups of coffee within a 24-hour period, while others, including the March of Dimes Foundation, suggest less than six cups but add, "the fewer the better."

The U.S. Food and Drug Administration cautioned expectant mothers in November 1980 that caffeine may harm unborn babies, citing a greater incidence of birth defects. Studies in animals have shown that birth defects occur when caffeine is given in amounts equivalent to 12 to 24 cups of coffee a day. Since the FDA's warning, little has surfaced to support it. In fact, a 1982 study conducted at Boston's Brigham and Women's Hospital involving 12,000 mothers revealed that cigarette smoking may be the culprit in some problems previously blamed on coffee. Unlike the Boston survey, smokers in the FDA investigations were not identified—a significant omission, since smoking has been linked with underweight babies and premature deliveries. The Boston research team acknowledged that there may be an increased risk of breech position and premature rupture of the membranes among women who drank 4 or more cups of coffee a day during the first trimester but concluded that "coffee consumption has a minimal effect, if any, on the outcome of pregnancy." Even so, the FDA claimed the size of the population monitored in this Boston study was not large enough to detect rare caffeine-related birth abnormalities.

Dangerous or not, caffeine remains in the bloodstream about twice as long in pregnant women as in nonpregnant women, and it freely enters the baby's circulatory system. Prolonged retention of this chemical, some researchers warn, may lead to a loss of appetite and poor eating habits.

Beverages	Caffeine (mg)
Cup of coffee	50–155
Cup of tea	9– 50
Glass iced tea	22– 40
Cup of cocoa	2– 40
Carbonated soft drinks	30– 65
Piece of chocolate	6– 35

Over-the-Counter Drugs	
Pain relievers	60–130
Cold medicines	20– 30
NoDoz and other stimulants	100–200

You can reduce your caffeine consumption simply by brewing weaker tea or coffee. Percolated coffee contains less caffeine than the drip type, and instant has considerably less still. Herbal and some other teas, along with 7-Up and other caffeine-free soft drinks, are alternatives. Although plain aspirin and acetominophen (such as Tylenol) contain no caffeine, all medications should be avoided during pregnancy. Definitely check first with your medical adviser before taking over-the-counter drugs.

Even though caffeine crosses the placenta and reaches the fetus, the jury is still out on its potential harm. Pregnancy provides you with a great excuse to change habits, and many women suffering from benign breast lumps find improvement when they cut out caffeine. Until more is known, you may want to minimize your intake of caffeine—to the equivalent of a cup or two of coffee a day—particularly during the first three months of gestation. "Women have everything to gain and nothing to lose by heeding this advice," claims the Center for Science in the Public Interest.

Over-the-Counter and Prescription Drugs: Avoid if Possible

Medications, including seemingly innocuous nonprescription drugs such as aspirin, should be avoided whenever possible during pregnancy. This is easier said than done, since many expectant mothers develop urinary-tract infections and other problems that often require treatment. The stumbling block in making an informed decision about practically all drugs is that the risks are theoretical, since only a handful of medicines are known to be teratogenic (causing deformation). Although most drugs cross the placenta with ease, there is not enough research to tell us about the potential harm to the unborn baby. Furthermore, just because a drug does *not* cross the placenta does not mean that it is safe.

"There is no way to prove that any substance taken by a pregnant woman does not cause birth defects," warns the U.S. Food and Drug Administration, despite laboratory animal studies that suggest some drugs are harmless. In fact, one animal species may not suffer from being exposed to a particular drug in utero, while another will. Such was the case in the thalidomide tragedy, which caused severe deformities to thousands of babies, most of them European. The sedative was believed to be nontoxic when tested on mice and rats, only later to be proved a teratogen in rabbits and monkeys. There is hope that by the time our children have children, much more will be discovered about various medicines. A new technique for testing drugs is in progress, whereby human fetal tissue is implanted in mice, enabling scientists to witness the effects of certain chemicals on human fetal organs outside the mother's womb.

Certain drugs should positively not be taken during the entire

maternity cycle; also beware of many remedies which may be dangerous at specific times during pregnancy:

● *Vitamins.* Excessive amounts of vitamins A and D may cause serious
deformities. Megadoses of vitamin C may cause dependency in the
newborn, and too much vitamin K can result in jaundice, possibly
leading to brain damage.
● *Hormones.* Estrogen, progestin and other hormones may cause
certain heart, limb and other deformities.
● *Antibiotics.* Tetracyclines may cause permanent discoloration of the
baby's teeth and also may retard skeletal development. Streptomycin
may result in deafness in the infant.
● *Tranquilizers.* Valium, Equanil and Miltown are among the popular
brands. If taken during the first trimester, they may cause cleft lip or
palate or other congenital malformations.

Don't self-medicate. Check with your obstetrician or midwife before
taking any medicine, even vitamins. If your medical adviser prescribes
a particular drug, get the answers to these questions:

(1) what are intended results, and how will it make me feel?
(2) generic and brand name?
(3) any known adverse side effects, including potential risks to me
and my baby or, if unknown, has any research *at all* been done on
safety of use during pregnancy?
(4) drug and nondrug alternative treatments, if any?
(5) interactions with other drugs, alcohol, food or tobacco?
(6) instructions on taking medications (before, during or after meals?
with water? with fruit juice? how much?).

● *Aspirin.* Drugs containing aspirin should be avoided throughout
pregnancy. Animal studies have shown that salicylates cause birth
defects. However, controlled studies using aspirin have not shown
proof of teratogenicity. Chronic, high-dose use of aspirin during the
last trimester—especially during the last two weeks—may prolong
pregnancy past 42 weeks and also may cause bleeding before and after
delivery.
● *Antihistamines and Decongestants.* Unfortunately it takes expectant
mothers longer to get rid of colds and other respiratory ailments. It's
not unusual for a runny nose to linger for 10-14 days instead of a
week. Although there is no conclusive evidence showing adverse
effects on the fetus, antihistamines and decongestant medicines are
best avoided. Try "natural decongestants" including camomile tea,
hot saline gargle (½ teaspoon salt to ½ cup of water), nose drops
and, of course, a vaporizer.
● *Motion-Sickness medicine.* To be on the safe side, stay away from

Dramamine and other drugs for motion sickness, especially during the first 12 weeks. However, there is no conclusive evidence of a relationship between use of Dramamine and major or minor birth defects. Also make sure that any doctor you see—from a dentist to a dermatologist—knows you are pregnant.

Several excellent resources listed in the Information Sources, which follow, can help you weigh the benefits and risks if you must decide about a certain drug treatment. Pregnancy-related problems such as constipation and morning sickness are discussed at length in "Common Discomforts and Some Remedies" (p. 47), along with advice about particular drugs. Medicines for more serious conditions, including diabetes and high blood pressure, can be found in "Anemia, Herpes, Toxemia and Other Complicating Factors" (p. 170). Whenever possible during these critical months of human development, avoid taking any drug that is not vitally important to you or your baby's well-being.

Information Sources

ADDITIONAL READING

About Your Medicines in Pregnancy, Labor and Breastfeeding, published by U.S. Pharmacopoeia. Contact USP, Publications, 12601 Twinbrook Pkwy., Rockville, MD 20852 for ordering and price information about this brand-new book.

"Alcohol Use During Pregnancy." A 20-page booklet reviewing human and animal studies. Available for $2.00 from American Council on Science and Health, 47 Maple St., Summit, NJ 07901.

AMA *Drug Evaluations,* by the American Medical Association and the American Society for Clinical Pharmacology and Therapeutics (New York: John Wiley and Sons, 1980).

"Calling It Quits." Ex-smokers swear by this booklet, which is full of suggestions on how to give up cigarettes. Available free from the Office of Cancer Communications, National Cancer Institute, Bethesda, MD 20205.

Physicians' Desk Reference for Nonprescription Drugs and *Physicians' Desk Reference.* Published annually by Litton Industries. These essentially provide the same information as that included in patient package inserts.

"Surgeon General's Advisory on Alcohol and Pregnancy," July 1981. 1 p. Available free from the Food and Drug Administration HFI-22, Rockville, MD 20857.

USP DI: Advice for the Patient. This 1984 dispensing guide is published by the U.S. Pharmacopoeia Convention. It includes guidelines for drug use during pregnancy. Available for $21.95 from USP, Publications, 12601 Twinbrook Pkwy., Rockville, MD 20852.

ORGANIZATIONS

American Foundation for Maternal and Child Health
30 Beekman Pl.
New York, NY 10022
This foundation, headed by Doris Haire, publishes articles on drugs, including a 4-page report titled "How the FDA Determines the Safety of Drugs—Just How Safe is Safe?" for $1.00.

Association of Birth Defect Children
3201 E. Crystal Lake Ave.
Orlando, FL 32806
Information about the morning-sickness drug, Bendectin, which is no longer being manufactured in the U.S.

Center for Science in the Public Interest
1755 S St., NW
Washington, DC 20009
Information clearinghouse with an interest in caffeine.

MEDLARS
National Library of Medicine
8600 Rockville Pike
Bethesda, MD 20209
MEDLARS (Medical Literature Analysis and Retrieval Service) is a computerized data base containing thousands of references to journal articles and books. A computer search can be done through 1300 universities, medical schools, hospitals, government agencies and commercial organizations. Sometimes there is a modest fee of $5.00; other times it is free.

National Clearinghouse on Alcohol Information
PO Box 2345
Rockville, MD 20852
(301) 468-2600
Telephone hot line.
Distributes free material and scientific studies.
Conducts a free literature search.

Pregnancy Research Branch
National Institute of Child Health and Human Development
NIH
Bethesda, MD 20205
Conducts and sponsors research.

Public Citizen Health Research Group
2000 P St., NW
Washington, DC 20036
Private organization that acts as a watchdog over the Food and Drug Administration and the pharmaceutical industry.

U.S. Food & Drug Administration
Office of Public Affairs
5600 Fishers La.
Rockville, MD 20857
This federal agency's experts can be contacted with specific questions about drugs and medical devices.

U.S. Pharmacopoeia (USP)
Drug Information Division
12601 Twinbrook Pkwy.
Rockville, MD 20852
Free pamphlets available; orders for their books *USP DI: Advice For The Patient* and *About Your Medicines In Pregnancy, Labor and Breastfeeding* must be prepaid. Free sample copy of *About Your Medicines* newsletter will be sent upon request.

COMMON DISCOMFORTS AND SOME REMEDIES

You may be lucky and experience only a few discomforts during your pregnancy. It is often easier to maintain a sense of humor and objectivity about these aches and pains if you know what provokes them. Here are known causes or, in some cases, theories, along with some remedies for these common aches and pains. To be on the safe side, avoid self-medicating. Don't decide to take calcium pills for leg cramps, for instance, unless you've gotten the okay from your physician or midwife. If a problem that's bothering you is not discussed here, check the following section, "Other Side Effects of Pregnancy," p. 57.

Backache. Your spine, the linchpin of your entire body, happens to be one of its weakest and most delicate structures. Your growing tummy gradually pulls it forward, causing considerable strain as your spine adapts to supporting the added weight of your baby. Other factors contributing to back pain, especially in the region between your pelvis and spine, are:

- pressure of the uterus on your lower back
- stretching of ligaments attached to your uterus

- relaxed ligaments supporting spinal column, because of elevated levels of progesterone
- normal softening of pelvic joints, which puts added strain on other joints and ligaments
- previous back injury.

Good posture is the most natural way to keep back pain to a minimum. Remember to keep your back from arching forward, whether you are sitting, standing or resting. Avoid any position that encourages your stomach to hang out, such as standing with your feet close together or wearing high heels. When lifting, don't bend at the waist but at the knees, putting your leg muscles to work rather than your back. Suggested exercises for backache are described in "Conditioning Exercises: What's a Kegel?" p. 68.

Heating pads, radiant heat or a shower with very warm water pulsating on your lower back may also help. Have a back massage with or without something like Ben-Gay. This will relieve not only soreness but tension. Swimming not only takes the weight off the spine but is relaxing.

Constipation. Two conditions necessary to keep your "pipes" in good working order are moisture and mobility. When you are pregnant, there is a reduction in both. Expectant mothers absorb water into their systems more efficiently and at a faster rate than before, making for drier, harder stools. The natural tiny muscle contractions in your intestines that push waste along (peristalsis) are relaxed by the higher level of the hormone progesterone. Intestines also expand, holding more waste in place. Add to that the partial blockage of your lower bowels by your expanding uterus, and it's understandable that your pipes get clogged. The food you eat and don't eat, even the prenatal multivitamins and iron tablets, can contribute to constipation.

Bulk-building laxatives contain a lot of sodium or sugar, which may increase the mother's blood pressure or cause water retention. This partly explains why natural remedies are preferred. Some experts suggest avoiding mineral-oil laxatives, which tend to interfere with the absorption of critical vitamins A and D. Herbal laxatives, specifically senna cascara, mugwart and aloe, are also not advisable. Castor oil may cause uterine contractions if taken near the end of pregnancy. Try some of these remedies, which are safe and generally pretty effective.

- Drink plenty of water or liquids (not just an extra glass) to keep the system moving. Very hot or very cold fluids tend to work best.
- Take natural laxatives, such as raw vegetables, whole-grain cereals, bran muffins, brown rice (the fiber acts as a sponge to

absorb water and other materials and hasten the movement of waste through the intestines). Eat cooked fruit, especially prunes, fruit juices and applesauce.

- Change your multivitamin pills if you suspect they are adding to constipation; it is possible to take tablets with stool softener.
- Drink herbal remedies such as plantago psyllium steeped in warm water for several minutes.
- Exercise, including walking, which helps to keep the digestive tract active.
- Have sex. Some say it may speed up peristalsis, pushing waste out faster.

Fatigue. Being constantly sleepy and tired during the first few months of pregnancy is one of the hardest adjustments you'll have to make. But with all the internal body-building, it's little wonder you're exhausted. Just seven days after conception, a cluster of cells is literally eating its way into the lining of your uterus to set up shop. It will take at least three months to get the machinery built, the placenta being the major component for the baby's support system. In addition to all this activity, hormones are also partly responsible for the weariness. After about the fourteenth week your energy level will rise again. Chronic fatigue will return during the last month or so. There is no question that you and your baby need rest, so don't feel guilty or lazy, but follow your body's craving for sleep.

- Even if you hate naps, take rest periods at least once a day.
- Go to bed earlier than usual and laze around in bed the next morning.
- Eat well, but lots of sweets and carbohydrates will slow you down after that initial spurt of energy.
- Watch your intake of coffee and other caffeinated foods.
- Take walks and get some regular exercise, which will actually give you more energy.

Headaches. Headaches usually signal that something out of the ordinary is occurring elsewhere in your body, generally for the same reasons as when you aren't pregnant:

- *Pressure headache.*   Anxieties, nervousness, worries
- *Frontal headache.*   Eyestrain, migraine (although many chronic migraine sufferers have a respite from these headaches during pregnancy)
- *All-over headache.*   Nausea, common cold, flu, hangover.

Headaches can strike anytime, but the one headache that typically hits expectant mothers during the first three months is associated with changing hormone levels and, possibly, increased activity of the pituitary gland.

Relief will depend on what is causing your head to hurt or throb. Once you figure out the reason, you probably can do something about it (too much close reading, dwelling on anxieties, drinking too much coffee, smoke-filled rooms or whatever). Don't reach for aspirin— even Tylenol, which is the preferred chemical, should not be taken without checking with your doctor or midwife. Aspirin should be avoided throughout the last trimester—especially during the last two weeks—because its anticlotting action may cause blood loss to the newborn and possible maternal hemorrhaging.

To help keep headaches at bay:

- get plenty of sleep (it helps keep your irritability and frustration thresholds high)
- eat regularly (no food for hours lets your blood-sugar level drop and may cause the temples to throb) and drink lots of fluids.

To relieve headaches once they start:

- work any tense muscles in your neck and shoulders by exercise or massage
- hold a cool, damp cloth on your forehead and behind your neck
- get some fresh air
- drink herbal concoctions
- get distracted, perhaps by taking in a movie.

Heartburn and Indigestion. During pregnancy, normal stomach acids tend to reenter your esophagus (the food pipe from your mouth to your stomach), resulting in a burning sensation in the lower part of your chest and sometimes in the bitter taste of stomach acid in your throat and mouth. The two culprits in heartburn and acid indigestion are the hormone progesterone and your uterus. In the process of digestion, food is passed down the esophagus to the stomach, to be broken down by acids and routed into the intestines, where nutrients are absorbed into your bloodstream. Progesterone relaxes the ringlike muscle-opening between your esophagus and your stomach as well as the tiny muscles in your intestines, which contract to shuffle the food along its way. The result is a mix of food and digestive juices sitting for a longer time than usual in your stomach, occasionally spilling back up into the sensitive lower lining of your esophagus. Toward the end of your pregnancy the condition may be aggravated by pressure on your stomach from your expanding uterus, coupled with the expansion of your lower ribs, which widens the muscle-valve opening into the stomach.

The best way to control this discomfort is to neutralize the acid in your stomach in order to keep it from burning your esophagus. Antacids should be used only after natural remedies have been tried, such as:

- paying attention to those foods that give you heartburn (pastrami for some, Indian food for others)
- avoiding coffee and cigarettes that may aggravate heartburn
- taking several small meals instead of three large ones
- sipping on carbonated drinks and consuming plenty of fluids
- lying down propped up; resting flat on your back often makes it worse.

If necessary choose antacids containing aluminum hydroxide (Amphojel), calcium carbonate (Pepto-Bismol, Tums), magnesium trisilicate (Gelusil, Am-T), magnesium carbonate or magnesium hydroxide (Di-Gel). These are less well-absorbed systemically; however, when taken for prolonged periods and/or in high doses, the chance of birth defects may increase. Don't get hooked on them because frequent use may delay absorption of nutrients in your diet.

Small quantities of antacids can help neutralize the discomfort, but be careful also of Rolaids, Alka-Seltzer and many other sodium antacids that contain aspirin and/or salt. It's wise to get your physician or midwife's recommendation for a particular antacid.

Hemorrhoids. Hemorrhoids or "piles" are nothing more than varicose veins in and around the rectum and anal canal. They affect many expectant mothers and are caused chiefly by pressure and progesterone. Progesterone relaxes the intestines, causing constipation, making you strain during a bowel movement. This hormone also dilates veins in your rectum, causing blood to pool and slowing down the blood's return to your heart. Flow becomes even more sluggish as your uterus expands and fills out your pelvis and your baby's head "engages," partially blocking circulation in the area.

Relief essentially comes from maintaining regular bowel movements (see "Constipation," p. 48) and finding ways to reduce the pressure on your rectum and anal canal.

- Get off your feet, with your hips raised, as often as possible; even put a pillow under your hips at night.
- Do exercises to keep the blood circulating.
- Don't strain when having a bowel movement; try placing your feet on a low stool or find some way to elevate them.
- Sit on a towel in a warm tub twice a day.
- Try Tuck pads (keep them refrigerated for extra relief).
- Try ice packs if you can manage to use them comfortably.

Beware of hemorrhoid ointments, sprays and suppositories.

Impatient Bladder. By the end of these nine months you will know the location of every ladies' room in town. From the very start, the hormone progesterone will relax the muscles in your urinary tract, causing fluids to pass more quickly through your system. At the same time your adrenal glands will alter your fluid balance, increasing the amount of urine. As your uterus enlarges and you enter the second trimester of pregnancy, it will rest more heavily on your bladder, congesting blood flow in the neck of the bladder. The amount of urine gradually decreases, but, because of uterine pressure and the subsequent limited bladder capacity, the number of trips to the bathroom stays about the same. In the final stretch, however, the trips may seem endless, as there is combined weakness in control and greater bladder pressure after your baby's head engages deeper into your pelvis. Some women find they go hourly and even leak a small amount of urine if they cough, sneeze, or experience a strong kick from the baby's foot or elbow.

Little can be done to reduce frequent urination, since you need fluids. In order to keep from having it wake you up at night, however, when the fluid that has collected in your ankles during the day moves to your kidneys, just reduce the amount you drink after 8:00 P.M.

Kegel exercises (described in "Conditioning Exercises: What's a Kegel?" p. 68) can help control incontinence, a problem that often bothers women after childbirth. This muscle toning not only can help you to regain bladder control but can be effective in preventing urinary-tract infections. However, some experts caution against practicing too much prior to childbirth because the pelvic floor may become so muscular that it is difficult to avoid an episiotomy, a small cut that enlarges the vaginal opening immediately prior to delivery.

Muscle Cramp, Charley Horse. Exactly what makes muscles in your legs and feet suddenly cramp up and pull remains a medical mystery. During pregnancy, it happens most often in the third trimester, usually at night, and could be due to any number of factors:

- too much or too little calcium
- fatigue
- calcium-phosphorus imbalance
- pressure on abdominal nerves
- sluggish blood circulation in muscles
- tension (when you are almost asleep and nerves make you suddenly jump awake, it can bring on a muscle cramp or charley horse)
- exercise you are not accustomed to

- pointing your toes (while stretching)
- not enough salt.

If you suspect your cramps are due to insufficient calcium—found in dairy products, dark leafy vegetables, molasses, tofu—eat more of these foods or, after checking with your obstetrical caretaker, try commercial calcium supplements. Take a 650 mg tablet of calcium lactate three times a day along with vitamin C, or, take 1 gram of a calcium supplement twice daily for two weeks.

To head off cramps before they get a grip on you, keep your legs warm, do not point your toes when you stretch or do exercises, try taking a warm bath before bed to relax tense muscles, maybe practice yoga, or try a light massage up and down your legs.

Here are ways to get rid of them once they've struck:

- rapid, firm, rigorous massage to the affected muscle
- straighten your leg and pull your foot toward you (or, if you can't reach your toes anymore, ask a friend to help). Never point your toes.

Expect a few minutes of pain before relief comes. Even after the intensity and pull subside a dull after-ache may remain.

Morning Sickness. Nausea and vomiting during pregnancy occur in fewer than half of all pregnancies. Morning sickness is something of a misnomer, since it can strike at any time of the day or night. It can range in severity from minor nausea that can be controlled by altering your eating habits, to severe vomiting and dehydration resulting in hospitalization. Morning sickness follows an erratic pattern for each individual woman; during one pregnancy you may experience no nausea, while in a subsequent pregnancy, it may be a different story.

No one is sure what causes morning sickness, but some theories are:

- The time frame when most women suffer from morning sickness coincides with the period from implantation (seventh day after conception) into the third month. During this time chorionic gonadotropin, the chemical messenger that secretes progesterone to maintain the lining of the uterus, is at its highest level. Nausea usually subsides by the fourteenth week, when the placenta begins to take over the job of producing progesterone.
- You are lacking crucial vitamins, especially B_6, and minerals.
- There is a shift in the hormonal balance, particularly with excess estrogen.
- There is a low blood-sugar level in the morning because of an empty stomach.

NATURAL REMEDIES

consume small, frequent meals

avoid going for long periods without food

drink fluids between rather than with meals

avoid tepid fluids and stick to very hot or very cold liquids

munch on crackers, dry toast or bread that has a touch of sugar on it before getting out of bed in the morning

don't jump out of bed, but get up gradually

try small amounts of apple or grape juice or carbonated drinks

avoid fried and greasy foods

avoid heavily seasoned foods

boiled egg, baked potato, lamb and chicken are best tolerated

be sure to get enough B_1 and B_6 vitamins (cereal grains, wheat germ, seeds, pork, liver)

try cooking with herbs such as wild yam root, raspberry leaf, peppermint, camomile, lemon balm, catnip

get fresh air, of course

In addition to these suggested remedies, there are gadgets such as elastic straps worn on each arm to pressure the acupuncture points that control nausea.

MEDICATIONS

B vitamins, specifically B_6 (also known as pyridoxine). 100 mg taken of B_1 (thiamine) once daily or a balanced B-complex vitamin are other alternatives. Such therapy should not be tried without first consulting one's doctor or midwife and only after natural remedies have been exhausted.

Most nausea drugs, such as Compazine, seem to be ineffective and have not been adequately tested on pregnant women. Bendectin is the *only* prescription drug approved for morning sickness by the U.S. Food and Drug Administration; however, in 1983 the manufacturer stopped making the anti-nauseant tablets. After being sold for 25 years, Merrell Dow said its decision was for non-medical reasons; the company's insurance premiums had soared, owing to hundreds of lawsuits alleging Bendectin had caused birth defects. The scientific research on Bendectin remains inconclusive and contradictory. A review of 250,000 births completed by the Centers for Disease Control and a study at the Boston Collaborative Drug Surveillance Program both implicate Bendectin as responsible for missing fingers, hands or feet. The drug is also suspected of causing stomach deformities, which sometimes can be corrected surgically. Several studies found no association between such birth defects and Bendectin. For women experiencing severe nausea, where the unborn child may risk being malnourished, hospitalization may be the only option in the absence of an effective anti-nauseant drug.

Shooting Pains. In the final month of pregnancy you may feel sharp, knifelike pains shooting along one or both sides of your groin, radiating down your thighs or traveling from the back of your pelvis down your leg. Your ligaments, bones and nerves can all be blamed for this harmless discomfort.

- Ligaments that support your uterus act like suspenders. Beginning at about the twentieth week and continuing through the thirty-second, they may cause some pain, probably the result of sudden contractions of one of the two round ligaments. If you have been sitting at your desk too long and stand up, pain may strike suddenly. Some women complain also of a stitch-in-the-side sensation.
- Near term, your pelvic bony structure softens and the front bones separate to make room for your baby's head to pass. You may feel a dull ache and/or shooting pains radiating down the front and inner sides of your thighs.
- At about the thirty-sixth week, or after your baby drops farther into your pelvis, you may feel a pinching sensation in your back, sending sharp pains down the back of your leg. This comes from your baby's head pressing on your sciatic nerve. Bring your knee up to your tummy and hold it there for a few moments till the pinching subsides.

For any shooting pains, you might try the pelvic-rock exercise (see "Conditioning Exercises: What's a Kegel?" p. 68).

Swelling, Edema. If your rings no longer slip easily on your fingers or if you notice your cheekbones starting to "disappear," chances are you are somewhere in the third trimester of pregnancy. Excess fluid in your body—bringing the total up to six liters—is responsible for the swelling in your face, hands, feet and ankles.

Fluid retention is necessary in pregnancy and has even been associated with good pregnancy outcome. Extra water serves to balance the increased blood volume and will keep you from going into shock after the normal blood loss accompanying birth.

During the first six months of gestation your accumulation of fluid is matched by an increase in your fluid "clearance" rate (those frequent trips to the bathroom). But by the thirtieth week the fluid buildup overtakes urination, causing puffiness, or edema. Edema is distinguished from simple swelling by its "pitting" nature. When you slip off your tennis socks, for instance, your ankles will be marked by the depression left from the pressure of their elasticized tops.

Although you may be releasing more water through lots of perspiration while pregnant, your body is still essentially a giant sponge. The sponge effect comes from rising levels of progesterone coupled with estrogen's effect on aldosterone levels, which makes your kidneys absorb more salt and water.

Remember, swelling and some edema are normal, and good for you. Severe edema, however, can signal serious complications, such as toxemia, otherwise termed preeclampsia. If your eyelids are very puffy and heavy, your cheeks shiny and the skin under your jaw swollen, notify your obstetrical caretaker.

In order to keep from holding too much fluid:

- cut down on salt, but do not eliminate it altogether
- limit your carbohydrates and fats and make sure you eat plenty of protein
- remove less-than-loose rings before they get uncomfortably tight
- lie down periodically with your legs up. Rest actually promotes fluid clearance, especially if you lie on your left (heart) side.
- do *not* take diuretics. Water pills, such as Pamprin, to reduce fluid retention or edema are not recommended. They may trigger a potassium deficiency, which can upset your electrolyte balance and may cause the placenta not to function properly. Absolutely no diuretics containing mercury should be taken. The U.S. Food and Drug Administration advises that diuretics do not prevent pregnancy-induced hypertension (toxemia), and that swelling (edema) usually needs no treatment other than such measures as elevating the legs or wearing support stockings.
- increase your water intake to eight glasses a day (not sodas). The combination of lying on the left side and consuming extra water is beneficial to pull fluid from puffy tissues back into the bloodstream to be excreted by the kidneys.

Varicose Veins. Varicose veins first appear as thin red squiggly lines just under the skin inside and in back of your calves or above the inside of your knees. These marks then often swell, standing out on your skin's surface as bluish or brownish veins and making your calves ache and throb after a long day, especially if you've spent a good deal of time on your feet. Varicose veins in your rectum (hemorrhoids) and vulva may fill up in the same way and for the same reasons.

Your circulatory system is designed to allow blood to flow evenly in all parts of your body, to and from the central pump, your heart. In your leg veins, for example, tiny valves are placed at varied intervals to open and close periodically regulating the return blood flow. When the hormone progesterone relaxes your smooth muscles during pregnancy, it also affects your veins, letting their walls stretch to accommodate more blood. The stretching of vein walls also means that these little valves will no longer close properly and blood will not return as efficiently to your heart and will collect in vessels from your waist down. The uterus also tends to slow up blood flow because it weighs on vessels in your pelvis, further obstructing the circulation route from legs to heart. Other factors involved are excessive weight gain and an inherited predisposition to varicose veins.

There are lots of tricks to counteract the pooling of blood and stimulate return flow:

- lie down on your left side
- prop your feet up whenever possible
- don't cross your legs
- avoid standing still; keep your legs and feet moving even if you just tense and relax your muscles, flex your knees and wiggle your toes
- avoid wearing anything that binds you around your upper legs such as tight elastic panties or a girdle
- wear support stockings, putting them on even before you get out of bed in the morning (buy one-half size larger than usual). If you have a prescription for them, save the receipt, because sometimes it can be applied to the medical deductible on insurance.
- avoid excessive weight gain
- wear walking shoes with lots of cushiony support.

Information Sources

ADDITIONAL READING

Positive Pregnancy Through Yoga, by Sylvia Klein Olkin (Englewood Cliffs, NJ: Prentice-Hall, 1981).

Safe Natural Remedies for the Discomforts of Pregnancy. Available for $1.25 from the Coalition for the Medical Rights of Women, 1638 B Haight St., San Francisco, CA 94117.

A Year of Beauty and Exercise for the Pregnant Woman, by Judi Mahon (New York: Lippincott & Crowell, 1980).

Also see "Warning Signs: When to Be Concerned" (p. 162).

OTHER SIDE EFFECTS OF PREGNANCY

Your complexion may clear up or, for the first time in your life, pimples may crop up. You may find your hair has more body than ever before or it may be limp and lifeless. Perhaps your contact lenses are giving you trouble. And your belly button is protruding. The good news about these weird side effects is that they come and go, and most of the time everything returns to normal after birth. Remember, your body—literally from head to toe—adapts to and rebels against the demands placed on it.

Appetite. Often one of the first clues of pregnancy is a strange metallic taste in your mouth. Sensitivity to smells and tastes may be due to fluctuating levels of estrogen and progesterone in your circulation, showing up in altered "thresholds" of sweetness, sourness, bitterness and saltiness. This is one explanation for dietary cravings and aversions. The various theories offered to explain particular food cravings are all rather shaky. A few we've heard are:

- the need for calcium (found in dairy products) and iron (a trace of which is found in chocolate)
- a demand for more calories
- boredom
- the body's reaction to stress and anxiety (based on the theory that stress triggers a need for sugar)
- nature's way of sweetening fluid to whet baby's appetite, so he/she will drink more nutrients.

Contrary to folklore, most experts agree that cravings do not signal a deficiency in those foods. That does not mean you should not indulge yourself occasionally, but be aware of worthless calories (milk shakes, for instance, at some fast-food joints are nondairy) and beware of bizarre food cravings. The urge to eat nonfood substances is a condition called "pica," which can seriously harm the developing fetus. Such cravings include the desire for ice, chalk, clay, coffee grounds, laundry detergent, cornstarch. Consuming any of these substances can interfere with your system's ability to absorb valuable nutrients and can lead to anemia, intestinal blockage, toxemia and other serious problems.

Breasts. Within weeks of conception your breasts will start to feel heavier, turn darker around your nipples, and occasionally tingle and throb. The initial soreness is due to engorgement of your veins by the rising volume of red blood cells and plasma in your system. This also causes fuller breasts and, possibly, protruding veins. Hormones are soon at work, too. In these large glands, progesterone results in swelling, and estrogen prepares your breasts for milk production. That throbbing sensation is probably from estrogen's stimulation of your milk ducts as well as from the expansion of breast tissue.

By the second trimester, your breasts are fully operational for nursing and sometime after the nineteenth week probably will begin to secrete a little bit of the filmy substance called colostrum, the forerunner of mother's milk. During pregnancy, a bra that provides support is a good idea, especially if you have large breasts to start with. Not only will it ease the discomfort of the extra weight, but it will help keep your nonmuscled breasts from stretching out too much. If your nipples are extrasensitive, try putting a little swatch of material or a Kleenex in your bra to cut down on the friction.

Coordination. You may feel more clumsy even before you carry extra "bulk." The fear of tripping or falling may cause you to be less surefooted. The mechanism responsible for some of the awkwardness, including bumping into things, remains a mystery, but researchers do connect it with changes in your neuromuscular system and reflex responses.

Ears. The "stuffy" ear sensation you sometimes experience after a long swim or in an airplane as it lands is similar to what you may feel if increased blood volume fills up blood vessels in your ear canals.

Eyes. Even your eyeballs temporarily change shape, because of increased water retention and elevated hormone levels. You may not see quite so clearly, and, if you depend on contact lenses, you might expect some difficulties during pregnancy. Your lens may not fit so well, and it is not uncommon for expectant mothers to resort to wearing glasses. Try cleaning your contacts several times a day if they cloud over more than usual. Your eye doctor or optician will be able to suggest specific types of eye drops or "tears," depending on the type of contacts you wear. This is a temporary condition, and most mothers find the symptoms subside after pregnancy.

Little floaters that some people frequently see in front of their eyes may turn into large spots during pregnancy. If they persist or you experience blurred vision, notify your health-care provider immediately.

Gas. That bloated feeling comes from the molasses-slow pace of your intestines. You may also have unconsciously swallowed some air while suffering from morning sickness, trapping gas in your digestive tract. To prevent pockets of gas from forming, avoid cabbage, beans, broccoli, corn, onions, sweet desserts.

Dizzy Spells. Your body is suddenly adjusting, making room for a new life, and the shift in gears may be jerky. You feel dizzy because of a decrease in oxygen-carrying blood to your brain. At the onset of pregnancy, your blood pressure falls, because blood is called down from your head and upper extremities to meet the demands of your now-hungry womb. Progesterone adds to the pooling of blood below the waist by dilating veins, and inhibits the blood flow's round trip to the heart. The distribution of blood is temporarily out-of-kilter, so in the first three months especially, any abrupt change in position—particularly from sitting to standing—can throw the adjustment of your circulation reflexes off-balance. Eating regularly helps to prevent dizziness. When you feel light-headed, sit down immediately and lower your head between your knees, taking several deep breaths so as to get the blood rushing to feed oxygen to your brain cells. If you experience frequent dizzy spells and actually faint frequently, notify your physician or midwife.

Heart Flutters. From time to time you might feel that your heart has temporarily turned into a butterfly, even when you are reading quietly in bed. These palpitations result from a brief acceleration of heart activity, which you usually feel as a flutter in your chest or, sometimes, deep in your throat. The general level of excitability of your heart tends to increase during pregnancy, perhaps because it has 30-40 percent more blood to pump, a quicker pulse rate, adding 10 to 15 beats per minute, or because your heart sits a bit higher, thanks to your expanding uterus. Occasional flutters can happen in any normal pregnancy, but if they become habitual, contact your health adviser.

Nose. Your nose may feel "fuller" because of additional blood sent to vessels in its mucous lining, and greater amounts of mucus may be secreted. It is best to stay away from nasal drops or sprays for relief. Instead, try mixing a half teaspoon salt with a half cup warm water and use it in a nasal-spray bottle.

The tiny blood vessels that line your nose are now more congested with blood, and can break at the least trauma. They are more fragile because of elevated levels of progesterone. Living in a particularly dry house can aggravate the problem, since the natural cleansing mucus in your nose will dry up, attach itself to the delicate lining and pull some of it off when you blow your nose. Treat your nose gently and keep your nostrils moist with a little Vaseline. To stop a nosebleed, tilt your head back and apply pressure to the bridge of your nose. If nosebleeds occur frequently or become severe, notify your doctor or midwife.

Insomnia. You might think that during the last few weeks before your baby's arrival your baby would be telling you to sleep...sleep! Strangely enough, the opposite is, in fact, true. Your metabolism rate actually speeds up as you near the homestretch, generating spurts of energy sometimes interpreted as the "nesting instinct," since the added energy is often spent in making final preparations for your baby and perhaps organizing and cleaning your house. Unfortunately, your metabolism doesn't know when night falls, so you may stay keyed-up and excited at night, perhaps dozing for two to three hours, then waking up, unable to get back to sleep. Maybe this automatic wake-up mechanism is designed to condition you for those 2:00 A.M. feedings. Add to that body changes such as fluctuations in your body temperature, frequent trips to the bathroom and pressure in your lower abdomen, not to mention your passenger, who is practicing the drums, and the possibility of falling asleep becomes even more remote. Just as you did not fight sleepiness early on, don't fight the lack of it toward the end. Your body will take all the rest it needs, and worry only keeps sleep at bay.

Stay away from sleeping pills. Most of these preparations contain antihistamines, which are not recommended for expectant mothers; another key ingredient, scopolamine, is not even present in sufficient quantity to produce drowsiness, according to *AMA Evaluations*. Everyone has her own tricks for insomnia; at least one of these should help:

- having an early dinner and avoiding hard-to-digest foods
- a very warm bath before bed
- a cup of hot milk (cocoa may keep you awake since it contains caffeine)
- lying on your left side, in running position, with a pillow under the right knee
- other pillow arrangements
- a hot water bottle or heating pad if backache interferes with sleep
- hot herbal teas
- a good book that isn't too exciting
- letter-writing or finishing some project
- counting sheep.

Nightmares. Since psychologists tell us that we usually dream about things we fear most, it is not surprising that expectant mothers have recurrent nightmares about difficult labor and losing their babies. These are often more vivid and frightening than your usual run-of-the-mill bad dreams, and come more frequently in that last, restless month before you give birth.

Stitch in your side. The two round ligaments supporting your uterus on either side can become strained, and you may feel a pull in your side. It generally goes away if you take a few minutes to lie down.

Pins and Needles. If your hands are swelling a good deal, you may experience a sharp, tingly pins-and-needles sensation running down your fingers from your wrists. The excess fluid in your wrists is putting pressure on tendons and nerves that bunch up there before spreading through your hands. That's why it seems to be worse in the morning after an overnight buildup of water and moving that joint so little. If the sensation is not coupled with swelling, you may be lacking in vitamin B, so check with your health-care provider.

Moods. Do you wonder why you are bouncy one moment and weepy the next? What makes you short-tempered? What causes those feelings of ambivalence and resentment about being pregnant? These emotional flip-flops are in large part biologically activated, specifically due to fluctuating hormone levels of progesterone in your system, which acts as a depressant. Excitement, anxiety attacks, identity crises, phobias, bad dreams and feelings of dependency are all quite normal mood swings for expectant mothers, and often for expectant fathers.

Perspiration. The combination of increased sweat-gland activity and heightened blood flow to your skin, generating more heat, will cause you to perspire more. This is especially true when your thyroid hormone activity increases, during the last three months.

Vaginal Discharge. Clear or whitish secretions from your vagina will increase, due to higher blood-flow volume to that part of your body. If the discharge becomes yellowish or smelly and/or makes you sore, you may have a vaginal infection. It is best not to wait until your next prenatal checkup but to call the medical clinic or doctor's office, because the physician or midwife may want to see you right away.

Pigmentation. Greatly elevated blood levels of estrogen and progesterone are believed to stimulate cells in your skin's surface that may produce a dark brown pigment from about the second month until shortly after birth. The areas affected are directly related to pregnancy and have nothing to do with sun exposure, although sunscreen can be effective in controlling such changes.

- The "mask of pregnancy" can range from small, yellow-brown spots to dark brown patches marching along the nose, cheeks or neck. For black women it is sometimes the reverse, showing up as whitish, depigmented areas. Small freckles of the mask may never disappear or may recur if you go on the Pill. One suggestion is to wear a sun block if you are at the beach or lounging next to a pool, or even around fluorescent lights at the office.
- A "linea negra," or dark line, may appear, running from the pubic area to the belly button, beginning at about the fourteenth week. This usually occurs only in white-skinned brunettes and deep-pigmented black women. This demarcation does fade, but not immediately after birth.

- The nipples and areolas often get darker around the third month.
- Tiny skin tags may spring up, usually from about the fourth month on, and often disappear after childbirth. These are in the form of tiny bumps thought to be the effect of hormones on nerve and blood cells.
- Warts, moles and surgical scars may temporarily darken.

Mild Rashes. More blood flow to the capillaries, dilated veins and increased sweat-gland activity combine to give a hot and clammy feel to your skin, especially during the second trimester, and may produce a mild rash or prickly heat.

Your skin may be hypersensitive to touch and to extremes in temperature, also believed to be related to the hormone-induced change in blood flow. Staying cool and dry should help. Loose-fitting clothes will relieve prickly heat, and lotion can reduce itching, although too much cream or ointment can actually aggravate the condition. Any unusual or severe rash should be checked by your physician or midwife.

Shortness of Breath. Being short of breath can be a sign of anemia, although most pregnant women experience it at sometime, especially as the due date approaches. The movement of your diaphragm, the muscle responsible for pushing your lungs up, then letting them down, so you can inhale and exhale, becomes restricted as your lower abdomen expands upward. This cuts down on your air supply, so even after the slightest exertion you may huff and puff. Lying down, of course, only makes it worse, since the force of gravity is no longer working in your favor. In order to sleep, just prop your torso up on a few pillows. If "lightening" occurs (the baby's head drops down in your pelvis prior to labor), you will breathe a sigh of relief, since those additional centimeters of space take some of the pressure off your diaphragm.

Uterine Contractions. Your uterus undergoes mild, irregular contractions, even in early months. By the second trimester they can be felt on the outside of your abdomen as it firms, then relaxes, corresponding to the tensing and softening of your uterus. Since Braxton-Hicks was the first to notice these, the contractions bear his name. Until the final month prior to delivery, Braxton-Hicks contractions are infrequent, sporadic and have no rhythmic pattern. In the last week or two, however, they will speed up, perhaps occurring at intervals of 10 to 20 minutes as your uterus practices for labor (see "Signs of Labor: True or False?" p. 213).

Unsteady Joints. If you feel wobbly in the final weeks, it is probably because the bones in your pelvis are separating slightly under the influence of the hormone relaxin, to give your baby a bit more room to pass into the birth canal. This loosens up the support you are used to leaning on.

Stretch (and Other) Marks. Stretch marks on white skin appear as thin pink lines, which eventually become dense white or brown and a bit wrinkled. On black skin they are more silver-gray in color. Most pregnant women get them, to a greater or lesser degree, according to how rapid or dramatic their weight gain is and if stretch marks run in the family. These squiggly stripes show up in the places where you stretch the most—breasts, thighs, tummy—because they come from weakened, elastic overextended skin fibers, pulled beyond the norm by the expanding uterus and extra deposits of fats and fluid. The addition of high progesterone levels makes stretch marks appear more readily than if you were to gain the same amount of weight while nonpregnant. Cocoa butter and lotions are recommended for the itching and pulling sensation that accompanies stretch marks, but no lotion or cream will prevent them from appearing.

Elevated estrogen levels, along with the increased expansion of blood vessels, are responsible for yet another skin phenomenon: vascular "spiders." You will notice these, any time from the second to the third month, as spiderlike reddish spots under the surface of the skin, on your face, neck, upper chest or arms.

Teeth and Gums. Your teeth and gums will need special attention throughout the maternity cycle. Your baby soaks up your store of calcium at the same time that thyroid and parathyroid functions in your system increase calcium elimination. Lack of sufficient calcium can lead to brittleness and decay in your own teeth.

Owing to an increase in estrogen, which increases blood supply and dilates veins just under the gums, your gums will swell, becoming tender and forming small gaps between their surface and your teeth. Food and stale saliva collect here, forming plaque, leading to tooth decay and gum problems. The old wives' tale that you loose a tooth for every baby is just that—a tale—as long as you pay attention to dental and gum care.

For more information, refer to "Looking Good: Complexion, Hair, Nails," (p. 150). And if you are worried, refer to "Warning Signs: When to Be Concerned" (p. 162).

SEX: TRIMESTER TO TRIMESTER

Sex is often more spontaneous and enjoyable, now that you are free from concern about contraception, yet practically every expectant parent worries about hurting the baby. Your baby is like an egg in a bowl full of water, surrounded by layers of protection that can absorb extra weight and pressure. Many experts now say, "Do whatever feels comfortable from the day of conception to the day of delivery, provided no medical problems arise." This certainly is in contrast to prohibitions our mothers were given, like the advice in *Better Homes and Gardens'* 1949 *Baby Book:* "Intercourse shouldn't be indulged in at all during the last two or three months." But many obstetricians still recommend abstinence at least four weeks before one's due date. Those who rarely discourage sex during pregnancy contend that the psychological benefits of intimacy outweigh the remote risks.

The primary controversy that divides the medical community is whether sex increases the risk of premature labor. Several studies published in the early seventies suggest that orgasm late in pregnancy induces uterine contractions and may trigger preterm labor. Research by Masters and Johnson found that labor will not start just because of coitus but that sex may initiate or stimulate contractions if conditions for childbirth are ripe. Anthropologist Margaret Mead reported that some primitive cultures use coitus to help along sluggish labor. A survey of over 10,000 low-risk pregnancies conducted in Israel in conjunction with the National Institutes of Health concluded that those having intercourse "showed no increased risk of premature rupture of membranes, low birthweight, or perinatal death at any gestational age . . . Preterm delivery was no more frequent in those having intercourse than in those abstaining." In fact, this study actually showed better outcomes for those who did engage in sex, but the researchers attributed those results to other factors.

Infection is another underlying concern in the back of some doctors' minds, although no hard evidence exists. An analysis of 25,000 pregnancies nationwide by Dr. Richard Naeye of Pennsylvania's Hershey Medical Center spotted a relationship between those expectant mothers who had sex during the last month and amniotic-fluid infections, a condition that can result in infant mortality. Naeye hypothesizes that sperm may help bacteria penetrate the cervix and membranes; he cautions, however, against drawing specific conclusions. Much criticism has been leveled against this analysis; some say that most of the deaths were due to prematurity, not to amniotic infections. Other medical experts contend that chlamydia infection and other sexually transmitted diseases that were not diagnosed at the time of pregnancy may explain Dr. Naeye's findings.

Apart from these provocative theories, the reason some physicians discourage sex during the ninth month (and sometimes during the entire third trimester) is simply "not to take any chances because parents would blame themselves if something went wrong." Some discourage engaging in coitus if you are carrying twins or the baby is in transverse position, though there is no consensus about this either. In the chart below, the middle column describes the feelings of those who would advise abstinence for many medical conditions. You have to decide with your doctor or midwife what's best for you. Often when intercourse is not advised, orgasm achieved by masturbation is usually also included on the theory that it too may stimulate the uterus to contract.

No Restrictions	Maybe/Maybe Not	Abstinence
normal pregnancy	history of miscarriages	cervix begins to open (dilate)
	threatened miscarriage	
	previous preterm birth	bag of water breaks and/or blood shows when mucous plug is dislodged and the seal protecting the baby from infection is broken
	twins, triplets, etc., since uterus must sustain more weight	
	incompetent cervix (neck of uterus cannot bear baby's weight)	
	baby in breech or other than headfirst position	abdominal or vaginal pain, which could indicate premature labor, bladder infection or detached placenta
	uterine scar from surgery	vaginal bleeding
	hypertension (high blood pressure)	threatened premature labor

Even though the sexual revolution of the sixties cracked open the whole issue of human sexuality, this subject is often not brought up at prenatal checkups either by the health-care provider or the expectant mother. Several precautions rarely discussed include the following:

- Blowing air into the vagina is dangerous and should not be done at all during pregnancy since it can actually force air bubbles into the bloodstream, leading to embolism and stroke.
- Douching with a bulb syringe can also cause air embolisms. Check with your physician or midwife before practicing this type of hygiene.
- Alternating between anal and vaginal penetration is not advisable, because during pregnancy you are especially prone to vaginal infections. A condom or careful washing between entries reduces the risk of transmitting germs.
- Urinating right after intercourse is advisable to avoid getting a urinary-tract infection, since pregnancy creates an ideal climate for infection in your bladder and/or kidneys.

Every woman responds in a highly individualistic way to all the physiological and psychological changes she undergoes. As you might expect, there is no typical pattern of sexual behavior during the maternity cycle. Research by Masters and Johnson found an increase in sexual activities in the second trimester, but other studies observed a steady decline in all modes of lovemaking as pregnancy progressed. The authors of *Making Love During Pregnancy* describe four different patterns of sex drive, ranging from no change from month to month, to a steady increase through the final trimester. We've outlined some of the more predictable emotional and physical changes that affect one's interest in sex:

Stage of Pregnancy	Positive	Negative
First Trimester	Because no longer anxious to conceive, or because free from contraceptive use, more relaxed	Tired, nauseous and perhaps worried about miscarriage
Second Trimester	Increased blood flow to breasts and pelvis, increased lubrication (vaginal discharge), and elevated production of estrogen and steroids make some women feel erotically supercharged	More afraid of hurting baby because of greater awareness of his/her presence due to size and movements
Third Trimester	Sexual intimacy provides reassurance in relationship, particularly during the final weeks, when expectant mother tends to feel more vulnerable and dependent	Fatigue, physical discomfort, awkwardness, feeling unattractive

All expectant parents soon find that the man-on-top position is less than ideal, and need to experiment with other positions, such as woman-on-top, lying side-by-side facing each other, and front-to-back, with the male approaching from behind. *Making Love During Pregnancy* has sketches of these and many other positions. Without question, a sense of humor and plenty of dialogue between partners are essential for getting through the sometimes trying moments during pregnancy.

Factors to Weigh

Some uncertainties about sex during pregnancy continue to cloud the picture, but more and more medical experts now say, in the absence of certain complications, that you have the green light as long as it feels comfortable. Those who discourage intercourse several weeks prior to one's due date are usually concerned about the unlikely and unproven risk of premature labor or infection. No experts worry about a man's weight on the womb or that penetration causes harm to the fetus, since a woman's protective instincts provide adequate safeguards. Your body will let you know if you should stop; in the event of abdominal pain, bleeding or any signs of labor, notify your physician or midwife. (Don't be alarmed if your genitals remain swollen for a few hours after lovemaking; usually it is just taking longer for the increased blood flow to subside.)

For many, pregnancy is a worry-free time to enjoy sex, and an intimate, affectionate relationship helps get through the rougher times during those nine months.

Information Sources

ADDITIONAL READING

Making Love During Pregnancy, by Elizabeth Bing and Libby Colman (New York: Bantam, 1977).

Sex, by Michael Carrera (New York: Crown Publishers, 1981).

Information about herpes and other sexually transmitted diseases is included in "Anemia, Herpes, Toxemia and Other Complicating Factors" (p. 170).

CONDITIONING EXERCISES: WHAT'S A KEGEL?

Two sets of muscles undergo dramatic change during these nine months. Abdominal muscles stretch to accommodate your expanding uterus, and the muscles around your expanding uterus and around your vagina and anus soften to ease your baby's exit from the womb. Several simple exercises can help minimize backache and other common discomforts brought on by pregnancy. Other conditioning drills that maintain muscle tone also help expectant mothers to become aware of the intricate network of muscles that will be used during childbirth. The earlier you develop the habit of doing various conditioning exercises, the better, because by late pregnancy the abdominal muscles are already stretched, and it is difficult to start strengthening them. Other benefits of the prenatal exercises described here include improving circulation, enhancing posture and providing a feeling of strength and well-being.

You may want to consult with your own doctor or midwife about your overall fitness regime to get advice about specific conditioning exercises. Regardless of what drills constitute your workout, follow these guidelines:

- warm up slowly and don't overdo
- maintain a relaxed attitude
- keep movements controlled and rhythmic
- avoid any exercises that deepen the hollow of your back
- rest if you get dizzy and stop if you feel miserable
- don't get out of breath
- take time to cool down with exercises that return muscles and the heart rate to normal.

Keep in mind that your joints are unusually vulnerable to sudden movements that could damage them. The elevated levels of several hormones, including relaxin, soften ligaments and connective tissues, particularly in the pelvis, so take time to warm up and avoid uncontrolled, jerky motions.

All instructors and exercise books have their own ways of teaching the most basic drills, whether they be the pelvic rock or the calf stretch. Most of these exercises are harmless, but some experts worry about certain stretching and abdominal exercises, particularly sit-ups and double leg raises. If you are unaccustomed to doing sit-ups, many health professionals say it is not worth the risk of putting too much stress on your stomach muscles, because of the remote possibility that the placenta will detach itself from the uterine wall. Bonnie Berk, R.N., says, "The first 30 degrees of a sit-up are all back strain, and a pregnant woman needs to strengthen her abdominal muscles, not her back." Dr. Mona Shangold of Cornell University's Sports Gynecology Center suggests, "There is no reason that double leg lifts and sit-ups are bad unless you possibly have back trouble. . . . Since some women are unaware of a back problem, it is better to do roll-ups, with the knees lifted." To do a roll-up, lie on your back with both legs bent, and as you exhale, slowly lift your head and shoulders off the floor. Tighten your buttocks and contract your abdomen against your spine.

Books, cassette and video tapes, not to mention special prenatal exercise classes for expectant parents, can complement the conditioning techniques elaborated here. Swimming, tennis and many other sports activities are discussed at length in Chapter 3.

Kegels. In the 1950s, Arnold Kegel, a gynecologist, postulated that strengthening the muscles around the vaginal and rectal openings could correct urinary incontinence, an annoying problem that is often triggered by childbirth and the natural aging process. These "perineal" muscles work harder when the body is in an upright position, fighting the forces of gravity and pregnancy. Another benefit of conditioning the perineal area is learning how to relax and contract these muscles that will be used throughout each stage of childbirth. Immediately after delivery, perineal exercises enhance circulation, promote healing, reduce soreness and, equally important, help to regain normal muscle tone. Kegels, or the perineal squeeze, are considered the most important prenatal and postpartum exercise by many health experts because they:

- improve muscle tone and elasticity
- provide the necessary support for pelvic organs during pregnancy and postpartum
- protect against uterine prolapse
- prevent or reduce incontinence
- enhance sexual pleasure for both partners.

The beauty of this exercise is that it can be done in any position, anywhere, and no one can tell you're doing it. To become aware of the muscles involved, practice urinating teaspoon by teaspoon. Simply contract and release to stop and start the flow of urine. This also can be practiced during intercourse by tightening these same muscles around the penis. To get in the habit of doing a set of Kegels several times daily, many childbirth educators suggest that you do them when you brush your teeth or do some other daily activity. To make it effective, hold each perineal squeeze (without tensing your thighs or buttocks) for about eight to ten seconds. It takes practice.

While it may be wise to get acquainted with these muscles, some experts suggest you wait to begin practicing Kegels until after the baby is born. This school of thought theorizes that an episiotomy (a surgical cut enlarging the birth outlet at the time of delivery) is more likely if the mother's pelvic floor becomes overly muscular. (More details on perineal massage and episiotomies can be found on pp. 197 and 249.)

Pelvic Rock. This exercise is suggested for anyone suffering from lower backache, and can be accomplished in several positions. On all fours, arch your back like a cat, by rocking your pelvis upward and tightening your abdominal muscles and buttocks. Then allow your pelvis to drop gradually, but keep your back straight, with your abdomen and buttocks relaxed. Another position for the pelvic rock to release back tension is to lie on your back with your knees bent and feet flat on the floor. Tighten the muscles of your lower abdomen and buttocks to flatten your lower back against the floor. Also, an excellent way to check your posture is to do the pelvic rock by standing against a wall and pressing your lower back against it. This turns out to be an effective exercise for strengthening your all-important abdominal muscles.

Squatting. Penny Simkin, a prominent childbirth educator and physical therapist, regards squatting as second in importance only to Kegels. This exercise is beneficial for several reasons:

- maintains the mobility of muscles and joints in the lower-back region
- gets you in the habit of using your legs instead of bending from the waist, which is bad for your back
- increases the pelvic outlet (when practiced late in pregnancy), thus encouraging the baby to rotate and descend
- sometimes helps labor progress
- works with gravity and is often preferred to other positions for pushing during the second stage of labor.

Women who may want to try this position during labor need to practice it beforehand because of shaky balance and wobbly joints. Stand with your feet one or two feet apart. Keep your spine straight and, without bouncing, gradually lower your body, keeping your heels on the floor. To stand, push up with your legs to straighten the knees. (You may also want to refer to "Positions and Labor Equipment: From Squatting to Birthing Chairs," p. 224.)

Posterior Tilt. It's a good idea to check your posture frequently so you avoid getting a swayback. Simply lean back against a wall with your feet about eight to ten inches in front of it. Place your hand behind the curve of your spine and press the entire back against the wall, trying to eliminate the space at the small of your back. Keep your pelvis in its posterior-tilt position as you move away from the wall, and practice it until this posture becomes second nature. This proper alignment of the spine will prevent strain and enhance abdominal-muscle tone.

Tailor Press. This is one way to stretch tight inner-thigh muscles. Sit with your back straight and with the soles of your feet together and drawn as close to your body as is comfortable. Place hands either on your ankles or under the knees. As you exhale, work the muscles of your thighs to move knees gently toward the floor. The tailor press also eases tightness in the shoulders and upper back. Another exercise for toning the inner-thigh muscles is to assume a fencing position, with one leg bent and the other straight. In a smooth, controlled motion, lunge and return to the upright stance. Repeat on the other side with that leg bent.

Rib-Cage Lift. This will relieve pressure under your ribs and the feeling of shortness of breath, both of which are common during the last trimester. Place one hand on your hip; curve the other up over your head. Bend your trunk sideways, stretching with the overhead arm and pivoting over the hand on your hip. Change arm position and repeat on the other side. Another method is to lift first one shoulder and then the other as high as possible. Shoulder rotation not only helps reduce "tightness" of breathing but stretches the pectoral muscles (the primary muscles across the chest). Tight pectoral muscles frequently cause round shoulders and contribute to shortness of breath.

Calf Stretch. Vertical push-ups are most effective in stretching tight calf muscles, which are often caused by wearing high-heeled shoes. Face the wall an arm's length away, with your feet parallel to each other and hip-width apart. Place your palms against the wall and inhale. As you exhale, bend the elbows and try to touch the wall with your forehead, but keep your back straight and heels flat on the floor. Inhale and return to the original, upright position.

Whichever conditioning exercises you choose to practice, they should be both beneficial and enjoyable. Music may help you get in the mood to spend a few minutes doing these body mechanics. Your workout should be free of abrupt, exaggerated movements that could injure joints and ligaments. Also remember to avoid any exercise that causes excessive compression of the uterus or increases the curve of your spine. There's more on exercise in "Sports and Fitness: How Much Should You Do." p. 152.

Information Sources

ADDITIONAL READING

The Complete Pregnancy Exercise Program, by Diana Simkin (New York: New American Library, 1980).

Essential Exercises for the Childbearing Year, by Elizabeth Noble (Boston: Houghton Mifflin, 1976).

The Jane Fonda Workout Book for Pregnancy, Birth and Recovery, by Femmy DeLyser (New York: Simon & Schuster, 1982). Also available in double cassettes or double album.

Moving Through Pregnancy, by Elisabeth Bing (New York: Bantam, 1976).

Pre- and Post-natal Exercises. Wall Chart and Cassette. Poster with pictures of different techniques, from shoulder rolls to inner-thigh stretches. For information about prices contact BABES, 59 Berens Drive, Kentfield, CA 94904.

Suzy Prudden's Pregnancy and Back to Shape Exercise, by Suzy Prudden (New York: Workman, 1982).

SONOGRAM: IS IT WORTH THE PICTURE?

"It's twice as exciting as hearing the baby's heartbeat for the first time," claim many expectant parents, and you get a photo of "Junior in utero" for the baby album. Sonograms, or ultrasound scans, are fast becoming one of the most popular prenatal diagnostic tests. This screening technique works along the same lines as radar and sonar, by short bursts of sound waves that echo back when they hit the baby, placenta and other tissues. These sound waves are translated into an image of dots, which is then projected on a screen. A more sophisticated form of ultrasound, called "real time," can detect activity in the embryo's heart as early as six weeks, and even motion inside the vessels of the umbilical cord.

This high-tech equipment provides doctors with valuable information about the health and development of the baby and offers parents an exciting glimpse at what's happening inside. But, as with any new medical procedure, little is yet known regarding the possible long-term effects on the unborn. There is some disagreement in the medical community regarding the wisdom of routine use on those experiencing a trouble-free pregnancy as well as its repeated use on an individual woman. The debate intensifies, but first, let's look at what a sonogram can provide.

Ultrasound screening usually amounts to a crude physical examination of the developing fetus. It can show:

- *gestational age*—due date can be pinpointed by taking measurements of either the baby's head or the femur bone, which extends from the pelvis to the knee
- *growth rate* of fetus can be charted
- *twins, triplets, and so on,* can be detected
- *initial evaluation* in high-risk pregnancies
- *position of placenta* in the event of bleeding
- *location* of baby and placenta prior to amniocentesis to avoid accidental puncture by the needle

- *confirmation of breech* or other position of baby in relation to birth canal
- *certain birth defects*
- *viability*—if there is reason to suspect the baby is no longer alive.

If something shows up that your doctor does not understand or is concerned about, a radiologist trained in interpreting ultrasound images may be consulted. This second opinion, commonly termed "Stage 2," means another sonogram may be done with a medical team of specialists on hand.

Benefits Versus Risks

Diagnostic ultrasound has been widely used in obstetrics since the mid-seventies, too short a time to notice any long-term effects. The most ambitious study by Dr. E. A. Lyons involves a follow-up of 10,000 Canadian women and their babies exposed to ultrasound at all periods of gestation. When compared to 1000 of their brothers and sisters who were not exposed and a control population of 2000 other children, preliminary conclusions showed no obvious problems with those who were "sonocated" but noted a small but significant rise in the number of babies who were underweight at birth, though this was no longer the case by the time the children reached the age of five years. Surprisingly enough, exposed babies had a lower occurrence of childhood cancers than would be expected for the general population.

Up until a few years ago the medical community was so enthralled by the valuable information provided by ultrasound that it denied that the sound waves had any effect on the unborn child. Now more doctors seem to go along with the caution noted in a 1979 study, in which Dr. Padmaker Lele of M.I.T. suggested, "No diagnostic technique in which energy is radiated into tissues can be totally safe regardless of the power, intensity and biological conditions." Dr. Melvin Stratmeyer of the U.S. Food and Drug Administration's Bureau of Radiological Health worries about not only routine exposures but what he sees as a trend toward using higher intensities of ultrasound to get clear pictures of smaller organs.

Outspoken critics who claim we've often paid the price of indiscriminate use of new technology remind us of what fun it was at the shoe store to stick our feet on the X-ray machine to be measured. Of course, we now know X rays damage soft tissues. Those soft-pedaling the use of ultrasound want to see it limited to diagnosing problems caused by vaginal bleeding or for some other bona fide reason.

Besides the question of safety for the unborn baby, there is also a lack of standardization of instruments, which have varying degrees of energy output. Until better standards are established and until the cost of the procedure goes down, Dr. Charles Hohler, Director of Ultrasound at Arizona's St. Joseph's Medical Center, would like to see it "used in a more definitive fashion with defined goals in mind." However, Dr. Hohler would side with those favoring widespread use, assuring us that the medical community has a "good feel for the energy levels, which really are very small." In view of the valuable glimpse inside the womb, many doctors agree with Dr. Jason Birnholz of Harvard Medical School that "perhaps the most important aspect of routine obstetrical ultrasound is that it provides a means of reassuring a concerned parent that, at a given diagnostic level, everything appears normal."

Ways to Avoid Problems

(1) A sonogram session may cost between $70 and $250, depending on the length of the examination and where it is done. Double-check your insurance policy.

(2) The doctor or technician should be experienced and well trained. Misreading the scan can cause unnecessary worry to expectant parents; for instance, if the fetus is judged to be too small for its age during the third trimester without taking into account the variations in growth rates.

(3) If you are being screened in your doctor's office, ask how new the machine is. Older models tend to have higher dosages of ultrasound waves, which may pose a greater theoretical risk to your baby than more up-to-date machines.

(4) Sophisticated interpretation of a sonogram, Stage 2, should be done by a licensed ultrasonologist.

(5) Beware of services that offer ultrasound video movies of your baby in utero, at least until more is known about this relatively new obstetrical diagnostic test.

(6) When an ultrasound test is done before an amniocentesis is performed, expect the blurry image of the fetus to have a profound effect on you. As John Fletcher, bioethicist at the National Institutes of Health, says, this "shock of recognition" may have the effect of reducing abortions.

Factors to Weigh

Without question, ultrasound is a real breakthrough in science. Most likely the burst of sound waves during pregnancy is not altogether harmless, but if there is a good reason for looking at life inside the womb, the benefits outweigh the as-yet unknown effects on the child. Numerous sonograms during a single pregnancy probably should be avoided because of the possible cumulative effect of energy being radiated into the body tissues. Perhaps the most prudent course is to have this diagnostic test only when there is a valid medical reason.

Information Sources

ADDITIONAL READING

"Question of Risk Still Hovers over Routine Prenatal Use of Ultrasound," by Barbara Bolsen. *Journal of the American Medical Association (JAMA)*, 247: (April 23, 30, 1982), 16. JAMA is available at your doctor's office or at many major public libraries.

"Research in Ultrasound Bioeffects: A Public Health View," by M. E. Stratmeyer. *Birth and the Family Journal*, 7: (Summer 1980), 2. This journal is available at medical libraries.

BIRTH DEFECTS AND GENETIC COUNSELING

Every expectant parent worries, "Will my baby be normal?" Yet the odds are vastly in favor of your having a perfectly healthy child—only about 3 percent of *all* babies born in the U.S. have major genetic or congenital diseases. But this endangered 3 percent can often be helped significantly through surgery, sometimes even to the point of living handicap-free.

Genetic counseling, which essentially consists of a review of a couple's family tree with regard to the family's medical history, usually can rule out the possibility of inherited diseases. Sonograms, amniocenteses and other prenatal tests can detect many disorders before birth, including blood diseases and deformities of the brain and spine. The results of these tests can give prospective parents the opportunity to terminate the pregnancy or to prepare themselves emotionally and financially for a handicapped child. With today's new diagnostic and surgical capabilities, birth defects can be treated, even before birth (see "From Transfusions to Open-Womb Surgery," p. 184).

Advances in genetic research and new ways to detect birth defects remain mired in controversy. In addition to the abortion issue, parents of handicapped children argue that prenatal diagnosis fails to distinguish between mild and severe cases of genetic disorders. Organizations such as the Down's Syndrome Congress emphasize the positive side of raising babies with certain diseases and have formed watchdog committees to assure adequate medical care is available for babies with birth defects.

The origins of many birth defects are still a mystery. Some come from chromosomal accidents, others result from faulty genes and still others are blamed on environmental factors. New research suggests that a combination of causes may be responsible.

Nervous-System and Spinal Malformations

Usually the creation of the baby's central nervous system is uneventful. A minute, platelike arrangement called the "neural tube," which will become the brain, spinal cord and spinal column, is formed in the first few weeks of pregnancy. For some unknown reason, occasionally the vertebrae fail to develop around the spinal cord. These so-called neural-tube defects (NTD) vary in severity. Babies born with anencephaly (little or no brain), the most serious case, are either stillborn or die shortly after birth, while some of the babies with an open spine (spina bifida) can have average intelligence and, with surgery, live handicap-free.

A neural-tube defect appears in approximately one to two births per thousand, ranking as one of the most common birth defects in the U.S. The cause is not known, but combined hereditary and environmental factors are thought to play a part. One new theory suggests that folic acid vitamin deficiency may trigger susceptibility.

All fetuses produce a natural substance called alpha-fetoprotein (AFP) in their urine, which winds up in the amniotic fluid. Some of this protein is always absorbed into the mother's bloodstream. If there is an abnormally large opening in the baby's body, more AFP than usual will be found in the mother's circulation, which will show up in a simple blood test. The test must be done at the proper gestational age (between 15 and 20 weeks) in order to be reliable; otherwise, reports of false positive or false negative AFP levels could result. In fact, finding unusually high levels of AFP is *not* a sure sign of NTD; it can also indicate twins, a threat of possible miscarriage or other medical problems.

To avoid erroneous AFP results, which not only could cause unnecessary emotional stress but might prompt a decision to abort a normal child, follow-up tests are recommended if the initial blood sample is positive. Usually a second AFP blood test is done, and if that is high, a sonogram and an amniocentesis are undertaken. (These procedures are discussed in detail on pp. 73 and 82.) If this sequence of tests is conducted, it can diagnose virtually all cases of anencephaly and four out of five cases of spina bifida. A specialist trained in interpreting ultrasound images is sometimes able to gauge with a sonogram the degree of deformity, prior to birth.

Down's Syndrome

The "accident of nature" responsible for most Down's syndrome babies occurs at conception. Each human cell contains 46 chromosomes, which contain thousands of genes, the programmers of our mental and physical makeups. Each egg and each sperm cell, however, carries only half that number, 23 apiece, so that when they merge, only one complete new cell is formed—an embryo. In Down's syndrome, because of a prior error in cell division, either the sperm or the egg contained an extra number twenty-one chromosome so that together the three number twenty-one chromosomes contribute to the creation of the new body cell. That single genetic mistake, known as Trisomy 21, produces 95 percent of all Down's syndrome babies.

A baby born with DS may have a heart problem, a weak respiratory system, a higher susceptibility to disease and will always have some degree of mental retardation. Attitudes toward these children have changed markedly, and now, with early detection of vision and hearing problems, combined with the help of special-education programs, children with DS can develop good social skills and remain at home. Now surgery can correct facial abnormalities and structural problems such as heart defects.

Down's syndrome occurs in about 1 in 700 live births and appears most frequently in babies born to teenagers and mothers over 40. The chances of bearing a DS baby are approximately 1 in 1000 at age 29, for example, and rise to 1 in about 135 at age 39. (Incidences year by year among women in their thirties and forties are listed on p. 9.) No one knows why the chromosomal accident occurs, but X rays, infections, drugs, hormones and heredity are suspected. The high incidence of these babies born to mothers on either extreme of the traditional childbearing-year scale gives rise to speculation that Down's syndrome is largely age-related, particularly in respect to "older" women.

A sample of theories under investigation includes:

- *Age of egg.* A baby girl is born with a lifetime supply of eggs. As she ages, so do her eggs, which lose their ability to perform well.
- *Faulty natural selection.* Younger women conceive Down's syndrome babies just as often as older women do, but their natural-selection mechanism is more efficient, and they miscarry.
- *Frequency of intercourse.* The older a couple is, the less frequently sex is engaged in. This could create a longer time lag between when an egg is ready to be fertilized and when it actually is fertilized. A longer wait may affect the egg's skill in casting out unnecessary chromosomes.
- *Father's age.* Although about 30 percent of the time it is the father's sperm that contributes the extra genetic material, age is suspected only if he is over 50, perhaps 55. Even then his age ranks second in importance to maternal age.

Down's syndrome can be diagnosed before birth, by amniocentesis. Fluid containing fetal cells is drawn from the amniotic sac and is then analyzed for any chromosomal abnormalities. This prenatal test is generally limited to women 35 or older or those with family histories that might predispose their children to certain birth disorders (see "Amniocentesis: Risky or Not?" p. 82).

Inherited Diseases

While Down's syndrome comes from a mistake in the formation of chromosomes, a separate group of inherited birth defects results from the passing on of a specific faulty gene. These disorders can be contributed by one parent, as in Huntington's chorea, some dwarfism and forms of glaucoma. In the case of hemophilia, color blindness and childhood muscular dystrophy, the defective gene is transmitted only by the mother to her son. Sickle-cell anemia, Tay-Sachs and cystic fibrosis are examples of diseases that must be passed on by both parents.

Because a parent usually carries the faulty gene without ever knowing it, many prepregnancy and prenatal screening programs have been set up to perform "carrier tests" and offer genetic counseling. Amniocentesis can detect many of these disorders if pregnancy is already in progress. Two of the most common types of inherited birth defects are described below.

Sickle-cell anemia is a blood disease caused by a defective hemoglobin gene that forms red blood cells that take the shape of a crescent moon or the blade of a sickle. These abnormal cells sometimes create logjams, which block blood vessels, resulting in severe pain. Anemia sets in because the body does not produce red blood cells fast enough to compensate for the sickle cells prematurely destroyed. Sickle-cell anemia is marked by periods of well-being and stages of illness, often requiring hospitalization. There is no specific cure for this chronic disease, but antibiotics and other drugs control many of the infections, and these children can lead quite normal lives.

Sickle-cell anemia predominantly affects blacks. If only one parent has red blood cells that sickle, then the baby will have either normal red blood cells or be a carrier. Amniocentesis is now the preferred way to detect sickle-cell anemia, rather than testing samples of fetal blood or tissue.

Tay-Sachs is always fatal unlike cases of sickle-cell anemia, which can vary from very severe to mild. Particularly wrenching for parents of these babies is that they appear normal at birth, develop well for a few months but soon falter because of a missing enzyme. Their nervous systems begin to collapse, and in four or five years they die. Although for the population at large there is only one Tay-Sachs baby born per 90,000 births, the disease has a ten times higher incidence among Jewish parents whose ancestry traces back to Central or Eastern Europe. The disease-carrying gene is present in about 1 in 25 Jewish people and can be detected by blood and tear tests. However, measuring the enzyme level is complicated and must be performed only at specialized laboratories (see "Information Sources," p. 81). Since Tay-Sachs is a recessive-gene disease both parents must be carriers to pass it on. There is a one-in-four chance with each pregnancy that the child will be afflicted with this fatal disease when both parents are carriers. Tay-Sachs can be detected during pregnancy by amniocentesis.

A Word of Advice About Genetic Counseling

The cost and quality of all medical care varies and this is particularly true for the burgeoning new field of genetic counseling. If there is some risk of a birth defect, a counselor should not only evaluate your odds according to the laws of genetics but also explore possible treatment and care for a less-than-perfect baby. As with other specialists, expect to shop around. Ask your own doctor for a recommendation or call the ob/gyn or genetics department of a nearby university medical center. Your local March of Dimes chapter, the National Genetics Foundation and the National Clearinghouse for Human Genetic Diseases all offer a free referral service for reputable genetic centers. Health insurance policies do not always cover these sessions, and usually the hourly fee is not cheap.

One example of a comprehensive program is at Georgetown University Hospital in Washington, D.C., where physicians and geneticists team up to provide preamniocentesis seminars for prospective parents. After a basic rundown on chromosomes and a detailed explanation of the amniocentesis procedure, there is private counseling with each couple. Later, in the unlikely event that the test results indicate a baby with birth defects, the counselor presents the parents with their options—elective abortion or raising a handicapped child. If an expectant mother decides to carry the fetus to term, at Georgetown further counseling is available on how to care for a child with that handicap, psychologically and financially.

Here are some pointers on how to get the best information possible if you seek genetic counseling:

(1) First check your insurance coverage. Counseling sessions are not always included under the umbrella of prenatal care. If this is the case, centers often require payment on the spot. However, if a university happens to be doing research on a particular genetic disorder, the charge may be waived.

(2) Make sure there is interaction with your physician if the genetic

counselor is not an M.D. Incidentally, as of 1982, the American Society of Human Genetics has begun to certify geneticists and genetic counselors.

(3) Switch counselors if you are not satisfied or feel uncomfortable because of the underlying personal and emotional issues. In the November 1982 issue, *Parents* magazine cautions, too, that "research has found that, even at an unconscious level genetic counselors may be pressuring patients to make a certain decision based on their own, not the patients', values..."

(4) Repeat tests should be considered if there is any reason to suspect negligence on the part of the laboratory that did the analysis.

(5) If a fetus with birth defects is diagnosed, counselors should give equal play to the decision to terminate a pregnancy and the decision to raise a handicapped baby. They should suggest organizations that can provide emotional support to parents and also be aware of state and local financial assistance programs for handicapped children.

Other suggestions are included next, in "Amniocentesis: Risky or Not?"

Information Sources

ORGANIZATIONS

Down's Syndrome Congress
1640 W. Roosevelt Rd., Rm. 156E
Chicago, IL 60608
(312) 226-0416
Information clearinghouse and free literature.

March of Dimes Birth Defects Foundation
1275 Mamaroneck Ave.
White Plains, NY 10605
Contact your local March of Dimes chapter to find a reputable genetic-counseling center.
Provides prospective parents with information about birth defects, free of charge. Single-page information sheets are available free on thalassemia, cleft lip and palate, club foot, PKU (phenylketonuria), rubella and congenital heart defects.

National Clearinghouse for Human Genetic Diseases
805 15th St., NW
Suite 500
Washington, DC 20005
(202) 842-7617

Provides list of counseling centers in your area from their *Directory of Clinical Genetic Counseling Centers.* The list is organized by state and includes for each center what services it offers—biochemical and/or cytogenetic workshops—as well as the doctor's name.

National Genetics Foundation
555 W. 57th St.
New York, NY 10019
(212) 586-5900
The Foundation's Network Clearinghouse will refer you to its network of 60 university-based genetic centers, which provide diagnosis, treatment and genetic counseling.

National Tay-Sachs and Allied Diseases Association, Inc.
92 Washington Ave.
Cedarhurst, NY 11516
(516) 569-4300
Provides referral of the Tay-Sachs testing center closest to you.

Spina Bifida Association of America
343 S. Dearborn St.
Chicago, IL 60604
(312) 663-1562
Information on neural-tube defects and 100 local chapters provide support to parents with children with spina bifida.
Toll-free number (800) 621-3141 (in Illinois call [312] 663-1562) for advice, information and counseling.

AMNIOCENTESIS: RISKY OR NOT?

Amniocentesis (pronounced am"ne-o-sen-te'sis) can detect before birth most chromosomal abnormalities, including Down's syndrome and over 100 metabolic diseases, and identify the sex of the baby. "Amnio" refers to the protective sac surrounding the unborn child, and "centesis" means pricking. This diagnostic test is routinely offered to those pregnant women 35 or older, because certain genetic disorders increase with advancing maternal age.

A new method of detecting genetic defects as early as the eighth week of pregnancy may eventually replace amniocentesis. Instead of a needle, a small plastic catheter is inserted through the vagina into the uterus to withdraw a preplacenta sample. Similar to amniocentesis, ultrasound is used to guide the catheter to the specific site, known as chorionic villi. The chromosomal analysis can be done quickly, with results often available the same day. This prenatal diagnostic technique, called chorionic villus biopsy, is not yet widely practiced, and most likely it will be some time before expectant mothers can consider this option.

The strong acceptance of amniocentesis by the medical community has occurred partly because doctors want to protect themselves from being held liable for failing to offer adequate genetic screening to a woman who risks bearing a baby with birth defects. No one denies that this test relieves the anxieties felt by practically every expectant mother. But there are those who attack amniocentesis as an unnecessary, expensive procedure and others who characterize it as a "search and destroy mission." Some counter that this prenatal screening helps to prepare people emotionally in the event a handicapped child is diagnosed and argue that amniocentesis is not necessarily linked to the decision to undergo an abortion.

Apart from these legal and ethical arguments, the first questions many expectant parents worry about are: Does it hurt? How safe is it? Most women who have had an amniocentesis compare it to a simple blood test. The difficult part is waiting for the lab results, not the painless 15–30 minute procedure itself. Complications for the mother and her unborn baby are rare, provided a well-trained and experienced doctor performs the test. The government's Institute of Child Health and Human Development regards amniocentesis as "an accurate and highly safe procedure that does not add significant risk to the pregnancy."

The decision whether or not to undergo this genetic screening is predicated on your own personal convictions, your health-insurance coverage and one or more of the following conditions, the chief criterion being the family medical history of both you and the father:

- if there is a family history of Down's syndrome or inherited diseases such as hemophilia
- if you will be 35 years or older at the time of delivery
- if either you or the father has a genetic disorder
- if you have given birth to a baby with genetic disease
- if both parents are Jewish (to rule out Tay-Sachs disease)
- if both parents are black (to rule out sickle-cell anemia)
- if you have had multiple miscarriages
- if you and the father have Rh blood incompatibility (done in third trimester)
- if your physician suspects your baby has an open spine
- if the fear of bearing a child with a genetic disorder is placing great emotional stress on you.

What to Expect

Preamniocentesis counseling precedes the test. The medical history of both sides of the family will be reviewed; this is the best time to ask any questions you might have about amniocentesis. As with any medical procedure that carries some risk, you will be asked to sign an informed consent form.

Usually the procedure is not performed until the second trimester, ideally done between 15 and 19 weeks' gestation. By this stage the volume of amniotic fluid has increased and the fetus is still quite small, so there is a greater chance of having a successful "tap."

It is standard practice nowadays first to use an ultrasound scan (sonogram) to locate the position of the fetus and placenta (see "Sonogram: Is It Worth the Picture?" p. 73). This allows for more precise insertion of the needle through the abdominal and uterine walls. A small amount of amniotic fluid—15 to 20 ml, or about four teaspoons—is drawn to get enough fetal cells to study. At this stage in pregnancy this represents a small percentage of the total amniotic fluid—approximately 250 ml—which is replaced within three to four hours. The initial tap does not always retrieve cells that can be cultured; in that case, the procedure must be repeated. Several prominent experts advise that no more than two needle insertions or "taps" be done during one amniocentesis.

It takes between two and six weeks to grow the fetal cells in a culture and to complete the lab analysis. Some cells grow more rapidly than others which explains why some results are available earlier than others. Many expectant mothers find this waiting period stressful. There is added anxiety when the test results will not be finalized until the very end of the second trimester, providing less time to decide whether to have an abortion if an abnormal baby is diagnosed (24 weeks is the limit in some areas of the country for terminating a pregnancy legally).

Tests are always run for genetic disorders, but not for metabolic diseases, unless warranted by family history. The chromosome count reveals mental retardation and many physical malformations. Amniocentesis identifies the sex of the fetus, which is essential information if either parent is a known carrier of an inherited X-linked disorder such as hemophilia or muscular dystrophy. Female offspring are not affected by an abnormal X chromosome, but a male stands a 50 percent chance of inheriting such a disease.

The biochemical composition of the cells indicates any enzyme deficiencies that can lead to diseases and, in the case of parents with Rh incompatibility, whether the baby needs an intrauterine transfusion.

Amniocentesis is sometimes performed during the third trimester, usually after 32 weeks' gestation, in order to obtain cells to test for the maturity of the baby's lungs when early induction of labor or a cesarean section is considered.

Risks Versus Benefits

Many of the complications arising from amniocentesis have been eliminated, thanks to its increased use over the past 20 years. There has been a quantum leap in the number of trained doctors and technicians administering the test and in the number of laboratories and university hospitals specializing in genetics. The use of sonograms to observe the position of the fetus and the placenta also contributes to an improved track record.

Since the health of the mother and fetus are so closely linked, harm to one often results in harm to the other. In amniocentesis, however, any real danger would be to the unborn child. Most problems experienced by mothers are minor, such as mild cramping and spotting. Although rare, puncture of the placenta can prove life-threatening to the fetus. Some leakage of amniotic fluid is not uncommon, but if it persists the doctor usually will order bed rest and watch for fever, a sign of infection. Although chances are slight, leakage of amniotic fluid could become a major complication and result in a miscarriage. Other risks to the fetus include needle-puncture marks to the baby, dislocation of a hip and respiratory problems after birth, although these are also very unusual.

Two large studies, sponsored by the National Institute of Child Health and Human Development (NICHD) and a Canadian government investigation, each monitoring more than 1000 amniocenteses, found no difference in pregnancy outcome. The NICHD study showed that amniocentesis did not significantly increase the chance of a miscarriage. Two percent of the women experienced vaginal bleeding or leaking of amniotic fluid following the procedure. Both studies found that the number of amniocenteses done in a single pregnancy did not appear to be a major factor in losing the baby, but the Canadian inquiry warned against multiple taps, or needle insertions, during a single amniocentesis.

The only large country-wide investigation to cloud these findings is a 1978 British survey, which showed a very slight increase in miscarriage following amniocentesis. American and Canadian geneticists, however, believe the conflicting results between this study and the North American ones are because of procedural differences and human error.

More recent studies conducted at the University of California found no evidence of danger, although the authors of the UCLA survey concluded there is a small risk of miscarriage, estimated at 0.5 percent. Statistics borne out by all these studies range from completely safe to a risk factor of approximately 1.5 percent. Although there is no hard evidence to bridge the gap between these figures, the chance of amniocentesis causing serious complications to the mother or her unborn baby is remote.

Ways to Avoid Problems

Here are some suggestions on what you should know prior to scheduling an amniocentesis:

(1) Double-check your insurance coverage; amniocentesis is expensive, ranging in cost from $400 to $900. Find out if your policy covers everything (that is, preamniocentesis counseling, the use of ultrasound, follow-up genetic counseling).

(2) Know the track record of the person who will perform the procedure and the lab that will analyze the specimen. If it's to be your own obstetrician, ask, "How many of these do you usually do in a month?" Given a choice, opt for having it performed in a medical center, by doctors skilled in amniocentesis. Be sure to call the lab, too, and ask what its accuracy rate is and how long the analyses generally take to complete.

(3) Ask in advance what will happen if the first tap is unsuccessful or if the cells do not grow. How many taps would the doctor do during one amniocentesis? How quickly can you be rescheduled if the lab reports it needs a fresh specimen?

(4) Be aware of what the actual objectives of the test are. In addition to genetic disorders, many labs also include as standard procedure an analysis of the alpha-fetoprotein for neural-tube defects.

(5) Confirm that a sonogram (ultrasound scan) will be used immediately prior to the procedure, so as to avoid accidentally puncturing baby or placenta. In many hospitals now, a sonogram is even repeated immediately afterward to ensure the baby has not been injured by the test (see "Sonogram: Is It Worth the Picture?" p. 73).

(6) Find out what the procedure is for letting you know the results. What is the channel of communication between you and the lab?

(7) Be sure to make it clear to your doctor, the lab or to anyone else who has access to your file, if you do not want to know the sex of your baby. Otherwise, it usually will be included in the report to you. Incidentally, if the father wants to learn if it's a boy or girl and you want to be surprised, you must give legal consent to have the information released to him.

(8) If you live far from a medical center that performs and/or analyzes amniocenteses, consider making the trip to ensure a safe and accurate tap. Even if your obstetrician does the procedure, little is gained, since the specimen will still have to be mailed, which involves a delay; possible extremes in temperature may affect the cells' ability to grow in the culture.

Chances are that the lab results will be reassuring, but expectant parents should not construe the findings as a guarantee for a normal, healthy baby, since amniocentesis cannot detect all defects. One final note: Be prepared to feel the baby's first kick at about the time when you get the results back.

Information Sources

ADDITIONAL READING

"Amniocentesis for Prenatal Chromosomal Diagnosis." Free booklet describes the procedure, along with step-by-step photographs. Write to: Center for Disease Control, Chronic Diseases Division, Bureau of Epidemiology, Atlanta, GA 30333.

New England Journal of Medicine, "Prenatal Genetic Diagnosis of 3,000 Amniocenteses," 300 (1979), 157–163. This journal is available at medical libraries and many public libraries.

Obstetrics and Gynecology, "Follow-up of 2,000 Second-Trimester Amniocenteses," 56:5 (1980), 625–627. This periodical is available at medical libraries.

ORGANIZATIONS

March of Dimes Birth Defects Foundation
1275 Mamaroneck Ave.
White Plains, NY 10605
Or contact one of 800 local chapters nearest to you. The March of Dimes offers a list of medical centers with good reputations for amniocentesis and genetic counseling, from their "National Listing of Clinical Genetics Services." It acts as a referral to other organizations specializing in particular birth defects.

National Institute of Child Health and Human Development (NICHD)
National Institutes of Health
Bldg 31, Room 2A32
Bethesda, MD 20205
NICHD sponsors ongoing research on amniocentesis and prenatal diagnosis. They can tell you of their latest publications. Libraries, particularly university medical libraries, usually carry copies or you can get these government materials through interlibrary loan.

②

You and the
Medical Profession

OBSTETRICIAN AND/OR MIDWIFE?

Even if you have been seeing the same ob/gyn for years, it's wise to consider all your options before deciding on your birth attendant. Keep in mind that, often, when you select a physician or midwife, the decision on where your baby will be born may automatically be made.

The degree of choice depends a lot on where you live. A small community may have nurse-midwives delivering babies at the state-run hospital, but a neighboring city may have several hospitals with maternity units staffed only by doctors. Birth centers, some of which are run by nurse-midwives with a physician on call, with others managed solely by obstetricians, operate in many metropolitan areas. Lay midwives as well as some doctors and nurse-midwives will attend a home birth (see "Hospital, Maternity Center or Home Birth?" p. 96).

Fewer family practitioners are delivering babies these days, mainly because of costly malpractice insurance. Given the fact that there are about 30,000 licensed obstetricians and only about 3000 certified nurse-midwives, most likely you will be shopping around for an obstetrician with whom you feel confident and compatible. Owing to the revival of midwifery in the United States, however, many expectant mothers seek the services of midwives, and now some obstetricians hire certified nurse-midwives, who share responsibility for seeing the patients during pregnancy and provide continuous attention throughout childbirth.

> ## Physician versus Midwife Deliveries
>
> Physicians delivered 97.9 percent of hospital births in 1980, a slight decrease from the 98.1 percent level in 1979. In 1980, midwives attended 1.4 percent of all in-hospital deliveries, compared with 1.3 percent in 1979. Midwives continued to deliver more babies in 1980, both in and out of hospitals, although the number of these births is still small.
>
> (Source: *National Center for Health Statistics*)

Economics comes into the picture, too. In an effort to reduce employee health costs, some corporations, including Arco, Kodak, DuPont and Rockwell, offer coverage for care by certified nurse-midwives. Most health-insurance plans covering federal workers now reimburse for midwifery care. One common misconception, claims the American College of Nurse-Midwives, is that under the care of a midwife no doctor is involved; the fact is that every nurse-midwife is required to work in collaboration with a qualified obstetrician. And, unlike a lay midwife, whose credentials are based on experience, a nurse-midwife is a registered nurse who has had formal education and clinical training—one to two years' worth—in order to be certified as a midwife. Hostility exists between some lay and nurse-midwives, but nothing like the economic and professional rivalry between doctors and nurse-midwives.

OBSTETRICIAN	CERTIFIED NURSE-MIDWIFE*
Definition: "obstare" in Latin means "to stand by."	*Definition:* "midwife" means literally "with woman."
Cost: Average fee $3900 for prenatal and postpartum care and normal vaginal delivery.	*Cost:* Average fee $1200 for prenatal, delivery and postpartum care.
Insurance: Except for deductibles or copayments, obstetrical costs, including hospital bill, covered by most insurance companies.	*Insurance:* Hospital charges covered by most policies, but some insurers will not reimburse for care by nurse-midwife.
Training: 4 years' undergraduate, 4 years' medical school and 4 years' residency in hospital, Board certification requires additional specialty train-	*Training:* Average 3 years' nursing school, 1–2 years' practical experience in obstetrics plus 1–2 years' schooling in nurse-midwifery. Certi-

OBSTETRICIAN	CERTIFIED NURSE-MIDWIFE*
ing and passing board exams; voluntary recertification.	fication requires passing exams; voluntary recertification.
Philosophy: Varies from doctor to doctor; some are more, some less, "interventionist." Unlike nurse-midwives, obstetricians are trained surgeons, skilled in solving problems during pregnancy and complications during labor.	*Philosophy:* Consistently noninterventionist; regards childbirth as natural process; views role as "pair of helping hands" and wants mother to take active role in her prenatal care.
Bedside manner: Depends on individual; sometimes overworked and pressed for time; role may be "doctor knows best" or a partnership with patient.	*Bedside manner:* Generous with their time at checkups; usually continuous bedside attention throughout labor and delivery.
Types of practice: Private (solo) practice; group practice; resident in ob/gyn department of private or university teaching hospital or public health clinic; health maintenance organization (HMO).	*Types of practice:* With an ob/gyn in private practice; in maternity or birth center with physician backup; in city or state-run hospital where nurse-midwives are granted privileges.

*Comparison chart of nurse-midwives and lay midwives follows later in this section.

Choosing Your Doctor

If this is your first child, there is no way to predict what kind of pregnancy and labor you will experience. The unknown is one reason many women who are pregnant for the first time feel more secure under the care of an obstetrician. Here are some pointers on how to go about choosing your doctor.

First of all, even if you are satisfied with the ob/gyn whom you've been seeing, it is wise to make sure you share the same philosophy about childbirth. Routine gynecological checkups usually are straightforward, with a minimum of dialogue, unlike prenatal visits, when there never seems to be enough time for discussion. Talk with your doctor about issues that most concern you. If you haven't focused on hospital procedures (during these early weeks of pregnancy, probably you are still adjusting to the idea that you're pregnant, rather than thinking about final-trimester decisions), we've prepared a list of questions to help you. But first, a few words of general advice:

- *Sex.* A female ob/gyn is important to some women, but don't assume a woman doctor will be more supportive or understanding than her male colleague. At the same time, if you prefer a female doctor, your chances of finding one increase every year.
- *Age.* Don't jump to the conclusion that a doctor in his or her thirties or forties will necessarily be more open-minded than an older M.D. who has kept pace with technology and changing philosophy.
- *University hospital affiliation.* Doctors at such hospitals are keeping themselves up-to-date on the latest obstetrical developments and may be more inclined to opt for "high-tech" maternity care.

If you are starting from scratch, talk first with others, including your family practitioner or internist, to get some names. If you are new in town, check with the hospital that has the best reputation and get a list of its residents. Also try contacting a childbirth-education group, the local chapter of the La Leche League or write to the International Childbirth Education Association for local contacts (see "Information Sources," p. 95).

Before you line up face-to-face interviews, which can be intimidating, call each office and ask the receptionist or nurse to tell you a bit about the doctor's views on childbirth, the average length of time for office checkups, and the ball-park price for prenatal care and delivery. Ask where the doctor has hospital privileges and whether he or she has been certified by the American Board of Obstetrics and Gynecology. Board certification does not guarantee excellence, but if doctors are not certified, that's probably a mark against them. Anyone who gets huffy when asked about credentials is probably someone to avoid.

In addition to relying on others' recommendations and your own intuition, once you find out which hospital(s) the doctor is affiliated with, call the maternity unit. If you are keen on trying a birthing chair, it is important to know whether the hospital has the right equipment or permits such nontraditional approaches to childbirth. By talking with other mothers, too, you will get an idea of the reputation of the hospital nurses and the care your newborn will get in the nursery.

An interview with a prospective physician should reveal a lot. It will be obvious if the obstetrician seems annoyed with your questions or gives stock answers. Your attitude during these interviews will help set the tone. Choose a firm but nonthreatening approach. Instead of questions that may make a doctor defensive, such as "What percentage of your patients have a cesarean?" you might ask "What circumstances necessitate a C-section?" After all, as one obstetrician volunteers, "If his cesarean rate is high, he's going to lie anyway."

Take notice if you feel uncomfortable asking questions or hesitate getting the doctor to explain something again because you don't understand. The next nine months and the intimate hours you will spend with your doctor during childbirth demand a good relationship, a comfortable and trusting partnership. Be yourself and don't compromise.

It is important that each of you understands what the other expects. Here are some questions that you may want to raise during the interview to get a feel for the obstetrician's philosophy and temperament.

(1) Should I abstain altogether from drinking alcohol?

(2) During the last trimester, is it okay for me to continue to play tennis or jog?

(3) Can you suggest a particular childbirth method?

(4) Do you or the hospital have any restrictions on when my husband (or labor coach) can be with me?

(5) What types of pain-killers do you prefer?

(6) If I decide I want a Leboyer delivery, is that possible?

(7) Does the hospital allow rooming-in (so you and your baby won't be separated)? Can the baby's father stay overnight at the hospital with us, and what about early discharge?

(8) How do you feel about inducing labor?

(9) What are your fees? Does that include lab tests? What if I need to see you more often; is that covered also? What about an estimate of my hospital bill? What expenses won't be covered by my insurance?

(10) What about your payment schedule? Do I pay a certain amount prior to my due date? (Often doctors require full payment prior to the seventh month or six weeks prior to delivery.)

Choosing a Midwife

Two modern versions replacing the "granny" midwife exist. The new lay midwife tends to be young and to have some college education but lacks formal medical training. Nurse-midwives work with a physician or in collaboration with a backup physician and provide not only prenatal through postpartum care but also routine gynecological exams.

CERTIFIED NURSE-MIDWIFE	LAY MIDWIFE
Definition: a medical professional; registered nurse who has completed further course of study and training qualifying her to practice midwifery.	*Definition:* a woman outside the medical profession who gives prenatal advice and assists in births.
Legal authority: Differs from state to state but usually can practice with physician backup and can carry emer-	*Legal authority:* Lay midwifery clearly legal in Texas, New Mexico, Washington and several other states but

CERTIFIED NURSE-MIDWIFE	LAY MIDWIFE
gency equipment, oxygen, pitocin (drug to stimulate contractions if labor fails to progress) and suturing equipment.	prohibited in most. Where legal, licensed midwives can carry oxygen but no drugs or suturing equipment.
Cost: Average fee approximately $1200 for prenatal through postpartum.	*Cost:* Fee ranges from $200 for attending birth to approximately $700 for all prenatal care and delivery.
Training: Average 3 years' nursing school, with 1–2 years' practical experience in obstetrics and 1–2 years' schooling in midwifery.	*Training:* Apprentice-style; learn from watching others deliver babies and gradually taking over themselves.
Philosophy: View childbirth as a natural process, with medical intervention only when necessary; some who practice with physicians are accustomed to using such "technology" as electronic fetal monitors.	*Philosophy:* Natural all the way, if at all possible; some regard their approach as "spiritual"; let mother do what she wants to do and lend support throughout pregnancy and childbirth.
Types of practice: With an ob/gyn in private practice, at a health maintenance organization, in city or state-run hospital, or in out-of-hospital birth center.	*Types of practice:* Since lay midwifery is illegal in many states, many midwives practice covertly. In other states, lay midwives work under supervision of a physician or licensed midwife.

Shopping around for a nurse-midwife is similar to scouting out a doctor with whom you feel comfortable and confident. By and large most certified nurse-midwives emphasize nutrition and are ardent believers in prepared-childbirth training. They are required to screen expectant mothers continually for signs of "high risk." This begins at the initial physical examination and continues throughout pregnancy and during labor. If a nurse-midwife suspects a problem, she will consult with the physician backup to determine if further tests should be run and/or if the woman's care should be turned over to the obstetrician. Word-of-mouth referral, particularly from mothers and other health professionals, usually results in good nurse-midwife selection. If you are having trouble tracking down a practicing nurse-midwife, simply write to the American College of Nurse-Midwives (see "Information Sources," p. 95). It will send you the names, addresses and types of practice of those midwives certified by the College in your area. Be sure to find out about the credentials of the backup physician and what choices you have on where you can give birth.

Also, inquire about whether your health insurance will cover prenatal as well as labor and delivery care. (Usually the backup obstetrician will sign the necessary insurance forms for reimbursement.)

Switching Doctors

The idea of getting acquainted with a new doctor or midwife in the middle of one's pregnancy might seem awful. You may have no other choice if you will be moving out of town. Dissatisfaction with your prenatal care is another reason for lining up a new physician or midwife. Or you may want to find another health adviser if you don't like the hospital or birth center where he or she has privileges. In either case it isn't as bad as it sounds, because few lab tests have to be repeated and, if you are in the second trimester, frequent office checkups usually don't begin until the seventh month.

After a trouble-free delivery, most parents feel indebted to the M.D. or midwife who attended the birth. It is a missed opportunity not to have a satisfactory doctor-patient relationship. If your health-care provider shuts off questions or forces you to go along with decisions about tests or treatment, consider switching doctors. Or, if you are just ill at ease with his or her bedside manner, talk with other women to find out how they get along with their obstetricians. Most likely you will hear how healthy a partnership with a physician or midwife can be.

The decision to switch doctors and get your medical record can sometimes be difficult and intimidating. Here are some ways to make it easier.

(1) Get recommendations for several doctors and/or nurse-midwives.
(2) Make preliminary calls to the office receptionist to find out where the doctor has hospital privileges, get an estimate for charges for the rest of your prenatal care and ask any other major questions on your mind.
(3) Don't notify your current doctor yet.
(4) Double-check your insurance policy to make sure of your coverage.
(5) Shop around, by interviewing other physicians either over the telephone or in their offices. Try to explain why you are unhappy with your care; the doctor's reaction should tell you a lot. Questions you might want to ask are outlined on p. 92.
(6) Once you have selected a doctor or midwife, have your medical record transferred to your new birth attendant. Usually you need to make the request in writing or sign an authorization form.
(7) Straighten out your medical bill. If you paid all or a portion of it in advance, this may be a problem if you think you are due a refund. First contact the bookkeeper, and if the issue of a refund

becomes sticky, don't let the problem be thrown back to the office receptionist but talk directly to the doctor.

If you run into any problems getting your medical record transferred or your money back, the best place to get help is by contacting the county or state medical society. The American Medical Association says in its 1982 code that a patient's medical report should not be withheld for any reason, even if the individual has not paid a bill. The local medical society usually needs between 60 and 90 days to settle a billing dispute.

Before you see your new physician or midwife, call to make sure your record has been received, to avoid having duplicate lab tests and other medical procedures performed.

Information Sources

ADDITIONAL READING

Directory of Medical Specialists (published by Marquis Who's Who, Inc.). Organized by specialty (i.e., ob/gyn) for each state, city; names in alphabetical order, and gives academic and professional credentials along with age and other miscellaneous information.

NAPSAC Directory of Alternative Birth Services and Consumer Guide (published by National Association of Parents and Professionals for Safe Alternatives in Childbirth [NAPSAC], PO Box 428, Marble Hill, MO 63764). Lists midwives, birth centers, home-birth programs and natural-childbirth doctors by state. Available for $5.95 from NAPSAC.

ORGANIZATIONS

American College of Home Physicians
664 N. Michigan Ave., #600
Chicago, IL 60611
Provides referral service of physicians who attend home births.

American College of Nurse-Midwives
1522 K St., NW, #1120
Washington, DC 20005
Provides names, addresses and types of practices of certified nurse-midwives in your area.

American College of Obstetricians and Gynecologists
600 Maryland Ave., SW
Washington, DC 20024
Free pamphlet titled "Ob/Gyn, The Woman's Physician" is available. Send self-addressed, stamped envelope.

American Medical Association
535 N. Dearborn
Chicago, IL 60610
Your county or state medical society can help you in the event you
have difficulties obtaining your medical record or getting a refund.

ASPO-Lamaze
1840 Wilson Blvd.
Arlington, VA 22201
Provides referrals of physicians who support Lamaze childbirth.

International Childbirth Education Association
PO Box 20048
Minneapolis, MN 55420
Provides referrals of health professionals and parents committed to
family-centered maternity care.

HOSPITAL, MATERNITY CENTER
OR HOME BIRTH?

Although most babies are born in hospitals in the United States—99
percent in 1980—home-birth services and out-of-hospital maternity
centers continue to attract expectant parents from all socioeconomic
levels. "Hospitals are not good enough to provide an environment
suited for a peak experience of one's life, nor for the birth of a family,"
writes Shirley Kitzinger in *Birth at Home.* Many hospitals, bowing to
consumer pressure, are trying to make maternity wards more like
home. Both the American College of Obstetricians and Gynecologists
and the American Academy of Pediatrics are adamantly opposed to
home births, arguing that "labor and delivery, while a physiologic
process, clearly presents potential hazards to both mother and fetus
before and after birth. These hazards require standards of safety which
are provided in the hospital setting and cannot be matched in the
home situation."

Maternity centers offer a compromise for expectant couples torn
between the intimacy of a home birth and the security of a hospital.
These alternative delivery facilities are usually managed by certified
nurse-midwives and are located within minutes of a major hospital and
backup physicians. Basic resuscitation supplies not easily transported
for home births are available at most maternity centers. Most doctors
are concerned about the overall safety of even the licensed birth
centers, for several reasons. They are skeptical of nurse-midwives'
ability to assume primary responsibility as the birth attendant and
believe that in the event an emergency cesarean needs to be performed,
even a five-minute drive isn't worth the risk.

Safety is the pivotal issue in this debate. Many doctors warn: "Why flirt with danger and take any chance?" Out-of-hospital advocates maintain that most pregnancies are uncomplicated and continuous medical screening can spot high-risk mothers, who would benefit from hospital specialists and high-tech equipment, particularly at a regional perinatal or "Level III" center. Most obstetricians believe complications during labor can happen suddenly, without warning, while midwives who attend out-of-hospital births claim life-threatening situations such as a prolapsed umbilical cord are rare. Moreover, proponents of home births cite numerous studies that show out-of-hospital deliveries are safer, owing to the absence or reduced use of common obstetrical procedures. They argue that the tendency of hospitals to interfere with the normal childbirth process (for instance, restricted mobility during labor, artificial induction or stimulation of labor, expulsion of the placenta too soon after birth) poses a greater risk to a mother and her baby. Many obstetricians admit there is abuse and overuse of certain obstetrical practices and procedures but insist that a controlled hospital environment with electronic fetal monitors and other equipment and an experienced staff trained to respond to emergencies is the only safe place to give birth. Moreover, they claim some institutions are becoming more progressive by offering in-hospital birthing rooms to low-risk patients. These conflicting arguments are articulated by three expectant mothers who give their reasons for choosing their birthplace:

(hospital)	"I want the security of knowing everything is there just in case. . . . Yes, I am steering the ship but know that there is a captain on board along with an experienced crew."
(birth center)	"I want the freedom to call my own shots in an environment that is safer than at home. I don't want to risk delivering my first baby on a doctor's timetable."
(home)	"I don't know how my labor will go, but I want to feel relaxed and in control, which is why I want to be comforted by family and friends in my own home."

About 10 to 20 percent of all women in labor will experience some problems, according to many physicians. This figure is supported by about the same percentage of mothers who plan to have their child born at home or at a birth center but end up transferring to a hospital because of unforeseen complications, such as failure to progress during labor.

Studies and statistics don't help settle the score on the question of whether birth at home is safe. The highest number of home births in Europe is found in the Netherlands. One Dutch doctor claims there is no proof that delivery at home is safer than in the hospital but says there is proof that the selection of low-risk and high-risk pregnancies is possible to a great degree.

Medical Criteria for Out-of-Hospital Birth

- no heart disease, diabetes or other serious condition
- no more than 35 years of age (some centers say 40) for first-time mothers
- no family history of genetic disorders
- no multiple births
- no previous uterine surgery, including cesarean (although some obs and midwives support certain women who want to attempt vaginal delivery after cesarean)
- baby in head-first position (some doctors and midwives will turn a breech or deliver a breech)
- labor must start spontaneously after 37 weeks' gestation and prior to the end of 42 weeks

---

After all, what matters is not national statistics but your health, philosophy, individual situation and trust in your obstetrical caretaker. This comparison chart may help you work through still other considerations, such as cost and insurance.

HOSPITAL	MATERNITY CENTER	HOME BIRTH
Cost: Average cost for ordinary vaginal delivery and hospital stay $1500–$3000 (prenatal care not included).	Average cost for all prenatal care and classes, labor and delivery and postpartum care $600–$2000; however, if you deliver at hospital because of complications, you may wind up paying two sets of fees.	Cost with birth attendant may range between $200 and $800; nurse-midwife home birth service, which includes all prenatal and postpartum care, comparable in cost to birth center; often extra charge of $100 for birth attendant to help midwife.
Insurance: Except for deductibles, usually insurance will cover hospital bill.	Out-of-pocket expenses may be higher than hospital if insurance does not cover nonhospital maternity care.	No coverage; however, often physician backup sends in claim to insurer.

HOSPITAL	MATERNITY CENTER	HOME BIRTH
Environment: Impersonal, rigid policies and obstetrical procedures; mother viewed as patient and birth seen as medical event; ultimately doctor and hospital staff make decisions.	Personalized care in homelike setting. Teamwork approach between parent(s), midwives and perhaps physician. Health-care team observes and provides support. Pregnancy seen as natural, healthy.	Most familiar setting. Primary responsibility rests on expectant mother in consultation with birth attendant. Greatest degree of autonomy. Birth often regarded as spiritual event.
Equipment: Medical equipment readily available; staff accustomed to dealing with emergencies.	Some emergency equipment at center; physician backup arrangement; usually advance arrangement with nearby hospital and ambulance service.	No emergency equipment usually, except oxygen; reliance on rescue squad; often difficulties gaining admittance to hospital if under care of a lay midwife.
Prerequisites: Insurance coverage or sizable deposit in advance.	Required to attend childbirth classes; take an active role and interest in prenatal care.	Patient must take initiative to find birth attendant, sometimes labor assistant too, and to organize necessary supplies; some home-birth services require a childbirth-education course.
Labor companion: Father or labor coach usually only person allowed with mother.	Siblings, relatives and friends allowed to witness birth.	Anyone can be present at birth.
Rooming-in: Separation of parents and newborn; often restrictions on when baby can be with parents.	Round-the-clock rooming-in with parents.	No family separation during or after birth.

Which Hospital Is for You?

Hospital maternity wards are changing constantly. As more women insist on "informed consent" and participate in the decision-making process during childbirth, more hospitals are bowing to consumer pressure. Enemas, intravenous hookups and other procedures that used to be standard hospital policy are often left up to the patient and her doctor. Birthing chairs and private visitation rooms for grandparents and siblings demonstrate an effort by hospitals to accommodate wishes of parents. Nontraditional maternity suites, where the emphasis is on family-centered care, can be found at many hospitals; however, like birthing chairs, some are unused showcases. It pays to find out about the hospital where you plan to deliver, and if it doesn't suit your needs, choose another one even if it means you have to choose another obstetrician or midwife.

Here are some general characteristics for different types of hospitals; of course, policies and obstetrical practices vary not only from one institution to another but also from community to community.

Teaching or University Hospitals. These are usually large, well-equipped institutions, with expert care immediately available (neonatalogist, cardiac surgeon and so on). Residents and medical students handle the bulk of patient care, as they are on duty around the clock and will care for you until your personal doctor arrives. In a university hospital, there is sometimes a conflict between the objectives of "practicing" medicine, carrying on research and caring for the expectant mother. The teaching hospital does provide an ideal birth place for the high-risk expectant mother who needs the benefit of sophisticated technological equipment and where the staff stays up-to-date on the latest research and obstetrical techniques. These hospitals often offer birthing rooms for low-risk mothers-to-be.

Small Community Hospitals. These hospitals, though they obviously lack large maternity units, nevertheless tend to honor individual preferences. Nursing staffs and supervisors often exhibit a more flexible attitude than in big hospitals. Birthing rooms are sometimes available, too, and labor-room nurses may be able to follow one woman from the time she is admitted through her delivery—or at least may spend considerable time with her. Small hospitals deliver fewer babies and may be less experienced in dealing with high-risk pregnancies.

Public Hospitals. Usually, the larger the facility, the more difficult it is to challenge established policies and procedures; yet you may have more say if the hospital offers family-centered birthing rooms. As economic limits have an impact on where you deliver, likewise economic levels also have an impact on the quality of care you will receive. A discrepancy between care afforded private patients and low-income women, otherwise termed "tracking," often occurs here, as it sometimes does in large teaching or university hospitals.

Private Hospitals. This broad category includes physician-owned hospitals; nonsectarian hospitals (run by a board of physicians and nonmedical members), which are usually for profit; and religiously affiliated hospitals (such as Catholic, Seventh-Day Adventist, Jewish, Methodist). Catholic facilities, for instance, tend to be more conservative and slow to change, though they generally support family-centered maternity care, which may include the option of delivery in a birthing room, and there are often restrictions on fallopian-tube ligation.

Hospitals now are more willing to answer probing questions from expectant parents. If your questions are brushed aside or sidestepped, that is probably a clue that a particular hospital may not be so flexible or adaptable to parents' needs. A hospital tour is usually offered, but the nursing staff often suggests that you wait for your orientation in the maternity ward until the final month or two of your pregnancy. That's too late to settle on what hospital best suits your needs and desires. It is a good idea, then, to ask your doctor about the hospital or hospitals where he or she has privileges. Some obstetricians are relatively powerless regarding hospital policies, but others have a lot to say about the care and treatment you will receive. "Standing orders" include routine procedures such as enemas and shave, use of IV (intravenous fluids), fetal monitors and types of medications during labor. Ideally you and your doctor can discuss in advance what kind of labor and delivery plan you want, and make sure it is compatible with the hospital policies (see "Final Countdown Checklist," p. 193).

Suggested Questions for Evaluating a Hospital

(1) Are hospital tours available?
(2) Who is allowed with me during labor *and* delivery? (Does it matter if we aren't married?)
(3) Are there restrictions on the involvement of my labor coach?
(4) Are IVs standard practice in the hospital or is this left up to the individual physician?
(5) Are different positions permitted during labor and/or delivery?
(6) Does the hospital allow Leboyer birth?
(7) Is there a birthing room? What are the restrictions and how often is it used?
(8) In the event of a cesarean, is my coach allowed to be present?
(9) Is breast-feeding allowed immediately after birth?
(10) Is rooming-in allowed? Day and night? In private rooms only?
(11) Do fathers have 24-hour visiting privileges?
(12) Is the hospital approved by the Joint Committee on Accreditation of Hospitals?

Sometimes better responses are elicited if inquiries are made over the telephone to the head nurse of the maternity ward or by pulling aside a hospital nurse rather than asking questions about controversial hospital procedures during the formal tour of the facility. Another approach is to ask to look at the hospital policy manual.

Choosing a Home-Birth Attendant

Just as other mothers-to-be should shop carefully when choosing their obstetrician and hospital where they will deliver, the same applies when selecting a freestanding maternity center or a home-birth attendant. Of course, the number of physicians or nurse-midwives who are willing to attend and experienced in home births may severely limit your selection.

The only other option is to rely on the underground network of lay midwives, where the burden of verifying experience and training (which licensure does through its minimum standards) rests on the expectant mother. Doris Haire, an outspoken critic of most hospital maternity wards, argues that hospitals *should* be required to "provide staff privileges to all midwives qualified to practice by national certification, state licensure, or local authority, and to provide the same obstetric backup presently provided for obstetric residents and junior staff." Haire believes "such a statute would reduce the number of women seeking obstetrical care from lay midwives unqualified to provide such care."

The International Childbirth Education Association 1979 medical and nonmedical criteria for birth at home include:

(1) Home-birth clients to be personally comfortable with their decision to give birth at home and to be low risk.
(2) Attendance by certified midwives or physicians in consultation with obstetric and pediatric specialists.
(3) Written, formalized set of criteria and procedures for consultation with, and referral to, backup physicians and other professionals.
(4) Written, formalized set of criteria and procedures for referral and transport to backup hospital.
(5) Written statement to home-birth clients, informing them if backup services (see 3 and 4) cannot be formalized.
(6) Home within short distance of a hospital (10 miles away maximum).
(7) Prenatal health care and education program.
(8) Home visit with family's consent during prenatal program.
(9) Advance instruction concerning preparation of home to ensure necessary labor and birth area, bedding, supplies, equipment and transportation.
(10) Arrangements for newborn evaluation and examination and

follow-up to ensure required screening tests and laboratory work performed.

Approximately one out of three first-time mothers who plan to give birth at home ends up at the hospital, so it is important prior to labor to discuss with your birth attendant hypothetical situations such as: What happens if my bag of water breaks but contractions don't follow? Is there a time limit that you adhere to on the length of the first and second stages of labor? Each physician and midwife has his or her own guidelines. Many birth attendants insist that their clients take childbirth classes specifically geared to those couples planning home births. Certified nurse-midwives are specialists in normal birth; however, some will deliver a breech baby (nonvertex position) either because they are confident of their ability and a physician is standing by or because they are pressured into it by a mother who refuses to go to the hospital. Twins or a previous cesarean don't fall under the definition of normal birth, but here again some midwives and doctors will assume the role of "lifeguard" at such home deliveries.

Discussion with your prospective home-birth attendant should unscramble these areas of confusion to avoid possible misunderstandings later in pregnancy or during labor. Furthermore, this is a good way for you to assess the experience and philosophy of your health-care provider.

Choosing a Birth Center

Freestanding maternity centers exist in almost every state. The majority of these warm, homelike facilities, which provide both maternity and gynecological services, are staffed by certified nurse-midwives in collaboration with physicians licensed in obstetrics and pediatrics. Some birth centers operated by obstetricians come under fire by midwives for being "mini-hospitals" that are not committed to a natural, family-centered birth experience.

Every birth center has its own risk assessment for screening expectant mothers. Some facilities with Blue Cross insurance coverage will not accept women over 35 or allow a mother with a previous cesarean to attempt an out-of-hospital vaginal delivery; yet other centers will open up their services to such expectant parents. Women who fail to attend childbirth-education classes and don't take an active interest in prenatal nutrition may be dropped from some programs.

Many facilities, such as New York City's well-known Maternity Center, have been in operation for years and can boast of very low infant-mortality rates. But Eunice Ernst, the head of the National Association of Childbearing Centers, cautions: "The birth center concept does *not* wear a halo." Ernst believes licensure and certification or accreditation should be number one on the list of requirements for birth centers. Here are some features you should look for when evaluating such a birthing place:

(1) Policy manual of routine and emergency care of the mother and her baby, until discharged by the center, during pregnancy, birth and postpartum.

(2) Adequate physician backup and arrangement with nearby hospital in the event of complications.

(3) Licensed birth center, provided the state public-health department has established regulations governing such institutions.

(4) Center carries malpractice insurance.

(5) In-depth medical record, which serves as a legal document and is vital if mother is transferred to hospital.

(6) Emergency equipment including oxygen, intravenous fluids and resuscitation devices.

(7) Diagnostic equipment, such as a sphygmomanometer to measure contractions, and auscultation equipment to listen to the fetal heartbeat.

(8) Infant mobile incubator if no perinatal transport system is available.

(9) Infant warmer in case of emergency or at mother's request.

(10) Clean, well-kept, well-lit facility.

Of course, choosing a freestanding birth center means you are also choosing your own birth attendant affiliated with the center. Some of the guidelines suggested earlier for selecting a home-birth attendant may help you evaluate credentials and experience.

Information Sources

ADDITIONAL READING

Childbirth: Alternatives to Medical Control, by Shelly Romalis (Austin, TX: University of Texas Press, 1981). Explores different birth settings.

The Complete Book of Midwifery, by Barbara Brennan and Joan Rattner Heilman (New York: E.P. Dutton, 1979). Nurse-midwife within hospital birth setting and other "progressive" changes occurring in some hospitals around the country.

Immaculate Deception, by Suzanne Arms (New York: Bantam, 1981). Recounts horrors of giving birth in a hospital.

In Labor: Women and Power in the Birthplace, by Barbara Katz Rothman (New York: W. W. Norton, 1983). Home-birth advocate condemns hospital maternity wards.

The Place of Birth, by Shirley Kitzinger (New York: Oxford University Press, 1978). Explores various birthplaces but primarily looks at home births.

The Rights of the Pregnant Patient: How to Have an Easier, Healthier Hospital Birth Together, by Valmai Howe Elkins (New York: Two Continents Publishing Group, 1976). Discusses various obstetrical procedures as well as patient rights.

Shared Childbirth: A Guide to Family Birth Centers, by Philip Sumner and Celeste Phillips (St. Louis: C. V. Mosby, 1982). Includes list of family-oriented maternity-care hospitals throughout the country.

ORGANIZATIONS:

American College of Home Obstetrics
664 N. Michigan Ave., #600
Chicago, IL 60611
ACHO publishes newsletter and provides referral service of physicians who attend home births.

American College of Nurse-Midwives
1522 K St., NW
Washington, DC 20036
Provides a referral of certified nurse-midwives who will attend home births or who are affiliated with a birth center.

National Association of Childbearing Centers
Box 1, Route 1
Perkiomenville, PA 18074
National organization that suggests guidelines for birth centers and serves as an information clearinghouse.

Home Oriented Maternity Care (HOME)
PO Box 450
Germantown, MD 20874
HOME does not teach birth attendants but has discussion groups around the country for those planning a home birth; publishes newsletter and a fine birth manual.

Informed Homebirth
PO Box 788
Boulder, CO 80306
Teaches midwifery skills and provides referral service of birth attendants near where you live.

Joint Committee on Accreditation of Hospitals
645 N. Michigan Ave.
Chicago, IL 60611

Provides information about particular hospitals and whether they are accredited.

Maternity Center Association
48 E. 92nd St.
New York, NY 10028
One of the oldest birth centers in the U.S., with an excellent reputation; publishes numerous pamphlets and newsletters.

National Association of Parents and Professionals for Safe Alternatives in Childbirth (NAPSAC)
PO Box 428
Marble Hill, MO 63764
Publishes "Directory of Alternative Birth Services."

The Alternative Birth Crisis Coalition (ABCC)
PO Box 48371
Chicago, IL 60648
Provides legal help to home-birth attendants; ABCC also publishes monthly newsletter available to its members.

LAMAZE VERSUS OTHER CHILDBIRTH-PREPARATION METHODS

Childbirth-education classes for expectant parents are flourishing. Birth handbooks, teaching manuals, films, slide shows are all in great demand. There is even the Prepared Childbirth Game, which is designed to help the father-to-be develop his "observation and response skills" during labor and delivery. The term "prepared" is now used more frequently than "natural" childbirth, the latter being something of a misnomer, connoting no training or practice.

Most of us have heard of Lamaze and perhaps of several other methods. As we've learned, the differences between them are subtle (although the proponents of each method will argue vehemently that their approach is quite different from others). All courses try to dispel the misconceptions and anxieties about birth. Most teach specific breathing patterns and muscular-relaxation techniques, train the father or a friend to be the mother's labor coach and discuss medical procedures such as the use of electronic fetal monitors and medications during labor.

Classes usually meet four to eight times, during the final trimester of pregnancy. Many organizations now offer a *free* introductory course that covers nutrition, fetal development and other questions that demand answers early in pregnancy. This preliminary prenatal class provides an opportunity to see whether you feel comfortable with that method's philosophy. Practically every program prepares expectant parents for labor by relying on its own unique recipe, but each recipe contains seven common ingredients, outlined below.

(1) *Combating the"Fear-Tension-Pain" syndrome.* Most childbirth teachers embrace the theory that mystery and misinformation cause fear about birth, which triggers tension and contributes to pain. Consequently, you will learn what to expect during all stages of a normal labor and delivery.

(2) *Relaxation techniques.* Most instructors believe that the ability to relax the muscles is crucial to a comfortable delivery and helps the woman conserve her strength through labor. Various sight and touch techniques are taught for identifying tension and keeping muscles relaxed.

(3) *Breathing techniques.* A set of breathing patterns is established for each stage of labor. These respiratory exercises are aimed at helping you "ride the wave" of pain for each contraction, either by distracting you from the pain or by aiding you in accepting it. It is still a subject of debate whether chest or abdominal breathing is preferable during childbirth.

(4) *Exercises.* Conditioning drills, and sometimes nonstrenuous body-building exercises, are taught. These are intended to complement your breathing and relaxation techniques (see "Conditioning Exercises: What's a Kegel?" p. 68).

(5) *Labor coach.* Your husband or partner plays an important role throughout the training program as well as during labor and delivery. He (or she) helps time contractions, touches and massages your body, deals with hospital personnel and serves as a "verbal anesthesia," giving you support and encouragement.

(6) *Hospital preparation and medication.* Instructors brief you on what to pack for the hospital as well as routine admission procedures. Some discussion is devoted to explaining different medications and the effects of analgesics and anesthetics in the event of a complicated or unduly difficult labor.

(7) *Postpartum and infant care.* Some time is spent on your newborn's needs, breast-feeding and postpartum recovery.

Expect to fend for yourself in two critical areas that often receive superficial treatment; namely, items 6 and 7. Since most courses stress the nonanesthetized state, the discussion on medications and pain relievers is often skimpy. A common complaint regards childbirth teachers who paint a rosy picture about "natural" or "painless" labor and gloss over what to do in the event of complications and/or problems during childbirth (see "Drugs During Childbirth," p. 236). Many childbirth classes concentrate on the mother and neglect to prepare you for the basics regarding newborn care. You may want to consider going to a local Red Cross class if you are not familiar with handling young infants.

Comparisons Between Lamaze, Kitzinger and Other Methods

It is the philosophical and psychological slant that produces most of the distinctions between the different approaches. Most of the prepared-childbirth programs fall into one of these two categories:

Psychophysical School (Bradley, Kitzinger and others). As the name implies, this category, which is the oldest approach to prepared childbirth in this country, relies heavily on the laboring mother's psychological state. The chief components are a positive, spontaneous mental attitude toward the birthing process, coupled with some breathing and relaxation techniques. This approach is based on Dr. Grantly Dick-Read's theory, often referred to as Childbirth Without Fear, that women have been negatively influenced by their cultural conditioning and that it is necessary to arrest the fear-tension-pain chain reaction. The other well-known psychophysical methods are the Bradley Husband-Coached Childbirth and Kitzinger or "psychosexual" program.

Psychoprophylactic School (Lamaze). Prophylactic means to be "on guard." Lamaze is the most popular childbirth method that falls into this category. The central thrust of this structured approach is to control the pain of labor through stimulus-response conditioning. For each contraction (stimulus), the mother is taught to respond automatically with learned breathing patterns or relaxation techniques. Unlike the psychophysical philosophy, specific responses are designed to divert the mother's attention from pain.

We've drawn up further comparisons between the two schools of thought in the following chart:

	Psychoprophylactic **LAMAZE**	*Psychophysical* **BRADLEY, KITZINGER** **AND OTHERS**
Basic Philosophy	This structured method stresses learning to control and deflect the sensations of pain during childbirth.	This individualized approach emphasizes a calm, relaxed and flexible attitude so you remain spontaneous.
Breathing and Relaxation	Use specific breathing patterns and muscular-control techniques during various stages	Rely on passive concentration yet remain attentive to signals from your body and concen-

	Psychoprophylactic LAMAZE	Psychophysical BRADLEY, KITZINGER, AND SO ON
	of labor; take one contraction at a time and don't think about how many more are to to come.	trate on what is actually happening as the baby moves down the birth canal.
Labor Coach	Husband or labor coach is encouraged to provide support throughout labor and has a checklist of responsibilities.	Husband is crucial in the Bradley method; Dick-Read, Kitzinger and others encourage mother to have a support person.
Drugs and Medical Intervention	Informed consent is important prior to using fetal monitors, drugs and so on during labor and delivery.	Rapport with your birth attendant is stressed; rejection of drugs is assumed and use of pain-killers is usually not discussed.
Criticisms	Bradley, Kitzinger and other proponents argue Lamaze deprives mother of the sensual and psychological experience of giving birth.	Some criticize this school as being too passive, mystical or introspective for such a major physical event.

Besides these childbirth methods, there are dozens of others, many of which are a combination of both schools. For example, some "modified-Lamaze" classes incorporate Shirley Kitzinger's colorful imagery about birth and many of her massage techniques. Each instructor has her own philosophy and style of presentation (most classes are taught by mothers or nurses), which sometimes overshadow the particular method; however, most of the approaches described below are quite different from the big three—Lamaze, Bradley and Kitzinger.

Hospital Classes, Red Cross, YWCA and So Forth. Hospital-run programs provide an opportunity for expectant parents to get to know a few of the staff members connected with the maternity ward and become more familiar with the medical center. These classes are criticized for failing to discuss alternative options to a conventional medically managed hospital delivery (that is, no electronic fetal monitors, different positions during labor). Red Cross chapters sponsor a set of classes consisting of an abbreviated Lamaze program and infant care. Local childbirth-education groups, some of which are not affiliated with ASPO-Lamaze (ASPO stands for American Society for Psycho-prophylaxis in Obstetrics) or other national childbirth organizations, offer general classes as well as courses on preparing for a home birth, cesarean and sometimes classes for the deaf. The YWCA, community centers and some county recreation departments also offer classes.

Leboyer "Gentle Birth." Eliminating the "birth trauma" by avoiding common delivery-room practices is the principal ingredient of this approach. Leboyer method is not an alternative to any of these childbirth approaches, but it is a supplement (see "Leboyer and Other Nontraditional Deliveries," p. 114).

Yoga. This childbirth preparation emphasizes physical fitness. The program starts early in pregnancy, when expectant mothers master breathing patterns, relaxation postures and a series of exercises designed to enhance muscle tone and litheness. Meditation is a principal component with some yoga instructors.

Inner Bonding. Couples are taught how to "make contact with their unborn baby." Expectant parents learn how to interpret and respond to their baby's movements and moods. Playful touching games, music and other sounds, meditation and sensory stimulus are some of the techniques. Prenatal bonding is closely linked to visualization.

Visualization and Biofeedback. An expectant mother is encouraged to picture what she wants to happen (that is, to have a positive childbirth experience), not what she does not want. Some teachers regard visualization as the way to achieve greater self-awareness and stronger emotional ties to the baby in utero, while others view it as a stress-reducing and relaxation technique. A new tool for handling labor is biofeedback. Largely by suggestive images—for example, visualizing the warmth one feels when lying on a beach—an expectant mother learns that her nervous system can enforce a relaxed state of mind. With the help of other mental exercises and sometimes a biofeedback machine, a mother-to-be can master the technique of keeping her relaxed response steady during a contraction.

Hypnosis. A tranquil, trancelike state during labor while the mother is still able to respond to directions and questions is the objective of hypnosis during childbirth. Expectant mothers often begin small group classes by a professional hypnotist or receive individual instruction about three months prior to delivery. Hypnosis can be so effective that some have used it instead of anesthesia in the event of an unexpected cesarean; however, some people cannot be hypnotized.

Acupressure or Zone Therapy. Different techniques are used; for instance, a laboring woman uses a special comb that she squeezes into the palm of her hand just below the fingers, to ease the intensity of contractions. While there are no formal classes, acupressure is easy to practice, although this approach does not work for everyone (see "Information Sources, p. 112).

Cesarean Preparation. Most courses inform expectant parents about types of incisions, anesthesia, postoperative discomforts and postpartum adjustments. Another type of class primarily trains those mothers who have had a cesarean to attempt a vaginal delivery. Owing to the number of national organizations that offer cesarean classes, make sure you know what material will be covered before you sign up.

Home Birth. All programs review basic obstetrical information about the stages of labor and discuss supplies and emergency backup systems. Some classes have a strong ideological or spiritual orientation, while others cover more practical material.

Don't wait until the fifth or six month of pregnancy to shop around for a course, because many classes fill up well in advance. Here are some considerations when choosing a particular method and course:

(1) *Free early-pregnancy class.* Many childbirth-education groups offer introductory courses to answer questions of particular concern during the first trimester. This is a good way to sample an organization's childbirth program.
(2) *Enroll early.* Even if you change your mind and decide you would prefer a different course, usually you can get your money refunded, provided you cancel two to four weeks before the class starts.
(3) *Class size.* Try to find a class that is small—ideally, no more than eight couples.
(4) *Cost.* The price for most childbirth classes that run six to eight weeks ranges between $30 and $70. Fees tend to be lower in some parts of the country and considerably higher in New York City and other major metropolitan areas. Some community-health clinics, local Red Cross workshops and women's centers offer workshops free or for a nominal charge. In the case of Lamaze, classes offered by Preparing Expectant Mothers (PEP), where nonmedically trained mothers teach, will be about $25, in contrast to $40 and up, charged by ASPO-trained instructors.
(5) *Rapport with your instructor.* Find a teacher with whom you feel comfortable. Being on the same wavelength can be far more important than what childbirth method you choose. Try to meet your instructor prior to the beginning of classes to see if there is

good chemistry. Another approach is to watch one of her workshops before your session gets under way.

(6) *Alternative: self-taught.* If you have a scheduling conflict or other problems in taking a childbirth course, and if you are eager to do so, consider teaching yourself. Most organizations (listed next, in the "Information Sources") have manuals describing in detail all the conditioning techniques. One popular book, *Six Practical Lessons for an Easier Childbirth,* by Elisabeth Bing, maps out the Lamaze method step by step. Cassette tapes of relaxation and breathing exercises are also available. To boost your confidence and understanding, get some additional coaching by a friend who has taken a similar course and had a great childbirth.

Information Sources

ADDITIONAL READING

Acupressure: *Natural Childbirth, the Eastern Way,* by Wataru Ohasi (New York: Ballantine, 1983).

Biofeedback: *New Mind, New Body-Biofeedback,* by Barbara Brown (New York: Harper & Row, 1980).

Bradley Method: *A Husband-Coached Childbirth,* by Dr. Robert Bradley (New York: Harper & Row, 1974).

Dick-Read: *Childbirth Without Fear,* by Dr. Grantly Dick-Read (New York: Harper & Row, 1959).

Inner Bonding: *The Secret Life of the Unborn Child,* by Thomas Verny (New York: Simon & Schuster, 1981).

Lamaze Method: *Awake and Aware: Participating in Childbirth Through Psychoprophylaxis,* by Irwin Chabon (New York: Delacorte, 1974).
Thank You, Dr. Lamaze, by Marjorie Karmel (New York: Dolphin, 1965).
Six Practical Lessons For An Easier Childbirth, by Elisabeth Bing (New York: Bantam, 1969).

Psychosexual: *The Complete Book of Pregnancy and Childbirth,* by Shirley Kitzinger (New York: Knopf, 1980).

Visualization: *Creative Visualization,* by Shakti Gawain (Mill Valley, CA: Whatever Pub., 1978).

Yoga Method: *Positive Pregnancy Through Yoga,* by Sylvia Klein (Englewood Cliffs, NJ: Prentice-Hall, 1981).

ORGANIZATIONS

The following national organizations provide a referral service, listing instructors who teach their particular method where you live:

American Academy of Husband Coached Childbirth
PO Box 5224
Sherman Oaks, CA 91413
(Bradley method)

American Society of Clinical Hypnosis
2400 E. Devon
Des Plaines, IL 60018
(Physician hypnotists)

ASPO-Lamaze
1840 Wilson Blvd.
Arlington, VA 22201
(Largest Lamaze organization)

Cesarean Connection
PO Box 11
Westmont, IL 60559
(Cesarean classes)

Cesarean Prevention Movement
956 Spaight St.
Madison, WI 53703
(Vaginal delivery instead of repeat cesarean)

C/SEC
66 Christopher Rd.
Waltham, MA 02154
(Cesarean classes)

Home Oriented Maternity Experience
P.O. Box 450
Germantown, MD 20874
(Monthly meetings nationwide)

Informed Homebirth
Box 788
Boulder, CO 80306
(Home birth training)

Midwest Parentcraft Center
627 Beaver Rd.
Glen View, IL 60025
(Gamper method)

National Association of Childbirth Education
3940 Eleventh St.
Riverside, CA 92501
(Lamaze method)

National Childbirth Trust
9 Queensborough Terrace
Bayswater, London W2 3TB
England
(Kitzinger method)

Read Natural Childbirth Foundation
1300 S. Eliseo Dr.
Greenbrae, CA 94904
(Dick-Read method)

Other good sources for information about what methods are taught where you live include the International Childbirth Education Association, PO Box 20048, Minneapolis, MN 55240 and the Nurses Association of the American College of Obstetricians and Gynecologists, 600 Maryland Ave., SW, Washington, DC 20024. If you want to deliver at home or at a birthing center, write to the International Association of Parents and Professionals for Safe Alternatives in Childbirth, PO Box 267, Marble Hill, MO 63764. Another good bet is to ask your doctor, midwife or, better yet, parents, who can give you firsthand recommendations about individual childbirth instructors.

LEBOYER AND OTHER NONTRADITIONAL DELIVERIES

Usually the first minutes following birth resemble automobile racing when the car pulls into the pit stop for inspection. In most delivery rooms experienced hands cut the umbilical cord, administer silver-nitrate eye drops and clean, weigh, measure and sometimes footprint the newborn before handing the baby over to the parents. A gentle but conventional delivery with fewer clinical procedures, reducing the separation time between the baby and parents, is now practiced by many midwives and some obstetricians (see "Eye Drops and Other Procedures Immediately After Birth," p. 253). Leboyer delivery and the highly controversial underwater birth go considerably beyond immediate mother-child contact, or "bonding." Both methods seek to provide an in utero environment to comfort and soothe the newborn baby.

Leboyer: Pros and Cons

Leboyer gentle birth strives to minimize the trauma of the baby's exit from the womb. This technique is a far cry from the cold, bright, noisy surroundings typical of delivery rooms. It provides:

- a dimly lit, quiet room
- skin-to-skin contact with newborn massaged and stroked while on mother's abdomen
- umbilical cord not cut until after it stops pulsating
- warm-water bath, with baby's head and buttocks cradled in father's hands.

Leboyer clearly provides a calmer birth setting, enhances mother-child togetherness and involves the father, particularly in the bath ritual. Flexibility is another advantage, since this style of delivery can be discontinued if the baby's physical condition requires immediate medical attention. One of the drawbacks is that not all babies are enchanted with the bath, which, after all, separates the newborn from its mother. Heat loss and hypothermia are concerns frequently voiced about the bath, as well as fear of infection from dunking the freshly cut umbilical cord. While some experts say there is an increased probability of infection, Leboyer advocates suggest that extra handling by the parents exposes the baby to "family bacteria," thus making the newborn more immune to those in the hospital. Delayed cord clamping is another subject of debate, which is discussed in "Eye Drops and Other Procedures Immediately After Birth" (p. 253). Apart from some of these medical reasons, many health professionals discount Dr. Frederick Leboyer's theory. As midwife Kay Matthews writes in *Family Health,* "Having great faith in Mother Nature, I think it unlikely that she would produce offspring unable to withstand the crisis of birth in good physical and emotional condition. . . . Babies are new and unique human beings, ready and prepared to enter the world. I wonder if all this dark and quiet and warm water may not be confusing? And after all, there is a time to be born."

Since many physicians and hospitals do not approve of or allow the immersion of the newborn in water, modified Leboyer, including dimmed lights and sometimes immediate skin-to-skin contact, is a popular alternative. Many couples select music to play at the time of birth, to complement the relaxed and joyous mood. For those born by cesarean, sometimes the Leboyer bath is given several hours later, when the mother can watch more comfortably and enjoy it.

Leboyer Versus Non-Leboyer Babies

Both sides of this debate can cite studies supporting their positions. According to a survey of 120 Leboyer babies, at birth these infants were more relaxed and responsive. A multi-year follow-up study found Leboyer children were exceptionally adroit with their hands, began to talk at an earlier age, displayed less trouble feeding themselves and with toilet training and had higher-than-average IQs. A 1980 Canadian study of 50 women found Leboyer babies were neither more responsive nor less irritable, nor any different in temperament or behavior, at 8 months. (One interesting footnote to this study: The mothers' labors were shorter in the group planning a Leboyer delivery. The researchers suggest the physical progress of labor may be influenced by women who have a positive attitude and expect a good childbirth experience.)

Underwater Births

Accidental and planned births underwater are not as rare as you might think, particularly in parts of Europe and Russia. Mini–swimming pools and bathtubs are frequently used by laboring women to help the mother relax and relieve painful contractions. A maternity clinic outside Paris reports labor sometimes progresses so quickly that the baby is unintentionally born in water. Moscow's Scientific Research Institute for Physical Culture, which has been studying underwater deliveries since 1963, says, "This method reduced the mother's pain and babies born under water took naturally to water." Barring complications, underwater delivery may be the most peaceful technique, since the baby leaves the amniotic sac, or bag of water, and enters another fluid environment.

Factors to Weigh

Many mothers say the best aspects of Leboyer method are twofold: It encourages the father's handling of and bonding with the baby and reduces, via the bath ritual, the parents' fear of bathing their infant at home. Even though some health professionals express concerns about infection and heat loss, no study has established that Leboyer infants run a greater risk of such complications. This alternative to conventional delivery is available if you choose to have your baby at home, at most birth centers and in some hospitals. The decision, like so many other childbirth issues, is a personal one. If you want a Leboyer birth, make the arrangement in advance with your doctor or midwife, so you won't be surprised during labor to learn that the hospital doesn't permit anything but the conventional delivery. As for underwater delivery, expect some difficulty lining up a birth attendant.

Information Sources

ADDITIONAL READING

Birth Without Violence, by Frederick Leboyer (New York: Knopf, 1980). Photographs and sparse but hard-hitting prose contrast Leboyer and conventional delivery.

Handbook for Underwater Birth, by Rima and Steve Star. Available for $5.00 from PO Box 10205, Austin, TX 78757.

ORGANIZATION

**National Association for Advancement of
Leboyer's Birth Without Violence
PO Box 248455
Coral Gables, FL 33124**

For further information, refer to "Bonding and Rooming-In: Overrated or Not?" (p. 278).

AFTER CESAREAN: NATURAL BIRTH

The 1916 dictum "Once a cesarean, always a cesarean" no longer holds true in modern obstetrics. Yet the state of the art is still a long way from being "Once a cesarean, always a vaginal." Even in carefully selected groups of mothers (in other words, the best bets) who have tried, the American College of Obstetricians and Gynecologists (ACOG) reports a success rate in vaginal delivery after a prior cesarean of only 50 to 60 percent, although that rate is likely to rise as more women and their physicians try it. Statistics are higher at certain hospitals where vaginal deliveries are officially sought rather than avoided. VBAC (pronounced *vee*-back), short for vaginal birth after cesarean, received sanction in 1982 by the official licensing organization for obstetricians after being recommended by the government's National Institute for Child Health and Human Development. With the security of established guidelines behind them, doctors are now free from fear of legal action if they depart from what was formerly recognized as "standard obstetric practice"—namely, a repeat cesarean after a previous C-section.

The American College of Obstetricians and Gynecologists has suggested the following guidelines for VBAC, although individual doctors and hospitals have their own criteria for deciding who should attempt a vaginal birth.

(1) The reason for your cesarean should have been a nonrecurring one, such as fetal distress.

(2) Your uterine incision is horizontal (low transverse), not the classical or vertical cesarean incision. You must have medical records to prove it, since the scar on your abdomen won't necessarily match the one inside.

(3) You are carrying only one baby, weighing less than 8.5 pounds, and it is in a head-first (vertex) position.

(4) You have access to continuous electronic fetal monitoring throughout labor.

(5) Your hospital has necessary blood supplies and the delivery room is adequately staffed in the event a cesarean is necessary.

Each individual pregnancy must be evaluated to decide whether to attempt a VBAC, but some doctors automatically recommend a repeat cesarean if the first one was performed because of "failure to progress" or "relative cephalopelvic disproportion," while other physicians are more open to trying a vaginal delivery. Nancy Wainer Cohen, author of *Silent Knife*, who has had two VBACs, the last one at home, emphasizes the need for a laboring woman to be in a relaxed environment and claims that continuous monitoring, intravenous hookup and other hospital procedures make an expectant mother feel like an intensive-care patient.

Risks Versus Benefits

If you fall within the guidelines recommended by the American College of Obstetricians and Gynecologists, you will already have met rigid criteria and considerably whittled down the possible risks of VBAC. Below are a few of the remaining risks, as well as some of the benefits.

Risks in trying VBAC	Benefits of VBAC over Cesarean
• cesarean scar may split open—the incidence of uterine scar rupture (from all types of incisions) is between 0.6% and 1.24%; chance of a low-transverse scar reopening is about 1 in 100; in event of rupture,	• VBAC is safer than repeat cesarean surgery—specifically, less blood loss and reduced chance of infection. • fewer anesthesia-related complications.

Risks in trying VBAC	**Benefits of VBAC over Cesarean**
risk of death for the mother is "almost nonexistent," says ACOG, and "relatively small" for the baby.	• emotionally satisfying and gives mother opportunity to get over feelings of disappointment, guilt or failure resulting from previous cesarean.
• long, hard labor may not be successful, resulting in a repeat cesarean, which may be very disappointing to you.	• husband or friend can participate more in labor and delivery.
	• no postoperative pain.
	• more rapid recovery and return home.

Special Planning

VBAC advocates emphasize that if you decide to try it, you must be informed, educated and determined. Expect to interview many obstetricians, not just a few, and find out their VBAC success rate. That should rule out those physicians who give only lip service to VBAC and become either nervous or simply impatient after six hours or so of labor. Obstetricians with a good track record are likely to have the attitude that a woman who wants a vaginal delivery will have one unless there are indications that she needs another cesarean. Also check out the number of attempted and successful VBACs at your hospital and find out if any particular policies might require your doctor to intervene even if labor is progressing normally.

Other suggestions for you to consider include enrolling in a good childbirth-preparation class, ideally one designed just for VBAC mothers (now available in some cities). Equally important is getting rid of the emotional baggage from your last delivery and confronting fears and uncertainties such as how well you can cope with painful contractions. Another important ingredient, advises Nancy Wainer Cohen, who first coined the term "VBAC," is to find a woman knowledgeable about childbirth to be with you during labor. "If you were climbing a mountain," Cohen says, "you would probably choose a mountain guide," not only for guidance but for reassurance.

Factors to Weigh

The decision about whether to attempt a vaginal delivery is both a medical and personal one. Even some mothers who meet the medical criteria say they would rather plan a repeat cesarean from the very beginning than risk having their hopes dashed in the end. Others—who have failed—have said they are glad they tried; now they'll never wonder, "What if. . . ?" Of course, if you plan on a VBAC, you can change your mind beforehand or during labor. Although some risk to you and your baby exists, the likelihood of your scar's splitting open or of newborn death is very remote. Many physicians confess that although a cesarean is safe, it is just not in the same league as vaginal birth.

Information Sources

ADDITIONAL READING

Silent Knife: Vaginal Birth After Cesarean and Cesarean Prevention, by Nancy Wainer Cohen (South Hadley, MA: J. F. Bergin Publishers, 1983).

"Vaginal Delivery in Patients With a Prior Cesarean Section," by Justin Lavin, M.D., et al., *Obstetrics and Gynecology,* 59 (February 1982), 135–148. This medical journal is available at hospital and medical libraries.

ORGANIZATIONS

Cesarean Prevention Movement
PO Box 152
Syracuse, NY 13210

VBAC
10 Great Plain Terrace
Needham, MA 02192

③
Financial and
Other Life-Style
Questions

FATHER TO FATHER

If, as a father, you are going to read one section, this should be it.

No one can say that if you are not totally involved with the mother's pregnancy and childbirth you will not be a good father. "Both cross-cultural studies and studies of American men have shown that there is no relationship between participation in childbirth and later involvement with the child," according to the authors of *The Father Book*. However, the same modern culture that pressures the new mother to be a superwoman also pressures the father to be a superman. To succeed in a career, *Business Week* urges you to spend 60 hours a week climbing the corporate ladder. To succeed as a lover, *Esquire* says you have to pump iron, wear designer jeans and learn how to cry at the movies. And now, childbirth educators would have you believe that your child may not feel welcome in this world unless you become the Vince Lombardi of the delivery room.

Adjusting to Pregnancy

During the nine-month maternity cycle you, too, will be experiencing a variety of new feelings. Often it takes awhile for the "news" to sink in and right now you may have mixed feelings about becoming a parent. You may think you've made a mistake in starting a family; you worry about how the life-style of the two of you will be altered and how your circle of friends might change with the baby's arrival. Your wife or companion may have a bedside table full of books about pregnancy and childbirth (or perhaps just this one) which she has read religiously every evening since pregnancy was confirmed, yet you can't seem to get all that interested. No need to feel guilty about such thoughts. It is to be expected that it takes time to come to terms with future fatherhood. Remember, it is her body that is going through dramatic and unusual changes, not yours. If you were the one who is actually going to have a baby seven or eight months from now, you might be doing a lot more studying than she is.

By the end of the first trimester, though, when you can actually hear the baby's heartbeat and feel it move, you will probably be more involved. During the second and third trimesters some fathers experience weight gain, stress, possibly nausea and food cravings. Such symptoms are referred to as "couvade syndrome" or brooding in the sense of a hen watching her chicks. On the other hand, some men react with pangs of jealousy. Your ego may begin to suffer because everyone seems to pay more attention to the mother-to-be and her cargo than to you. After all, your job is over for the time being. Still, there are a few subtle things you can do so at least you aren't excluded from the conversation. Try referring to the mother's condition as "our pregnancy" and say "we're pregnant." Read "Month-by-Month Developments," p. 16. Any additional reading will also pay off in understanding and patience when they are needed.

If your self-esteem suffers a bit during pregnancy, keep in mind that at times the mother-to-be too will lack confidence. As her body changes shape, it is natural for her to feel that she is no longer sexually attractive. Her ego will need boosting, and you are the only one who can do it. Try some exotic things together; maybe buy some sexy underwear (it worked for us). On this subject, "Sex: Trimester to Trimester," p. 64, may address some unspoken concerns.

Participating in Your Child's Birth

Ideally, your level of involvement in the actual childbirth should be based on both your feelings and those of the mother. If you have strong feelings against participating in any way and the mother feels comfortable enough about getting through labor without you, she, together with the health-care team, will probably get along fine. But you may be missing something very special. The same culture that pressures you to be a superman has also made it acceptable for you to experience the extraordinary feelings that can come only from watching your child enter the world.

If you have any inclination at all to participate in the birth, learning more about it will help you to decide. Any fears you may harbor are likely to be based on lack of information or simply on misinformation. To aid in making a decision:

- Talk to other fathers who were present during their son's or daughter's birth.
- Go along to a prenatal check-up and don't sit in the waiting room reading old copies of *Reader's Digest.* Go into the examination room, meet the doctor or midwife and ask questions, even if they seem stupid. And be sure to listen to the baby's heart beating through the stethoscope or doptone device.
- Go along to a local childbirth-preparation group and arrange to attend at least one hour of class. This can usually be done free of charge. Just don't be overwhelmed by the information overload you may encounter.

If you decide to attend childbirth education classes, discussion about the stages of labor will give you a notion of what to expect, as well as a working vocabulary of medical terms. If you think the time spent on socializing during the class is a waste, bear in mind that hearing other men voice the same fears and uncertainties you have been experiencing can be helpful. You may find that many of the tasks suggested for the labor coach, such as fetching ice chips, are to keep you from feeling bored or useless. Your chief responsibilities—and they are important—boil down to these:

- being a companion essentially a non-professional who can offer support and comfort to the mother as well as share in her joy
- ensure that the medical staff follows the mother's wishes about positions during labor, use of pain-killers and other medications and so on. (Both of you should work out ahead of time your feelings and philosophy about these decisions.)

Much of what you will be doing will be for yourself—watching and participating in the birth of your child. Specific suggestions begin on p. 215 in "Typical Birth: Stages of Labor."

If you decide not to attend childbirth classes but still want to be present for labor and delivery, you may have a problem. Many medical facilities will allow the father to witness the birth only if he attended classes.

Staying at the Hospital Overnight

If you are going to attend the birth of your child (and maybe even if you aren't), you may want to consider staying overnight at the hospital while the mother and baby are recovering. If the mother pays more for a private room, many hospitals will bring in an extra bed and let you spend the night. You may find it a great little vacation, even though the facilities will be far from those at the Ritz. The additional benefits will include the following:

- You and the mother will have more time to share your initial excitement over your baby.
- You can give the mother more care and attention than can be provided by the hospital staff, and you can certainly sneak in some tastier food than the hospital provides.
- You can attend mini-hospital classes on infant care and feeding, which allows both parents to go up the learning curve together; as a result, this will make you both feel more comfortable about diapering and bathing your baby once you get home.

Dealing with Unspoken Fears and Anxieties

Insomnia during the last month or two of pregnancy is a common complaint among expectant mothers and also a problem for prospective fathers. Anxiety over the financial responsibilities of a family usually seems to be most intense just prior to the due date and during the first couple of weeks after the birth. In addition to concerns about paying bills or job security, fears that center on childbirth are inevitable.

The worry "Can she count on me during labor?" can be allayed considerably if you do a little reading. Start with "Typical Birth: Stages of Labor," on p. 215, which contains tips on what you can do at specific points during labor; for instance, watch for signs of hyperventilation, apply counterpressure in the event of backache, give encouragement and frequent progress reports during the pushing phase.

Another common fear is "I'm afraid about being alone with her at home during labor." The best thing to do is review the two brief sections "Warning Signs: When to Be Concerned," p. 162, and "Signs of Labor: True or False?" p. 213. As soon as the "bag of water" breaks and/or contractions begin, don't hesitate to pick up the phone and call the doctor for advice about how to proceed. If, during labor, the two of you feel uneasy being alone go ahead and make a trip to the hospital even though you might be told to return home if it's the very early stage of labor.

It's easy to wonder how you will react to the sight of blood and worry about fainting in the delivery room. The best prevention is to go watch films of vaginal and cesarean deliveries (childbirth organizations as well as the Red Cross and YWCA have free film showings in most communities). Also go to a bookstore or library and look at graphic pictures of babies being born. During labor, remember to eat and if you don't want to leave the maternity ward to run out for a bite, see if the nurse can have a food tray sent up for you. If you feel woozy, don't keep it a secret; the hospital staff is experienced in dealing with this type of situation. In the event of an unexpected non-emergency cesarean, you would be positioned near the mother's head and drapes would obstruct your view while the abdominal and uterine incisions are made. (More about surgery on p. 260.)

The thought "Will my child be normal?" crosses every expectant parent's mind. It cannot hurt for you to think through alone, or preferably with your partner, how you might handle the situation if your baby were not normal or didn't survive. Getting such worries out in the open will melt away much of the apprehension and also lay the foundation of better communication. You may want to refer to "Premature Babies and Other Newborns Needing Intensive Care," p. 270 and "If Your Baby Dies," p. 275.

The last worry to address is what to do if you are without professional help and the baby's head can be seen in the birth canal or if contractions are strong and less than two minutes apart. Step-by-step instructions on what you should do are outlined in "Emergency Childbirth: How to Deliver Your Baby," p. 257.

Taking Time Off with the Family

The first days at home can be emotionally and physically difficult for a new mother (see "Blues and Depression: It's Not All in Your Mind," p. 313). If it is possible, you may want to consider taking time off work for a few days once the baby comes home from the hospital. Although this is not practiced widely, child-care leave for fathers is becoming more commonplace. A 1981 survey conducted by Catalyst Career and Family Center found that 9 percent of the top U.S. corporations offered paternity leave. As late as 1978 there were virtually no companies addressing this issue. However, Catalyst believes that corporate policies in the future will handle paternity leave within a general category called "personal leave of absence" to help eliminate any stigma that may be associated with paternity leave.

Besides getting a break from work, there are other reasons for staying home:

- You may find child care more enjoyable than the mother does, and you may be better at it. The maternal instinct is by no means proven, and most evidence points to the fact that women are better at taking care of babies only because they are more likely to be given that responsibility.
- By learning how to take care of your baby together, you are less likely to defer to the mother for every little question that may come up, and will find yourself experiencing the rewards of solving problems yourself.
- If the mother knows that you will be around to help her adapt to and share these new responsibilities, you will have a companion who will be more relaxed about parenting and with whom it will be a lot easier to live.

Mood swings, even the "weepies," are not unique to mothers; fathers also may be vulnerable to postpartum blues. It's easy for a father to feel frustrated or inadequate in satisfying the needs of his baby by himself or in conjunction with the mother. Dr. Martha Zaslow of the government's National Institute of Child Health and Human Development suggests that these symptoms in men may also be provoked by hormonal changes. If the strain or exhaustion gets to you, remember to heed the advice frequently given to new parents... just take one day at a time.

Information Sources

ADDITIONAL READING

At least a dozen sections in this book may be especially useful. The following would be relevant if you intend to participate in the birth:

"Patients' Rights and Informed Consent" (p. 200)
"Typical Birth: Stages of Labor" (p. 215)
"Positions and Labor Equipment: From Squatting to Birthing Chairs" (p. 224)
"Electronic Fetal Monitors: Pros and Cons" (p. 232)
"Drugs During Childbirth" (p. 236)
"Long Labor: Let the Sun Set Twice?" (p. 246)
"Forceps-Assisted Delivery" (p. 251)
"Eye Drops and Other Procedures Immediately After Birth" (p. 253)
"Cesarean: What Every Expectant Mother (Father) Should Know" (p. 260)

To help you with other decisions which should be made jointly, refer to:

"Breast and/or Bottle?" (p. 283)
"Circumcision: Not a Medical Decision" (p. 287)
"Help During Week One!" (p. 297)
"Sex: Intimate Questions" (p. 330)
"Car Seats, Cribs and Other Essential Equipment" (p. 341)
"Emergencies and First Aid" (p. 362)
"Child-Proofing: From Poisonous Plants to Popcorn" (p. 402)

Earth Father, Sky Father: The Changing Concept of Fathering, by Arthur and Libby Colman (Englewood Cliffs, NJ: Prentice-Hall, 1981). Emphasizes the importance of cultivating nurturing aspects of your own personality and suggests how to develop your own style of fathering.

Expectant Fathers, by Sam Bittman and Sue Rosenberg Zalk (New York: Dutton, 1979). Discusses various stages of pregnancy, range of feelings and experiences during birth.

The Father Book, by Rae Grad et al. (Washington, DC: Acropolis, 1982). Describes anxieties of and pressures on expectant fathers and discusses various experiences such as a father's fainting during a film on childbirth. Provides different views on whether or not to coach during labor and also problems that might arise during labor.

Pregnant Fathers, by Jack Heinowitz (Englewood Cliffs, NJ: Spectrum, 1982). Advice to expectant fathers on how to cope with their feelings, and what issues they can expect to confront during and immediately after childbirth. Stresses the importance of communicating with one's partner.

ORGANIZATION

The Fatherhood Project
Bank Street College of Education
610 W. 112th St.
New York, NY 10025
Clearinghouse provides information on support resources for fathers. Send stamped, self-addressed envelope to receive free material.

HEALTH INSURANCE: WHAT WON'T BE COVERED

It is difficult to generalize about health-insurance policies, since they vary in cost and coverage depending on whether you have a group or individual plan and whether it is with Blue Cross/Blue Shield, a private insurer or a prepaid health maintenance organization. That's why you need to reread the fine print and talk with your employer or insurance agent so you are clear on what is and what isn't covered. Even if you are already pregnant and it would be impossible to upgrade your coverage, it is better to know what your coverage consists of.

Most doctors' (and some nurse-midwives') fees and hospital charges will be covered if you have group "basic protection" and/or major medical insurance. Of course, if you have major medical protection only, you must figure on the deductible you must pay or possibly the coinsurance payment, which usually ranges from 20 percent to 80 percent. The majority of policies cover most of your bills for prenatal appointments, lab tests and whatever else your physician deems medically necessary, although some insurers reserve the right to evaluate the appropriateness of certain procedures. Labor and delivery-room charges and the cost of your hospital stay in a semiprivate room are normally covered by your policy. Find out exactly what charges are insured by your health plan by comparing it with the two checklists below.

Expenses Usually Covered	Expenses Often Excluded
prenatal checkups	pregnancy test
lab tests	prenatal vitamins
sonograms	genetic counseling
amniocentesis	childbirth-preparation classes
medications during labor	out-of-hospital birth center
electronic fetal monitor	private hospital room
delivery-room charges	newborn exam by pediatrician
birth attendant's fee	circumcision
cesarean birth	television and phone calls
anesthesiologist	infant formula, etc., in "newborn pack"
newborn hospital care	six-week postpartum checkup

If you are not yet pregnant and if your individual maternity coverage is skimpy, discuss your options with your insurance agent; but the best route may be to rely on your savings instead of buying additional protection. If you are pregnant, supplementary insurance will not be an option because of the usual nine-month waiting period and an exclusion for preexisting health conditions—in this case, pregnancy. Furthermore, since most insurance policies provide similar outpatient, hospital and surgical benefits, some of the gaps in your coverage cannot be filled at any price.

Two-career couples with different employee health plans may still be underinsured in certain areas; however, the strengths of one policy may make up for the shortcomings of the other. Often the second group policy picks up where the first one leaves off, enabling you to get up to 100 percent reimbursement for covered maternity expenses.

If you shift from full-time to part-time work, are temporarily unemployed, quit or leave your job, chances are that you will lose your health insurance. Check with the personnel department about converting your group plan to an individual policy, but remember that your premiums will increase and your coverage will be less comprehensive.

Individual policyholders should make sure not to let their insurance plans lapse. Usually the grace period for paying your premium is 31 days. If you pay your own premiums directly, try to arrange to pay on a quarterly or an annual rather than a monthly basis, because it is cheaper.

Check on the time limits for filing claims, and also find out when you have to notify your insurer of your baby's birth in order to claim benefits.

You are bound to have lots of questions about your maternity, postpartum and baby-care coverage; luckily, there are many people to call for answers. For questions about

- your group plan: ask your employer, labor union or trade association
- your individual plan: discuss with your insurance agent
- paying bills and filing claims: ask at the doctor's office, hospital, midwifery service or birth center
- legal rights or problems with claim settlement: contact your State Insurance Department.

While you are scrutinizing your health insurance, try to get in the habit of reviewing your policy each year. When it comes time to renew your plan, see if it is up-to-date. Some policies adjust to inflation better than others, so make sure your benefits have not been outdistanced, advises the Health Insurance Association.

Information Sources

ORGANIZATIONS

Health Insurance Association
1850 K St., NW
Washington, DC 20006
Information clearinghouse.

State Insurance Department
Check directory assistance for the toll-free number. If you write your state insurance commissioner, give the name of your company and your policy number, but don't send your policy.

WORKING BEFORE AND AFTER: SAFEGUARDS AND SCENARIOS

From a helicopter above the San Diego Freeway, the radio broadcaster sprinkled her traffic report with the news that her obstetrician's latest prediction was she would be at the hospital within a day or two. The anchor then made a plug for the radio station's contest to guess the baby's sex and weight. Many women work up until they feel the first contractions, either to keep the paycheck coming in or to stay busy. "I loved all the attention, and besides, I would've gone crazy waiting, particularly because I was three weeks late," admitted an attorney. Other expectant mothers quit, often to have the time to satisfy their "nesting instincts" and to refuel prior to the big event.

What's Safe or Unsafe

The prevailing view in the medical community is to stick with your job, provided you have a trouble-free pregnancy and the work environment poses no danger to you or your baby. The American College of Obstetricians and Gynecologists (ACOG) advises that "if the patient continues in good health, feels well, and the pregnancy proceeds normally, there is generally no reason why a normal working schedule cannot be continued until close to the expected date of delivery." But there are those who think these ACOG guidelines are too lax.

What worries some obstetricians is that since pregnancy is no longer viewed as sickness, many working women insist on their "wellness" and deny feeling tired and run-down. Chronic fatigue and stress can increase the risk of premature labor, claims Dr. Calvin Hobel, who is involved in the University of California's prevention of preterm delivery at the Harbor Campus. A by-product of stress is the release of catecholamines, essentially a higher level of adrenaline; according to Hobel, this causes "uterine irritability" and may stimulate contractions. His advice to expectant mothers is to get in the habit of resting periodically each day to regain strength and avoid stress. For high-risk pregnancies, most health professionals will urge women to get off their feet for at least three hours a day. Ideally, pregnant women should avoid jobs requiring them to stay in the same position for long hours, either sitting or standing, not so much to prevent varicose veins and swollen ankles but so that plenty of blood is routed to the placenta.

Further caution was signaled by a study conducted at the Lackland Air Force Base obstetrical clinic during the seventies. About 200 pregnant women who continued on active duty until the day of delivery were compared to an identical number of expectant mothers (many were military wives) who had the option of not working or of reducing their work responsibilities at any point during pregnancy. Despite the similarities in age and other characteristics, the active-duty patients experienced more complications. Of note was a twofold increase in pregnancy-induced hypertension, commonly called toxemia or preeclampsia, and a fivefold increase in premature labor. These findings, like practically all studies, should be viewed not as conclusions but as theories.

Most obstetricians and midwives do not regard working while waiting as risky provided you avoid physical overexertion and are not around environmental toxins. Lifting, pulling, climbing and heat exposure are the principal hazards that fall into the category of physical stress. The list of gases, chemicals, fumes, dust and other hazardous substances is much longer and, unfortunately, continues to grow. Two federal agencies, the National Institute for Occupational Safety and Health (NIOSH) and the Occupational Health and Safety

Administration, establish safe levels of exposure for lead, mercury and other environmental toxins, but, as one company doctor warns, that's the safety threshold for adults, *not* for the developing fetus. It's important, if you are working in an industrial facility or factory, to meet with the company doctor or nurse as soon as you know you are pregnant. You may be transferred to another site or be given a different job during the entire gestation period to ensure less risk for yourself and your unborn baby. In the ACOG-NIOSH report *Guidelines on Work and Pregnancy*, it is suggested that often it is better to scale down job responsibilities than to move to a less-demanding one that is unfamiliar.

There are warnings for women in specific occupations. Hairdressers and beauticians should be aware of hair-spray resins, hair dyes and solvents of nail polish (not to mention being on their feet much of the day). Artists need adequate ventilation, at the very least, to reduce paint fumes. Typesetters and those with other jobs that require time spent in front of word processors (VDTs, or visual display terminals) should have their employers check with the manufacturer to make sure the machine does not emit radiation (most VDTs are not believed to pose a risk to the developing fetus). X-ray technicians, nurses and hospital staff members need to transfer jobs during pregnancy in order to avoid radiation, chemotherapy and viral infections, as well as anesthesia and other gases.

The National Institute for Occupational Safety and Health, at the main office, in Washington, D.C., or at its regional offices, has consultants who can answer any specific questions you might have about work exposure to various toxins and stresses (see "Information Sources," p. 139, for the address). You should make your own job evaluation, perhaps keeping an hourly diary for a day or two, noting tasks performed and materials handled, and volunteer seemingly trivial details to your obstetrician or midwife.

Checklist

_____ number of hours plus overtime
_____ amount of time sitting or standing
_____ opportunities to rest besides coffee breaks
_____ physical work such as lifting boxes
_____ noise level in the office or factory
_____ average temperature as well as highs and lows
_____ commuting time to and from work
_____ pressure due to deadlines or work load
_____ chain smokers in the work area

These are all important factors which you must consider with your health-care team when making the decision to remain on the job during the nine-month cycle.

Maternity Leave and Legal Rights

The 1978 Pregnancy Discrimination Law sounds tough: You cannot be fired or denied a job simply because you are expecting a baby, and employers must treat pregnancy in the same manner they would any other medical condition. This amendment to the Civil Rights Act provides some protection against losing your earning power, but ultimately the extent of your legal rights is dependent on your own employer's policies.

If you work for a company that offers temporary disability insurance, you are in luck; you are entitled to the same benefits as any male employee. But businesses that don't offer disability plans are not required to institute them. The same applies to employee sick-leave programs and health insurance. Large corporations with set policies usually will be fairly straightforward regarding maternity benefits; however, small companies with unwritten guidelines may be a different matter. The law applies to employers of 15 or more people, and often, in the case of small companies with unwritten policies, your benefits may depend on the goodwill of your boss.

Here's what you *are* and *are not* entitled to under the 1978 law:

- Pregnancy and pregnancy-related conditions must be treated like any other disability or medical condition, but employers are not required to establish benefit programs if none exist. (Some states provide temporary disability insurance if you are not covered by your employer.)
- You are entitled to the identical medical coverage and paid disability leave as that offered by the employer for other disabilities; however, the paid medical leave and maternity absence may be too short. See if you can use your accrued vacation time and unused sick-leave days to maximize your period of maternity leave.
- Maternity benefits must be paid to employees' wives whenever spouses are covered for other disabilities.
- You have the right to be reinstated in the same job when you return to work if there is a company policy that no seniority is lost due to disability or sick leave, provided the job is not abolished. If there are no such guarantees where you work, it will depend on your boss whether you will retain the same job along with fringe benefits.
- You cannot be forced to give up your job by a specified month of your pregnancy and stay away until a certain time after your baby's born, although the Supreme Court ruled that an airline can force a stewardess to take maternity leave without pay because her pregnancy could incapacitate her and jeopardize

passengers in the event of an emergency. This type of blanket policy is most unusual.

- Your employer cannot deny you a raise or promotion because of pregnancy, but it is difficult to prove discrimination unless there is an automatic salary adjustment and/or promotion schedule.
- You are entitled to an extended leave of absence if other employees have taken sabbaticals, returned to school or traveled for several months or more.
- You cannot be denied a job simply because you are pregnant; however, employers may refuse to hire a pregnant woman on the ground that the workplace may be hazardous.

Each year more companies are getting accustomed to having pregnant women on the payroll and are adapting to mothers in the work force, but discriminatory practices still exist in every type of occupation. Even if you don't run into any problems arranging maternity leave and, perhaps, an extended unpaid leave of absence, keep good records to be on the safe side. Put down in writing your agreement with your employer, and even though the company probably will keep track of your sick days, it's not a bad idea to maintain your own file.

If you believe you have been denied a raise because you're pregnant or if your job has been abolished when you return to work after your baby's born, you can get help from a variety of government agencies and private organizations. There are several avenues for obtaining free advice about discrimination questions.

DISCRIMINATION: DO YOU HAVE A CASE?

(1) Regional Equal Employment Opportunity Commission (EEOC) offices have lawyers who are on call, referred to as "Attornies-of-the-Day," who will answer questions and provide free legal advice on filing a discrimination complaint.

(2) Your state or local fair-employment-practices agency, sometimes called the human rights commission, may be able to help you faster than the federal EEOC.

(3) Even if you are not affiliated with a union, local labor-union representatives are familar with pregnancy discrimination questions and may be useful to contact.

(4) Legal Aid Society, the Women's Legal Defense Fund and other private, nonprofit organizations often offer free counsel (see "Information Sources," p. 139).

Maternity-Leave Scenarios

No perfect strategy has been devised for deciding how and when to inform your employer about your pregnancy and whether or not to return to work. Some choices are outlined below.

- When should I tell my boss?

    Scenario 1: Be up front and inform your supervisor soon after your pregnancy is confirmed. If you are feeling under the weather, you don't have to make excuses, and perhaps you can rearrange your schedule to accommodate flexi-time, particularly during the first trimester.

    Scenario 2: Wait until about the fourth month, when the likelihood of miscarriage is past, and by that stage in your pregnancy, you may be further along in deciding about whether or not to return to work.

    Scenario 3: You are on the verge of being promoted or a salary increase is in the pipeline and you don't want to miss out; however, this can backfire in the sense that your employer may be miffed if your job requires increased responsibility and within a few months you will be taking time off and may not return.

- When should I start my maternity leave?

    Scenario 1: If you want to have time off before the baby is born, some disability plans will provide for paid leave to begin two to four weeks before your due date; of course, that free time may dissolve if you are early.

    Scenario 2: If you have some pressing job responsibility or are simply eager to keep working up until delivery, probably your doctor or midwife will certify your expected date of delivery at 42 weeks rather than 40; after all, it's an educated guess that is known only ex post facto.

    Scenario 3: You want to remain on the job as long as you're feeling fine but want to cut down on your hours. See if you can cut down to working three days a week or part-time. But be sure this won't make you lose your group health insurance!

    Scenario 4: You want to quit (permanently), so consider using up your accumulated vacation time and sick leave during the final month(s). Make sure you arrange with the personnel office to convert your group health-insurance policy to an individual plan if you have no other coverage.

● What about discussing the long-range job picture?

Scenario 1: If you are positive that you don't plan to return to work after your baby has arrived, tell your boss and volunteer to help train your successor.

Scenario 2: If you are uncertain about what to do, keep your options open and tell your employer you are investigating child care, and discuss possible options such as part-time work, job sharing or doing some of your work at home. Promise to keep him or her informed of your plans once you map them out.

Scenario 3: If you intend to take a short maternity leave and then return to work, discuss with your employer a variety of choices regarding the length of time you take off. Keep in mind that if you have a cesarean you may want a bit longer to recuperate; furthermore, it is not uncommon for you to have a change of heart when it comes time to choose between staying at home watching your baby grow and resuming your full-time job.

Scenario 4: Some mothers know in advance that they want to take two or three months, and others are interested in an extended unpaid leave of absence lasting half a year or longer. Find out what your employer's leave policy is generally. See if the company is willing to go along with such an arrangement, but remember, many companies may be wondering if you will return to work for only a short time if a second child is contemplated.

MISCELLANEOUS ON-THE-JOB TIPS

● If you feel nauseous, see if you can arrange to come in later in the morning or try flexi-time.
● Try to avoid working lunches, and use the time to refuel, particularly when fatigue strikes during the first trimester.
● Don't skip meals, and as insurance against empty-calorie snacks, keep a stash of food such as raisins, nuts and crackers, at the office, or bring a thermos full of yogurt and fruit or hard-boiled eggs, cheese, bananas and other fruits that require little refrigeration.

- Watch the office cocktail parties with regard to booze, and don't let hors d'oeuvres replace a meal.
- Those fluorescent lights may change your skin pigmentation. If you notice a mask of pregnancy, consider wearing sun block to work.
- Chairs with armrests can make an enormous difference in taking the strain off your back, and the backrest should be low enough to support your pelvis.
- Periodically prop your feet up on a stool, file-cabinet drawer or wastepaper basket during the day.
- If you are sitting down or are on your feet a lot, take five-minute breaks to get the blood circulating. For instance, rotate your ankles by making circles if you have been at a desk for hours.
- Try not to keep your legs crossed for long periods of time.
- Practice Kegel exercises in the elevator and do the pelvic tilt against a wall each time you go the restroom (for details see "Conditioning Exercises: What's a Kegel?" p. 68).
- Airlines often require a letter from your doctor saying it is okay for you to fly during the final month or two. Check with your travel agent in advance of your trip, since regulations change all the time.
- Low-heeled shoes or flat soles are recommended during the third trimester, to lessen the shift of the weight-bearing angle.

Returning to Work

If your income is not essential to the family budget but your identity and self-esteem are closely linked with your professional pursuits, join the crowd of mothers who are torn between their children and work. Part of the conflict is that women are bombarded by so many choices, particularly deciding whether the rewards of a career are worth the necessary 8- to 10-hour daily separation from their babies. Some working mothers seem to thrive on the dual nature of their lives, such as a physician with twins who has a live-in nanny, a maid and a backup sitter for the weekends. Many women, however, cannot afford such costly child care or are not as relaxed about being absentee parents.

Reassuring research may reduce some of the pangs of guilt. Countless studies have shown no adverse effects on infants and toddlers who receive high-quality child care. Researchers observing children from three months to three years of age who had been entrusted to day-care centers for eight hours a day found these youngsters still showed a strong preference for their mothers and were neither more aggressive nor more cooperative than young children of full-time mothers. The government's National Institute of Education claims that children of working mothers do as well in school as those of mothers who stay at home, although it is not known why. Nonetheless, plenty of pediatricians, psychologists and mothers argue against regular surrogate care, at least during the first six months, and prefer to see mothers remain with their babies until the second or third birthday. Even those with strong opinions about what's right admit there is no conclusive evidence. As Dr. Niles Newton, of Northwestern University Medical School says, in order to draw conclusions, "we have to look at how these people are going to grow up and interact with their own families."

The degree to which a mother's attitude about herself affects her child's development is acknowledged now more than ever; certainly many working women believe their children gain in terms of independence. But perhaps in the near future the endless struggle to justify the dual role will be unnecessary. In her book *This Is Judy Woodruff at the White House*, Woodruff writes,

> Eventually I hope we'll see the day when mothers will no longer be called upon to defend their decision to continue working any more than fathers are today. Neither will it be considered remarkable for a father to take a leave of absence from his job to raise his children, as ABC newsman Ted Koppel did while his wife attended medical school. It's worth noting that Koppel's career didn't suffer, as evidenced by his position as anchorman of ABC's *Nightline* newscast.

Timing Your Return

According to Catalyst, an organization that serves working women, most mothers return to their jobs before their babies are 4 months old. This time frame coincides with the maternity leave offered by many employers, although more generous options are available, such as those at AT&T, Procter & Gamble and other companies that permit an unpaid six-month-care-for-newborn leave of absence. Unfortunately, prolonged maternity leave is not realistic for many professionals, since projects won't wait, clients won't wait and sometimes employers won't wait. Besides fear about losing one's job, it's understandable why women worry that time off may mean being passed by at promotion time on the ground they aren't serious enough about their careers.

If you have a real choice about timing, there are conflicting views about when to return to the office. Some suggest getting back to work within the first eight weeks after the baby is born, so the child doesn't become accustomed to having mother around during the day. Others theorize that a child should get used to a babysitter or play-group environment before 7 or 8 months, an age when separation or "stranger" anxiety usually occurs. Another school of thought is to wait until this phase has passed, so the child will have developed another layer of security.

Another approach, regardless of how much time you take off, is to ease the transition by working part-time at first. Phasing in gradually, even working at home initially, can help out a lot, especially if you want to continue to breast-feed. But don't count on your baby's nap time to get your work done, and definitely line up someone to watch your child at least some of the time you are working at home.

Not all jobs are well suited for mothers, as in the case of a trial lawyer unable to set courtroom dates. In many occupations, though, it is possible to get more control over your schedule by negotiating flexi-time, compressed work weeks or perhaps a four-day week. Flexibility in one's work life provides room to maneuver in such unavoidable situations as having to rush your child to the doctor. Reliable child-care arrangements that are convenient and give you peace of mind as well as a backup babysitter are equally important. Dorothy Rich, president of the Home and School Institute, finds that people who are good organizers manage to arrange their lives so they can survive on the job and still find time to spend with their children. Many studies support the conclusion that working mothers spend almost as much "quality" time interacting with their children as full-time parents.

Factors to Weigh

Working during pregnancy may be an economic necessity rather than individual preference. In either case, make sure you and your physician or midwife take time to evaluate the safety of your work environment and job responsibilities. Chronic fatigue and stress should not be ignored. Otherwise, a normal woman with an uncomplicated pregnancy and a normal fetus faces "no greater potential hazards than those encountered in normal daily life in the community and may continue to work without interruption until the onset of labor and may resume working several weeks after an uncomplicated delivery," according to the American College of Obstetricians and Gynecologists.

Although the Pregnancy Discrimination Law prohibits unequal treatment, it guarantees little. Don't hesitate to contact your local Legal Aid Society or union to get free advice on how to deal with your employer to ensure that you get the maternity benefits to which you are entitled.

The decision on whether or not to return to your job after the baby is born is difficult to make. Many women have no idea how they will react to motherhood, and it's not unusual for one's loyalites to a career to be superseded by those to the new arrival. Pamela Daniels and Kathryn Weingarten, authors of *Sooner or Later: The Timing of Parenthood in Adult Lives*, concluded that mothers who returned to work soon after the birth of their children experienced not guilt, but "a profound sense of loss." It is not uncommon to have a change of heart and decide you want to scale back your job responsibilities or spend a lot more time at home. Part-time work, job sharing or a home-based career may be possible alternatives. By all means don't try to prove to yourself and others you are a "Supermom"; rather, march to the beat of your own drummer. Certainly, more and more mothers are succeeding with full-time work and, in some cases, also managing successful breast-feeding (see "Back on the Job and Breast-feeding," p. 326).

Information Sources

ADDITIONAL READING

The Balancing Act: A Career and a Baby, by Sydelle Kramer (Chicago: Chicago Review Press, 1976). Several professional women who have children share their thoughts.

Career and Motherhood, by Alan Roland and Barbara Harris (New York: Human Sciences Press, 1979). The conflict between mothering and working is explored.

How to Have a Child and Keep Your Job, by Jane Price (New York: St. Martin's, 1979). Interviews with working parents and their families, along with suggestions about child care and related issues.

The Job-Sharing Handbook, by Barney Olmstead and Suzanne Smith (New York: Penguin, 1983). Explores range of job-sharing possibilities that are economically viable.

Managing Your Maternity Leave, by Meg Wheatley and Marcie Schorr (Boston: Houghton Mifflin, 1983).

Mothers Who Work, by Jeanne Bodin and Bonnie Mitelman (New York: Ballantine, 1983). Good reading for working mothers who need a shot in the arm.

Sooner or Later: The Timing of Parenthood in Adult Lives, by Pamela Daniels and Kathryn Weingarten (New York: Norton, 1982).

Working Mother. Monthly magazine. To subscribe, write: PO Box 10609, Des Moines, IA 50336.

The Working Mother's Complete Handbook, by Gloria Norris and JoAnn Miller (New York: Dutton, 1979). Interviews with 150 women, who discuss the benefits of working along with material such as "Pacing Your Career," and so on.

ORGANIZATIONS

Catalyst
14 E. 60th St.
New York, NY 10022
National clearinghouse on two-career families; information on working mothers, reentry into job market, child care and so on. Data base available to those with access to BRS terminal; publications available.

Equal Employment Opportunity Commission
2401 E St., NW
Washington, DC 20506
Regional offices and national office offer free advice on your legal rights and on filing a discrimination complaint.

National Alliance of Homebased Businesswomen
PO Box 95
Norwood, NJ 07648
Provides support network of professional contacts and also publishes annual directory and other literature.

National Council for Alternative Work Patterns
1925 K St., Room 308A
Washington, DC 20006
Clearinghouse on flexi-time, part-time and job-sharing opportunities.

National Institute for Occupational Safety and Health (NIOSH)
5600 Fishers La.
Rockville, MD 20857
NIOSH researchers, consultants and doctors study occupational hazards and conduct on-site health-safety investigations.

Occupational Safety and Health Administration (OSHA)
200 Constitution Ave., NW
Washington, DC 20210
OSHA investigates complaints and enforces safe working conditions in factories and offices.

Pregnancy Rights Monitoring Project
Women's Legal Defense Fund
2000 P St., NW #400
Washington, DC 20036
This private nonprofit group will give individual advice and will take individual cases to court.

Women's Occupational Health Resource Center
Columbia University

21 Audubon Ave., Third Floor
New York, NY 10032
Fact sheets on reproductive hazards; WOHRC will answer questions
about pregnancy-related hazards on the job.

Women's Rights Project
American Civil Liberties Union
22 E. 20th St.
New York, NY 10016
Refers you to local volunteer attorneys for individual cases.

SINGLE AND PREGNANT

Times are changing. At least one-fourth of young children live with a
single parent, and the U.S. Bureau of Census projects that by the late
1980s, the figures will be between 40 and 50 percent. Now more
working women are financially able to support a child. Other reasons
that make it easier—that does not mean easy—to rear a child alone
are that more support systems exist for single-parent families and the
high divorce rate means that a youngster growing up without a father
at home does not feel as out of place as formerly.

Still, single parents, particularly unwed mothers, often have to
contend with negative attitudes. Such terms as "nontraditional family"
or "alternative life-style" have not replaced the old vocabulary,
"broken home." "On the whole, in our society," write Elizabeth
Herzog and Cecelia Sudia in *Child Education,* "the one-parent family
has been viewed as a form of un-family or sick family. For a number of
reasons it would be wiser to recognize the one-parent family as a form
that exists and functions . . . such families can be cohesive, warm,
supportive and favorable to the development of children." Robert
Weiss, author of *Marital Separation,* says, "A number of studies suggest
that the greater participation of the children in the management of
the single-parent home and their greater closeness to the mother tend
to enhance their verbal skill."

Despite such claims about the positive aspects of one-parent families,
there is no denying that single mothers need a lot of support,
especially when work, finances or parenting get to be too much.
Relatives may have good staying power. Besides providing often-needed
doses of encouragement, a grandmother or uncle can wear many hats,
including that of disciplinarian. Beyond family members and friends,
numerous mutual-help groups have sprung up in response to the more
than eight million single-parent families. Organizations such as Parents Without Partners and Big Brothers/Big Sisters have local chapters
around the country. Churches and community groups may put you in

touch with other single parents; they also provide various services, such as inexpensive child care. Most working parents feel overextended from time to time, but that pressure is compounded for single parents, who often try to be two parents in one. Many experts say it is neither possible nor necessary to fill the role of the missing parent. "You cannot be everything—don't even try—just do your best," urges a never-married mother who has survived several crises involving her job and living situations. A friend, neighbor, relative, mutual-help group or even a therapist can be your sounding board. Sharing your concerns with other single parents most likely will give you peace of mind, too. For instance, if your baby is about 7 or 9 months old and gets upset every time you go away, it's natural to blame yourself or ask what's wrong; practically all children (regardless of whether they live with one or two parents) go through what's termed "separation anxiety," which is a normal and temporary stage of development.

In addition to building a secure, stable family environment and support system for yourself and your baby, another area that demands your attention is your "other life." Until a routine is fairly well established and the novelty of parenting wears off, you may not have much energy or interest in socializing with the outside world. Try to reserve time to meet your own needs. The happier you are, the happier your baby will be.

• *Your doctor.* Be up front with your obstetrician, starting with the first prenatal visit. If you sense the least bit of disapproval, don't hesitate to switch to another physician or a nurse-midwife. Every expectant mother needs solid emotional encouragement, and if you are alone, your obstetrician or midwife will play an even greater role in supporting you through these nine months.

• *Father's medical history.* If possible, get a rundown on any diseases or medical conditions that run in the father's family. That information should include his blood type and blood group. If you are a carrier of sickle-cell anemia or Tay-Sachs disease, the father should also take a carrier test to determine the chances of the disease affecting your baby.

• *Insurance coverage.* Does your policy cover your pregnancy? Unmarried women should be sure to have a special clause covering childbirth costs in their insurance plan. If you are separated from your husband, does your joint coverage still apply to you?

• *Hospital policies.* Signs saying "Husbands Only" frequently keep anyone else, including blood relatives, out of the labor and delivery rooms. Check hospital protocol well in advance. Even if your doctor allows someone other than a husband to attend the birth, the hospital may not.

• *Labor coach.* Take a friend or relative to be your partner in childbirth classes. It can be a real advantage having a mother as your coach, since she knows firsthand what you will be going through. If there is no one you feel comfortable asking, some prepared-childbirth classes provide trained labor coaches.

• *Cat owners.* Because there is always some risk that a cat carries a parasitic infection, toxoplasmosis, pregnant women are advised to stay away from their litter boxes. Perhaps a friend or some neighbors can help out, and in exchange, you can take out their garbage or do some yard work.

• *Backup transportation.* As your due date draws near, make sure you have at least two people "on call" to take you to the hospital or birth center.

• *Child support.* If you think you may sue for paternity, keep careful records of all your medical expenses and receipts for any baby clothes, diapers or equipment. Under the law, a child has the same right to financial support, whether born outside of wedlock or within a marriage. In 1973 the Supreme Court ruled that denial of support rights to "illegitimate" children was a denial of equal protection of the law. However, each state has its own statute of limitations (time limit) for establishing paternity.

• *Day care.* It may seem a long way off, but unless you can afford to take an extended leave of absence from work, start looking right away for a good child-care program that takes very young infants or line up a sitter who is experienced in caring for babies (see "Day Care, Live-Ins and Babysitters," p. 334).

• *Support system.* Perhaps the most important thing is to build a support group and be sure to let your friends help out, particularly during the more trying times of your pregnancy.

Dollars and Cents

Unlike other working mothers, whose incomes contribute to running the household, most likely your income represents the total family budget. Assuming you cannot afford not to work, child-care expenses take a sizable bite out of your salary. Here are some suggestions on stretching your hard-earned dollars:

● **Living Expenses.** Splitting the rent on an apartment or home with a friend, relative or another family offers benefits in addition to reducing monthly overhead; however, this living arrangement usually is not free of problems, as is the case with most roommates.

● **Health Care.** Family practitioners tend to be less expensive than pediatricians. Another way to shave your health bill and avoid paying as much as $20 per inoculation is to get your baby vaccinated at the local county health department. Inquire at the health department and community mental-health agency about other services and counseling. If your employer does not furnish health insurance, look into a health maintenance organization. While monthly premiums may be a bit higher than for other policies, there is usually no deductible for doctor visits or hospitalization. Parents Without Partners also offers in-hospital and excess major medical insurance.

● **Baby Equipment and Toys.** Secondhand cribs, changing tables, mobiles and the like can save you lots of money, and your baby will never know the difference. But make sure toys and furniture meet safety standards (see pp. 345 and 359). Also check with your hospital to see whether the personnel know about infant car-seat loan programs in your area, so as to avoid spending $60 or more for a brand-new one.

● **Child Support.** Most likely you will not qualify for various local, state and federal programs, such as WIC (Women, Infants and Children), which serve low-income families. Still, some government agencies may still be useful allies. Should the ex-husband, for instance, fail to meet his child-support payments, a divorced mother can enlist the IRS and other government agencies to try to collect what's due. Start by contacting the state office of child-support enforcement for help. Nonwelfare mothers sometimes have to pay a fee for the service to locate the delinquent father and make him pay. Some women find the mere threat of going to court to sue for child support is enough to convince the biological father to contribute financially; however, many single mothers don't want to have anything to do with their child's father. If you decide to establish paternity and petition for palimony or a lump-sum settlement, "be prepared for the worst," advises one mother whose case never went to trial yet who spent several thousand dollars in attorney fees. Never-married mothers may want to talk with the Legal Aid Society or the American Civil Liberties Union about palimony suits.

Information Sources

ADDITIONAL READING

The Complete Book of Child Custody, by Suzanna Ramos (New York: Putnam, 1979). Handbook of divorce, custody and single parenting.

Divorce Is a Grown-Up Problem, by Janet Sinberg (New York: Avon, 1978). Designed for preschool children; illustrated.

Going It Alone: The Family Life and Social Situation of the Single Parent, by Robert Weiss (New York: Basic Books, 1979). Positive discussion about strengths and advantages of single parenting.

Single Parent. Bimonthly magazine. To subscribe, write: Parents Without Partners, 7910 Woodmont Ave., Bethesda, MD 20014.

Single Parenting: A Practical Resource Guide, by Stephen Atlas (Englewood Cliffs, NJ: Prentice-Hall, 1981). Useful advice and encouragement to single parents.

Single Parents Are People, Too, by Carol Murdock (New York: Butterick Publishing, 1980). Discusses how to fight pangs of loneliness and feelings of inadequacy as well as offers practical pointers.

A Single Parent's Survival Guide: How to Raise the Children, by Leroy Baruth (Dubuque, IA: Kendall/Hunt, 1979). Parenting guide along with approaches for coping with misbehavior.

When You're a Single Parent, by Robert DiGiulio (St. Meinrad, IN: Abbey Press, 1979). Advice on how to enjoy being a single parent.

ORGANIZATIONS

Big Brothers and Big Sisters of America
117 S. 17th St. #1200
Philadelphia, PA 19103
Volunteers work with individual children, providing friendship and support.

Displaced Homemakers Network
755 8th St., NW
Washington, DC 20001
Women at least 35 years old can get help in finding job placement; write national office for local center nearest you.

Family Service Association of America
44 E. 23rd St.
New York, NY 10027
Programs designed to help families assist themselves.

Fatherhood Project
Bank Street College of Education
610 W. 112th St.
New York, NY 10025
New approaches for male involvement in families where mother has custody.

Parents Without Partners
Information Center
7910 Woodmont Ave.
Bethesda, MD 20014
Local chapters throughout the country aimed at never-married, separated, divorced or widowed parents; organizes support meetings and family activities. Call toll-free number for nearest chapter: (800) 638-8078. Publishes *Single Parent* magazine (see "Additional Reading") and other literature and offers in-hospital, excess major medical, disability and life insurance.

Single Parent Resource Center
3896 24th St.
San Francisco, CA 94114
Provides peer counseling and referrals.

Sisterhood of Black Single Mothers
1360 Fulton St.
Brooklyn, NY 11216
Emphasis on self-help for single black mothers.

Stepfamily Association of America
900 Welch Rd. #400
Palo Alto, CA 94304
Publishes quarterly newsletter and provides other resources.

Widow to Widow Program
58 Fenwood Rd.
Boston, MA 02115
Outreach programs to help widows.

Community organizations, including the YWCA, YMCA, local NOW chapters, as well as churches and civic groups, may put you in touch with other single parents.

MATERNITY CLOTHES:
FROM LINGERIE TO PONCHOS

You can find clothes to conceal or accentuate your expanding tummy, and if you work, exercise, disco or host black-tie dinners, fashions tailored for expectant mothers are there to be found. If you cannot find maternity leotards or an evening gown where you live, even the chic New York City maternity boutiques sell through the mail.

Of course, you can spend a fortune on maternity clothes or economize by sewing, borrowing from friends, wearing your husband's shirts and sweaters, or shopping for secondhand garments. Your lifestyle, particularly if you intend to stay with your job through the final trimester, will dictate the kind of wardrobe you'll want. Unfortunately, even if you need certain types of clothes for work, the IRS does not allow tax deductions for such business expenses.

The trick for most women is to try to buy dresses and slacks suitable for both spring and summer or fall and winter, since fuller clothes are needed for about six months, sliding from one season to another. This strategy is not always possible if the baby is due, say, around Halloween, when summer clothes are inadequate on brisk autumn days. Here are some suggested seasonal guidelines, which have to be adapted to your individual dressing habits and needs:

Fall/Winter Wardrobe	Spring/Summer Wardrobe
2 dresses	2–5 dresses
1–2 dressy dresses or evening outfits	1 dressy dress or evening outfit
2 jumpers	2–3 pairs of pants
2 pullover sweaters or tops	3–5 blouses or tops
2–3 pairs pants	2 pairs of shorts
3 blouses or tops	1–2 jumpers or sundresses
1 cardigan, jacket or shawl	1 bathing suit
1 winter coat, cape or poncho	

"Fashion mileage is the key," says Barbara Schlaks of Motherhood Maternity Boutique. Today's styles lend themselves to versatility, especially interchangeable blazers, skirts, slacks, tops and jumpers. Careful shopping for mix and match means you won't get tired of these clothes so quickly. Also think about staggering your purchases so you get a psychological boost from a few new things, particularly on those days when you are apt to feel down—sometimes depressed—about your 50-inch waist.

With a little imagination, lots of regular clothes can be worn.

Another advantage is that you might get some use out of these clothes long after your baby arrives. But keep in mind that the seams may give way around the armpits or hips, and elastic waistbands on pants and underwear may be stretched beyond repair. Some ways to supplement your "basic" maternity apparel include: tunic tops, oversized blouses and sweaters, drawstring or elastic-waist pants, kimonos, empire-waist dresses, long cardigans and shawls. Slacks and some skirts can be modified easily by sewing an elastic stretch panel in the front. The hemline is all that needs to be altered on some loose-fitting dresses. As for lingerie and other essentials:

● *Underwear.* For some women, regular bikinis are cut low enough to be comfortable throughout pregnancy, while full-size maternity panties may be a necessary expense for others. If you want something more exotic, try a G-string, which conforms comfortably to the expanding tummy. Your regular slips may be roomy enough, but remember that you run the risk of stretching the elastic and seams. If you plan to breast-feed, delay buying a couple of nursing bras until the final month, and keep the price tags on one of them in case the fit turns out not to be comfortable once your milk comes in.

● *Stockings.* Queen-size stockings are fine, but more expensive maternity support panty hose may help if you spend a lot of time on your feet. Avoid knee-high stockings or socks with tight elastic tops that restrict your blood circulation.

● *Sports clothes.* Be wary of shapeless maternity bathing suits if you are a serious swimmer. Many of these loose, sometimes strapless suits are impractical in the water. Maternity suits that cup over your belly may show off "junior" more than you'd like, but they are comfortable and definitely the new style these days. Bikinis work well for some pregnant women. Jogging suits with elastic waists may be good for racquet sports, and if you don't like the selection of tennis dresses at maternity shops, some specialty tennis stores provide custom-made maternity apparel.

Tips on Maternity Clothes

(1) Stagger your purchases so you have some new clothes at about the time that you are sick and tired of the old ones.
(2) Try to shop for maternity clothes at the start of the season, before the selection dwindles, particularly if you wear the more popular sizes.
(3) Beware of the sales pitch that certain stretch fabrics return to their original size. This may be true, but you may find these

maternity clothes either don't stretch enough during the final month or show every bump and curve of your pregnant body.

(4) Vogue, Butterick, Simplicity and McCall are a mere sampling of the maternity patterns available to you. If you don't sew, for a few dollars a seamstress at your nearby dry-cleaning store can make such alterations as putting an elastic stretch panel in a pair of slacks.

(5) Maternity clothes can be worn during the first couple of weeks after your baby is born, but chances are that you will want something fresh that will bridge the transition between your full-size and prepregnancy weights.

Your life-style and personal finances will of course determine what clothes you buy and how much you spend. While maternity clothes may seem like a waste of money, keep in mind that you probably will be wearing them for four to six months—about as much wear as some other clothes get. Another way to justify the money you spend is that they will be needed again if you plan on having more children.

Few working women are provided with special maternity uniforms, but there is a huge selection of imaginative and classic business clothes. If you cannot find what you are looking for, send away for catalogs (listed below), check the return policies and order through the mail.

Information Sources

ADDITIONAL READING

Newborn Beauty, by Wende Devlin Bates (New York: Bantam, 1981). Tips on dressing and ways to expand your existing wardrobe.

CATALOGS

Numerous mail-order catalogs are available. Take notice of such advertisements in many national women's magazines. Here is a sampling of free catalogs available on request:

Lady Madonna Boutique
36 E. 31st St.
New York, NY 10016

Mothercare-by-Mail
P.O. Box 228
Parsippany, NJ 07054

Motherhood Maternity Boutique
183 Madison Ave.
New York, NY 10016

Saks Fifth Avenue
Maternity Catalog
611 Fifth Ave.
New York, NY 10022

LOOKING GOOD: COMPLEXION, HAIR, NAILS

You are probably looking healthier and more radiant than ever before. Changes inside your body—for instance, more blood—help to give you a rosy glow. Sometimes, though, the internal activity can produce some unwanted changes on the outside. Stepped-up hormone production, increased blood volume and greater water and fat deposits can show up in a drier or oilier complexion, marks on your skin or a difference in hair and nail texture. As a result, you may have to adjust your beauty regime temporarily or begin some kind of routine for the first time.

Of course, your body's reactions to pregnancy will be different from any other woman's, but here's a brief rundown on the types of changes you might notice. With a little common sense and a few pointers from skin and beauty specialists, they are easy to control and, with the possible exception of one or two, will disappear after birth.

Complexion

Your complexion will usually take on a dewy, rosy look, but, because of hormone activity, may also turn dry and flaky in patches or oily, with acnelike spots. Keep dry skin moist with an extra-creamy lotion; keep oily skin clean and topped with a light moisturizer. If the acne is serious, seeing a dermatologist may be a good idea. Prescription topical antibiotics may be effective but should not contain any tetracycline, since it may be absorbed through your skin. A dry-ice treatment in the doctor's office to flake off the blemishes is another possibility.

Areas of darkened skin, the mask of pregnancy, may appear on your forehead, cheeks and upper lip. To help control darkening of the "tea stains," Dr. Zenona Mally, a Washington, D.C., dermatologist, advises avoiding sun exposure and wearing a #15 sun block (the strongest) whenever possible, since even fluorescent lighting can deepen the "mask." There is a good chance that it will fade away completely after pregnancy, though Dr. Mally has noticed that traces seem to remain on some mothers who return to the Pill.

Stretch Marks and Brown Patches

You may notice long, narrow pink lines on your thighs and/or abdomen. These are the result of a quick stretching of skin fibers from the rapid accumulation of water and fat. Not all women get them, and some believe that daily application of cocoa butter is essential. Others swear by a healthy dose of bath oil in the tub. A more expensive route is to buy special lotions that may cost as much as $20 for a secret mix of herbs and oil. Creams and lotions may relieve the itching sensation that accompanies stretch marks, but none will prevent them.

Brown patches may show up anywhere on your body but generally appear on wrists, hands, face and neck. Skin bleaching is a possible remedy. The U.S. Food and Drug Administration says that before marketing, over-the-counter fade creams are supposed to have been proven safe and effective but cautions against any that might contain mercury. Fade creams and skin bleaches containing mercury were banned in 1973, but to be safe, read the labels carefully.

Hair

Like your complexion, your hair may change for the better during pregnancy, although you may want to wash it more often simply because your elevated metabolic activity causes more blood than usual to circulate to the skin, making you feel hot and sweaty. The texture and body of your hair will probably follow the pattern of your skin: oilier and limp, dull and dry or just as healthy as ever. If you hair does become a problem, switching shampoo and creme rinse should do the trick, or you might treat yourself to a hair analysis at a large department store.

If your face becomes fuller, a different style or cut might be more flattering, or even a perm or change of color. So far no evidence has surfaced that the fumes or chemicals in either permanents or hair dyes are harmful to you or your baby, although it is possible that the chemicals could enter your bloodstream if there is a scratch in your scalp; many hairdressers will advise against dying hair during pregnancy.

Nails

Nails grow faster during pregnancy, but for reasons still unknown—perhaps a drain of certain vitamins and minerals—some women notice their nails are more brittle, sometimes developing deep ridges from side to side or even lifting up. You may want to treat yourself to a manicure and pedicure a couple of weeks before your due date.

Be sure to tell a dermatologist or any other doctor that you are pregnant. Don't wait for anyone to ask you, even if you think it's obvious. Your hairdresser also should be aware of what's cooking, and may tend to be more cautious about perms and hair dyes. This is an opportune time to pamper yourself, because you probably won't have such a luxury once your baby arrives!

Information Sources

ADDITIONAL READING

How to Look Good and Feel Great, by Bonnie Estridge (Secaucus, NJ: Chartwell Books, 1982).

Newborn Beauty, by Wende Delvin Bates (New York: Bantam, 1981).

The Pregnant Woman's Beauty Book, by Gloria Natale (New York: William Morrow, 1980).

A Year of Beauty and Exercise for the Pregnant Woman, by Judi McMahon (New York: Lippincott & Crowell, 1980).

For a fuller explanation of internal changes, see "Common Discomforts and Some Remedies" (p. 47) and "Other Side Effects of Pregnancy" (p. 57).

SPORTS AND FITNESS: HOW MUCH SHOULD YOU DO?

There's a modern-day belief that athletic women have an easier and faster labor. So far the evidence of the benefits of exercise during pregnancy is based primarily on anecdotal experience rather than hard data. The physically active expectant mother usually feels more relaxed with her body, and that lack of tension contributes to speedier deliveries, says one female obstetrician. Dr. Allan Ryan, editor of *The Physician and Sportsmedicine,* noted that women he observed to be in good condition saw childbirth as an invigorating experience, while those who weren't in shape said "Never again." Stamina and discipline also help women tolerate the stress of labor, which is, after all, an "athletic" event.

No one denies that physical activity increases a pregnant woman's overall cardiovascular capacity and her self-image, but many doctors worry about numerous theoretical risks to her child. A major concern is that exercise diverts the blood flow away from the womb to the working muscle. Animal studies on pregnant sheep, according to Dr. Lawrence Longo of Loma Linda University, demonstrate that moderate or heavy exercise may jeopardize the baby's oxygen supply and retard its growth in utero. Another potential risk is that physical exertion raises a mother's body temperature and, by virtue of its location, the baby is faced with the problem of heat elimination. Preliminary research on sheep indicates that the fetus is unable to dissipate heat at the point when the mother's blood needs to be diverted away from the womb to provide blood flow for the working muscle as well as to cool down her skin. To what extent the baby's metabolic and hormonal systems are affected by heavy or prolonged exercise is another unanswered question.

The medical community remains uncertain as to what and how much athletic activity is safe during pregnancy. The old school still cautions women to stick to walking and swimming. It's only natural for physicians to be conservative, because so little is known about risks to the baby. Furthermore, the schedules of most obstetricians and midwives don't allow them to exercise regularly, so they may be less interested in and informed about sports than you'd like. However, there are those who would encourage an expectant mother to continue her activities but suggest that the experienced horseback rider give up jumping or warn the professional scuba diver not to plunge more than 30 feet. If you scout around enough, you can always find a doctor who will tell you whatever you want to hear.

Should you go easy during the first trimester to avoid a miscarriage? Can you continue running through the ninth month? Any suggestions for the nonathlete? Before exploring these and other questions, let's put to rest one nagging fear: What happens in the event of a bad fall? Falling does not necessarily cause serious complications, because the fetus is in the most well-insulated part of the body—the uterine muscle and the bony pelvis—and is floating in amniotic fluid. It would take an extraordinary impact to upset a normal, securely implanted pregnancy. However, many doctors advise against vigorous physical activity until after the first trimester, when the risk of miscarriage decreases. But Dr. Donald McNellis of the government's National Institute of Child Health and Human Development claims: "The loss of early pregnancy has often been associated with prior exercise, with *no factual basis.*" Pregnancy-related complications such as high blood pressure or the placenta located near or over the cervix rather than high up in the uterus probably means it's wise to give up sports until after your baby is born. Many physicians would rule out exercise if an expectant mother is obese, is a heavy smoker, or is carrying twins, particularly during the final months, to reduce the risk of premature delivery. But, again, even if you don't fall into the high-risk category, there are many obstetricians who recommend that during the third trimester, you stop jogging and stay off the tennis court, based on the theoretical risk of premature rupture of your membranes.

If you are out of shape or essentially a nonathlete experiencing a normal pregnancy, doing stretching exercises and other conditioning drills geared specifically for mothers-to-be won't worry most physicians. Dr. Mona Shangold, head of Cornell University Medical College's Sports Gynecology Center, suggests supervised nonstrenuous body building or weight training for those not accustomed to exercise. "Ideally," says Dr. Shangold, "you should start exercising to become physically fit several years before you become pregnant, but at least a few months before you conceive." Concern that a nonathletic woman may not know what is a safe level of exertion for her or may not recognize her body's signals to stop explains why many doctors are reluctant to encourage athletic activities.

Ways to Measure Whether You're Overdoing It

Since every pregnancy is highly individual, it's impossible to say what is too much physical stress, but there is a batch of simple tests to judge whether you are pushing yourself too much. Check yourself from time to time, especially during the final months, when the demands of pregnancy leave you less energy for exercise.

(1) Pay attention to your body. If you feel wrung out, weak or faint, call it quits.

(2) Don't get out of breath. If you can carry on a conversation while exercising, probably you are not overexerting yourself, says Dr. Leon Speroff of the University of Oregon.

(3) Take your pulse when you're resting, by counting the number of pulsations during 60 seconds. Five minutes after exercising, take your pulse to make sure it is the same as the resting rate, suggests Dr. Joel Rosentsweig of Texas Women's University.

(4) Check to see that your pulse rate remains equal to 70 percent of 220 minus your age, recommends Dr. Mona Shangold. For example, a 30-year-old expectant mother should not let her pulse rate extend above 124 beats per minute.

(5) Be very cautious about competitive sports during pregnancy, because the urge to win may make you ignore or deny the symptoms that you're overdoing it, advises Dr. Donald McNellis.

Do have fun.	*Don't* play competitively unless your opponent is evenly matched to your level of skill at that time in your pregnancy.
Do rest if your normal exercise routine suddenly makes you more tired than usual.	*Don't* push yourself if you feel bad.

Do get out and breathe fresh air, stretch your legs, regardless of how lazy you feel.	*Don't* feel guilty or inadequate if you don't want to exercise, particularly when you are tired or sick during the early months and worn out during the last trimester.
Do rest if you get a muscle cramp, and if you resume exercise, use a different set of muscles.	*Don't* continue exercising if you have a stitch in your side.
Do make sure to adjust your caloric intake to meet the increased demands of physical activity.	*Don't* let yourself get dehydrated; drink plenty of fluids.
Do check your temperature after exercising, and if the thermometer registers over 101°, exercise at a slower pace and wear lighter clothing.	*Don't* get overheated or overdo.
Do enjoy the hot tub (Jacuzzi) if you like but keep it brief (see p. 6).	*Don't* take a long sauna, particularly during the first trimester (see p. 6).

The following opinions on participation in sports that range from swimming to scuba diving were the results of numerous interviews. Physicians, physiologists and individuals, including sports professionals and mothers, contributed. *These personal views are just that—they are not to be taken as recommendations.* It is essential that you consult with your doctor or midwife before embarking on a vigorous exercise program. The advice of your health-care team should be suited to your individual needs and based on your personal health history. In fact, many health clubs require pregnant women to produce written permission from their physicians before allowing them to take part in certain exercise classes and physical activities.

Dr. Donald McNellis of NICHD offers the general opinion: "Whether a particular sport is safe probably depends more upon the intensity of participation and the level of skill and conditioning of the participant than it does on the sport itself." In addition to health considerations, remain practical about your exercise regime. For example, before you sink $30 into a maternity bathing suit, think ahead about where you will swim once the summer is over. The more realistic you are, the easier it will be to follow through on staying in shape during these nine months.

Aerobics. Many exercise and dance classes are advertised as aerobic, and some pure aerobic programs, which yield respiratory and circulatory benefits, may be too strenuous. Check with the instructor about the workout and get the okay from your physician or midwife. It's a good idea to check your pulse periodically during the session. And, of course, if a particular drill doesn't feel right, pay attention to your body and sit it out.

Backpacking. Because your center of gravity will be further forward, backpacking may be easier for you now. It is wise to stay in shape during the week (weight training, walking or some other exercise) if you are planning to backpack on the weekends, because suddenly stressing your body is not a good idea. The main problem is that, as your abdomen enlarges, the use of the hip belt becomes impossible, so that all the weight must be carried on your shoulders. Day hikes may be better, but they still require sure footing.

Ballet. If you are an experienced dancer, the first thing you'll notice is the changing center of gravity. If ballet is something you think you would like to start during pregnancy, a beginner's class, which involves stretching and strong, subtle muscle control, will help get you in shape for childbirth. However, a prenatal conditioning program might be better.

Bicycling. This is great exercise, provided you don't overdo it, particularly pedaling uphill. Take time to get a sense of stability and balance. Consider readjusting the handlebars to avoid further back strain; racing bikes will prove uncomfortable (probably unworkable) toward the end of pregnancy.

Canoeing. If you are not experienced, condition yourself sensibly and stick to slow currents. Unlike flat-water canoeing, white water should be avoided unless you are an expert in fast water. One of the chief concerns is capsizing and getting hypothermia, thereby endangering the baby and yourself.

Cross-country Skiing. Cross-country skiing is essentially an aerobic sport, so you can follow the same guidelines discussed earlier, such as periodically checking your pulse rate. Also, be careful not to get overheated. Wear several layers of warm clothing and peel them off; as you cool down, put each layer back on.

Dancing. Disco to tap dancing should not pose any problems. Participation in dance depends mostly on your basic level of energy, skill and physical competence. Have fun as long as the steps or movements feel comfortable.

Downhill Skiing. The central concern about skiing is not a fall but a broken leg. This would mean being immobilized, which might increase the chance of an embolism. Some doctors advise not skiing at elevations above 10,000 feet, because of the reduced oxygen supply. One of the advantages of taking to the slopes is that your center of gravity shifts forward to compensate for the curvature of the back, which helps you lean into the skis.

Golf. Your swing may be more limited or jerky, though one mother says her protruding belly meant she stayed down with the ball and was "ten strokes better than before." The added weight of junior may mean you rely on the cart, particularly if you are not accustomed to walking the course.

Hiking. A walking stick may help balance you even on flat terrain. Weekend hiking is excellent exercise; it is sometimes suggested that jogging, swimming or some other fitness program be done during the week to ensure adequate conditioning. Remember to choose a hike that isn't too strenuous, particularly in the later months, when your stamina may be somewhat diminished.

Horseback Riding. An experienced rider can bounce around on the saddle and should not have any problem if she has a healthy, securely implanted pregnancy. Many physicians do recommend against jumping. Of course, this is not a time to break in a high-strung horse or expose yourself to situations that might cause your horse to shy or stumble.

Jogging. If you have been jogging prior to conception and are experiencing no problems during pregnancy, Dr. Kenneth Cooper, the author of *Aerobics for Women*, thinks it's fine to continue up to the sixth month. Other physicians don't bat an eye about jogging through the final trimester as long as the pace is comfortable. Your doctor or midwife should be consulted about your jogging regime. Make a point of doing a set of stretching exercises before setting out, and end each session with a cool-down period. Running is discussed separately.

Mountain or Technical Rock Climbing. Even if you are an experienced climber, your agility and skill are bound to be affected by your changing balance and decreased stamina. Falling is not only dangerous in terms of the possible distance and force with which that might happen, but also because tie-ins could limit the supply of oxygen to the baby during the time it takes for you to get back to a climbing position.

Racquet Ball and Squash. These racquet sports probably should not be played competitively during pregnancy. One problem may be finding partners to suit your game from month to month. The pace of squash may become too vigorous, and some players switch to squash doubles or tennis. An experienced player need not worry about the fast-moving ball and the chance of getting hit by her partner's racquet, but an injury is not what you need now.

Running. Experienced runners may continue running through the third trimester as long as they feel up to it, but some physicians will suggest walking and swimming instead. Dr. Kenneth Cooper recommends to his patients with normal, uncomplicated pregnancies to stop at the sixth month of pregnancy. Pay attention to your pulse and be careful not to get too overheated. Of course, this is not the time to run in shoes without excellent construction and padding, since your lower extremities need to support additional weight. As with all sports, consult your physician or midwife. To keep track of the latest developments with regard to pregnancy, watch for articles in *The Runner* magazine.

Sailing. While sailing in a large boat is comparable to taking a drive in the car, being in a small sailboat is a different story. Morning sickness may be either soothed or aggravated by the motion of a sailboat. Take care not to lose your footing on deck. And, of course, tight-fitting trapeze harnesses would be uncomfortable. Sun exposure should be protected against with tanning screens, particularly if you have a mask of pregnancy or other brown spots.

Scuba Diving. Physiologic changes such as first-trimester nausea and fatigue may impair a diver, and the wet suit will become too constricting. One survey of 200 women suggests that pregnant women limit their dives to a depth of 60 feet and to a duration one-half the limit of the U.S. Navy decompression table. How much danger decompression sickness poses for the mother and her unborn baby remains an unanswered question.

Skating. Ice skating or roller skating is a great activity, particularly if you have other children who can tag along with you. As pregnancy progresses, though, the weight of the fetus may interfere with your sense of balance. Bulky sweaters and coats may provide a bit more security in case you take a dive, but most falls don't have the force to do any harm. Because of the changing center of gravity, an experienced skater may have trouble making turns that were once easy. By the final months, the greatest ordeal may be reaching down to tie the skates.

Softball. As your stomach expands, catching ground balls, sprinting to bases and batting may be difficult. Playing softball for fun should be dandy so long as you make sure to keep an eye on the ball to avoid getting hit.

Stationary Bicycling. This is a good way to condition your legs, as long as you don't push yourself too hard or too long. Of course, there is no risk of falling, but don't let yourself get overheated. Flex your feet from time to time, to avoid getting muscle cramps. Check your pulse periodically, to help gauge if you are overexerting.

Swimming. Not only does swimming help maintain muscle tone, provide basic body conditioning and improve endurance, which all help with the stress of labor, but the weightlessness is terrific, especially when you feel like a beached whale. Swimmers should avoid challenging themselves to do another five laps if they don't feel up to it. Two precautions suggested by many physicians are not to dive, so as to avoid any unnecessary trauma to the abdomen, and not to jump into the water feet first, on the theoretical risk that a sudden surge of water up the vagina might prompt premature labor. Some doctors suggest abandoning swimming two weeks prior to your due date as insurance against infection, but numerous studies have proven that water does not enter the vagina, and any infection probably would enter via the ears or mouth. During the final month, you just need to pay attention to any body signals, especially if you notice a trickle of water down your leg after you've dried off. It's possible, although unlikely, that your bag of water broke while swimming and you didn't feel a thing. *Swimming Through Your Pregnancy,* by Jane Katz (New York: Doubleday, 1983), offers a week-by-week, trimester-to-trimester program of water-works exercises.

Tennis. Doctors disagree about whether it is risky to continue playing tennis during the last trimester, when the abdominal weight is substantial. More conservative physicians are concerned that repetitive bouncing and sudden starts and stops might conceivably cause premature rupture of the membranes; however, strong abdominal muscles most likely will provide adequate support to prevent this from happening. The other school of thought says that tennis is okay so long as your body doesn't seem to mind. Playing doubles, which are usually less strenuous, is another way to moderate your game. Other suggestions are to avoid an overhead smash, running backward for a deep lob and a serve that demands a well-arched back. Solidly built shoes with good padding are advisable to help carry the 20 or more extra pounds, and biking, body building or some other fitness program will improve your stamina and coordination on the tennis court.

Walking. Even back in the days when our mothers were told to stay home with their feet propped up, physicians recommended that they walk. Walking tones muscles and improves circulation. A brisk walk yields aerobic benefits, but even a saunter is better than nothing. The beauty of this physical-fitness regime is that it does not require a reservation for a court, finding a partner or buying special equipment, although a pair of sturdy shoes isn't a bad idea.

Water Skiing. Many doctors are not keen on this sport for expectant mothers, for fear that water may shoot up the vagina if the skiier goes down at high speeds with her legs apart. An experienced skiier who wants to continue this water sport can wear a tank suit with a wide, substantial crotch. Inexperienced skiiers probably should wait until after the baby arrives, because of the theoretical risk of repeated belly-flopping.

Weight Training. "Weight training is fine during pregnancy even if you never did it before," says Dr. Mona Shangold. Stronger back and leg muscles will help support the extra pounds acquired over the nine months, and stronger arm muscles will make it easier to carry heavier packages and, eventually, your child. Pay attention to your body and lift the amount of weight that seems like work but not too much work. . . . In other words, be careful not to overstrain.

Again, the views about these 25 exercise and sports activities are informational only, and should not be taken as recommendations to individuals.

Factors to Weigh

Exercise during pregnancy clearly carries the benefits of improving an expectant mother's overall cardiovascular capacity and of giving a healthy feeling of accomplishment. "You are priming your body and mind to meet the physical and psychological demands of labor," sums up Bonnie Berk, R.N. The drawback to pursuing prolonged or heavy physical activity is that we still lack basic information about uterine blood flow, "hot womb" and other effects of exertion on the unborn child. Expectant mothers continue to participate in research projects, and pregnant sheep keep pacing on treadmills, but conclusive answers are years away. At this point we are asking, "Is it safe to exercise?" but soon the question may be "What is the minimal amount of exercise needed to remain fit during pregnancy?" For now, common sense and moderation are about the only answers. And above all, consult with your doctor or midwife and, perhaps, an expert in sports medicine, to make sure that you are eating right, that you are not overdoing and that you and your baby show no signs of being compromised by your physical-fitness regime.

Information Sources

Research on exercise during human pregnancy is being conducted at medical centers throughout the country. These six are in the forefront:

Cornell University Medical College
Sports Gynecology Center
1300 York Ave. at 69th St.
New York, NY 10021

Department of Medicine
University of Oregon
Health Science Center
3181 S.W. Sam Jackson Park Rd.
Portland, OR 97201

Department of Ob/Gyn
Madison General Hospital
202 S. Park Ave.
Madison, WI 53715

Department of Ob/Gyn
M.S. Hershey Medical Center
Pennsylvania State College
Hershey, PA 17033

Department of Ob/Gyn
University of Vermont College of Medicine
Burlington, VT 05405

Pregnancy and Perinatology Section
National Institute of Child Health
NIH and Human Development
Bethesda, MD 20205

4

Major and Minor
Problems

WARNING SIGNS: WHEN TO BE CONCERNED

With all the odd changes taking place in your body, it is sometimes difficult to know which you can ignore and which signal a possible problem. Though you might feel like a hypochondriac, now is not the time to be a martyr about discomfort. If you experience any of the symptoms below, notify your doctor or midwife at once. Some are signs of approaching labor, but other symptoms could mean you or your baby need medical attention.

- vaginal bleeding or frequent spotting
- continuous abdominal pain not due to gas or constipation
- severe nausea or vomiting
- fainting spells
- blurred vision
- persistent headaches
- rash that doesn't subside within 24 hours
- chills or fever
- unusual or sudden swelling
- sudden weight gain
- unusual vaginal discharge
- burning sensation when you urinate
- trickle or gush of water from your vagina (this means your bag of water has broken and the seal protecting your baby from infection is no longer intact; see "Signs of Labor: True or False?" p. 213)

Don't ignore subtle muscle activity in your abdomen. If you notice painless tightening or hardening of your uterus that lasts about 30 seconds and occurs every 10 minutes or so even after you lie down for a while, call your health-care adviser. Although your uterus may just be "practicing" contractions, it is possible that you are experiencing preterm labor, which can be stopped if caught early enough.

Some expectant parents go a step further in self-care and buy a stethoscope. Babies' active and quiet times lengthen as they age, their lively periods characterized by accelerated heartbeats, according to a 1982 study published in *Obstetrics and Gynecology*. By periodically noting your own baby's movements and listening to the heart, unusual reductions in fetal heartbeat and activity can be detected early on.

If you are worried or concerned about something, don't brave it out. Pick up the phone and let your doctor or midwife decide if you need to be checked. The relief and reassurance you will probably get will be worth the call.

PROBLEM PREGNANCIES: MISCARRIAGE, ECTOPIC PREGNANCY, PREMATURE LABOR

Often worrisome symptoms such as spotting or bleeding, abdominal cramping or early uterine contractions come and go without causing any problems. Even though most pregnancies remain healthy and last for the proper 38 to 42 weeks, a sizable number are not trouble-free. Miscarriage, for instance, occurs surprisingly often, in approximately 20 percent of all known pregnancies. It is rare for a fertilized egg to grow inside a fallopian tube instead of the uterus, but such a tubal or ectopic pregnancy is life-threatening to the woman if it is not diagnosed promptly. Unlike a miscarriage and an ectopic pregnancy where there is little you can do to prevent them from happening, premature labor, if detected early, can be effectively suppressed for several weeks—even months—allowing the baby more time for development in utero. This is why it's so important to pay attention to your body's signals; by all means, call your doctor or midwife immediately if you suspect problems.

Miscarriage: Dispelling the Myths

It is natural to worry about miscarriage, particularly if you had difficulties conceiving. It is also normal to be bitter, deeply depressed and even overcome with guilt if you lose your baby, although some women feel a sense of relief. Little can be done to prevent a miscarriage from happening. Your chance of having another miscarriage is no higher than for women who have never been through the ordeal.

The medical term used is "spontaneous abortion," because it is often nature's way of telling you there was a problem with your pregnancy. Eighty-five percent of the time, miscarriages occur during the first three months of gestation, peaking at the second month, then decreasing to about 15 percent in the second trimester. If you are experiencing some bleeding in your first trimester, don't be too alarmed, but be sure to notify your doctor or midwife promptly. Less than half of these "threatened abortions" end in pregnancy loss.

In most miscarriages that occur during the first three months of pregnancy, the fetus is either genetically or anatomically abnormal. Another cause is a poor growth site in the womb; perhaps the placenta was not securely connected to the uterine wall. Some miscarriages that occur toward the end of the third month are the result of the transitional period of the embryo's support system. At this stage the corpus luteum (which is responsible for the baby's growth until the placenta takes over) shrivels up, and the transference does not always progress smoothly. Late miscarriage also can involve a less-than-ideal growth environment or be caused by hormonal imbalances or problems in the reproductive tract.

Early Miscarriage (prior to about 12 weeks)	**Late Miscarriage** (between 12 and 20 weeks)
"blighted" pregnancy due to genetic defect, virus or infection, maternal disease or possibly fetal malnutrition	structural abnormalities in mother's uterus or her cervix may be unable to support baby's weight
blood incompatibility between mother and baby	DES exposure when you were in utero is linked with reproductive-tract defects (still under study)
poor womb environment, perhaps due to immature uterine lining, faulty nesting by embryo or insufficient production of the growth hormone progesterone	infection, possibly because of IUD left in place
	hormonal problems such as thyroid-endocrine imbalance
	renal-hypertensive disease
	syphilis

The list of suspected environmental causes responsible for miscarriage continues to grow. The effects of radiation and smoking are well documented. Gas anesthetics are under investigation, with one study showing an alarming 30 percent miscarriage rate among operating-room nurses and a rate of 38 percent among anesthetists. New evidence points to a greater risk of miscarriage among wives of certain industrial workers, specifically those exposed to chemicals.

Most experts deny a cause-effect relationship between physical or psychic trauma and miscarriage. If a fetus is no longer alive, a fall or accident might trigger the miscarriage, but it is unlikely that physical injury was the cause of death. It is probably coincidental, since, in all but some late miscarriages, the fetus has died well before the miscarriage.

WARNING SIGNS AND AFTERMATH

The first sign of a possible miscarriage early in pregnancy is spotting or bleeding, usually bright red but sometimes dark brown, which may be accompanied by cramps. Usually the advice is to rest as much as possible and cut back on activities, including sex, though none of these measures is known for certain to make any difference. There is a high spontaneous cure rate for first-trimester threatened miscarriage, and the outlook is very promising if bleeding stops.

If bleeding persists and pain intensifies for more than six hours, most likely you will lose your baby. The embryo and placenta material may be expelled in what look like large blood clots. Because this can mean blood loss and possible infection, your physician or midwife will probably send you to the hospital, where you can be treated on an outpatient basis if there are no complications. If the miscarriage happens very early, all the contents of the uterus may be emptied, resulting in a "complete abortion." Later in pregnancy, in an "incomplete abortion," fragments may remain and bleeding may continue until the womb is clean or until the tissue is surgically removed by a D and C (dilation and curettage). This is often done on an outpatient basis.

A late miscarriage is more complicated, since the fully formed fetus is surrounded by a fair amount of amniotic fluid. Probably there will be a sudden gush of fluid when the bag of waters breaks, accompanied by contractions and followed by the premature birth of the fetus. Sometimes, if the body fails to expel the fetus after it dies, you may continue to carry it for a few weeks. Doctors disagree on the best medical treatment for a "missed abortion." Some believe that it is physically less dangerous to wait until you abort spontaneously than to have labor induced. Others counter that easing your emotional distress by getting it over with as soon as possible outweighs any physical risk.

Because it is important for you to know the reason for the miscarriage, try to screw up your courage and, if possible, gather up whatever your body has expelled and take it to your doctor. By examining the fetal and placental material, doctors can probably discover why you lost your baby, determine whether or not a D and C is necessary, and improve your chances for a positive outcome the next time.

Depression is a common reaction for many women. "I didn't get over it until I got pregnant again," says a mother-to-be. In addition to the mental anguish, your hormones and reproductive system are in an uproar. The time to conceive again, if you decide to, will depend on several factors. Preliminary research suggests that women who conceive soon after a miscarriage are more likely to miscarry again. This explains why some physicians advise waiting for six months, while others recommend going ahead after you have had one or two normal menstrual cycles. Equally important is waiting until you feel emotionally and physically ready.

Ectopic or Tubal Pregnancy: Outside the Womb

After conception, in a normal pregnancy, the fertilized egg travels from the ovary to plant itself in the lining of the uterus. But sometimes the egg settles elsewhere to grow, forming an ectopic (pronounced ek-top'-ik), meaning "out-of-place," pregnancy, as happens in about 1 out of approximately 200 pregnancies. Possible sites include the ovary, abdomen, cervix and, 95 percent of the time, the fallopian tube (tubal pregnancy). Since only the uterus is designed to nurture and protect a growing baby, an ectopic or tubal pregnancy is fatal for the tiny embryo and can endanger the woman's health as well.

The number of ectopic pregnancies is steadily climbing in the U.S. Researchers suggest that "fallout" from the sexual revolution of the 1960s and 1970s may be to blame, since the rate of these pregnancies, especially the tubal type, is high among women who have had more than one elective abortion or who suffer from chronic pelvic inflammatory disease, a condition often associated with gonorrhea. The higher general incidence appears to run in tandem with a wider use of IUDs, tubal-ligation procedures (which do not always prevent tubal pregnancies) and a growing number of older women with histories of ectopic pregnancies using fertility drugs. Because the fertilized egg is programmed to begin to grow after about six to seven days from conception, any condition preventing or delaying its arrival in the lining of the uterus within that critical period, such as scarred fallopian tubes or a hormonal imbalance, can result in an out-of-place pregnancy.

WARNING SIGNS AND AFTERMATH

Although it has buried itself in the wrong place, the ovum goes on to behave just as it should. But in about 8 to 12 weeks, as the embryo grows too large for its home, it must either be expelled and passed through the end of the tube or burst the tube itself. A ruptured tube leads to death for the embryo and great discomfort and internal bleeding for the mother.

The cardinal symptom of a ruptured tubal pregnancy is a stabbing or tearing pain striking suddenly and soon accompanied by other discomforts:

- *vaginal bleeding* or "spotting" that is scanty and dark in color, mixed with a "prune-juicy" fluid
- *diffuse lower abdominal pain,* either crampy and intermittent or continuous
- *abdomen tender* to the touch
- *shoulder pain* from the pressure of blood on your diaphragm.

If you have considerable internal bleeding, you may go into shock and experience hot and cold flashes, nausea, dizziness or fainting.

Your doctor can diagnose whether your pregnancy is ectopic or not by a pelvic exam, "belly check" and blood tests (low red blood count and high white count can indicate internal bleeding). An ultrasound scan can reveal whether your pregnancy is in your uterus, where it belongs (see "Sonogram: Is It Worth the Picture?" p. 73). Unfortunately, though, the symptoms of an ectopic pregnancy are easily confused with other mimicking disorders, such as appendicitis, which is responsible for about a 25 percent rate of error in diagnosis.

Surgery is the only treatment. The fallopian tube that has burst must be removed, or if it and the embryo are still intact, the tube can be "milked" of the embryo and preplacental material. Your hospital stay will be no more than ten days unless you have experienced severe internal bleeding, in which case recuperation time may be a bit longer.

Probably the thought of having an ectopic or tubal pregnancy, let alone surgery, never entered your mind. Postoperative recovery takes time, and in addition to your body healing, your hormones are being asked to shift gears abruptly to your prepregnant state. Feelings of anger, guilt and grief may get the better of you. Local childbirth-education organizations may have group sessions to provide emotional support, and you may also want to find out if there are "warm" lines available, which offer telephone counseling.

Premature Labor: Catching It in Time

Painless contractions before 37 weeks' gestation, often described as hardening or tightening of the abdomen, may signal premature labor. Such subtle muscle activity that occurs every ten minutes or so warrants an immediate call to your obstetrician or midwife. Other symptoms besides rythmic pelvic pressure include low backache, menstrual-like cramps and perhaps a vaginal mucous discharge. Contractions may either stop on their own, be suppressed by drugs or result in the birth of a premature infant.

Just why labor starts early remains unclear. Perhaps the womb has become an unhealthy home for the baby or something may be amiss with the still-mysterious mechanism responsible for giving labor its cue, making premature contractions just a matter of faulty timing. According to the University of California's Preterm Birth Prevention Program in San Francisco, likely candidates for premature delivery are expectant mothers carrying more than one child and those who have experienced previous second-trimester miscarriages or previous premature labor. Other characteristics include an age of under 18 or over 40 years, inflammation of the pelvis and kidneys, preeclampsia (toxemia), DES exposure and placenta previa, where the baby's major support organ is formed close to or over the opening of the cervix. Some research also implicates poor diet and stress as in part responsible. If you are expecting more than one child or have a history of miscarriage, the American College of Obstetricians and Gynecologists recommends the following ways to rest your pelvis and increase your chances of carrying to term:

- don't allow your bladder or bowel to become overdistended for long periods
- don't stand for a long time, as this congests pelvic organs with blood
- don't douche or have intercourse
- don't lift heavy objects or work with arms extended outward, since this puts a strain on your lower spine.

TREATMENT AND AFTERMATH

If premature labor involves rupture of the membranes, this usually leaves little choice but to deliver, because invading germs can enter the womb once the bag of water and mucous plug are gone, and infection is likely to endanger the baby. If early labor begins in a mother ill with toxemia or diabetes, contractions will be allowed to continue and the birth process is likely to be shorter and involve less pushing, since the baby is small and may slip out before the cervix is fully dilated. Because premies are especially fragile, forceps are often used to protect the soft head from the mother's bony pelvis. As extra insurance, a neonatologist and respiratory specialist will probably be standing by.

Except in cases of ill health or premature rupture of the membranes, the uterus provides the best environment for the growing baby, so the longer the fetus stays there, the better. Odds are about fifty-fifty that labor will stop on its own just with extra rest, and if it is caught early enough, those odds improve with drug treatment. Although the use of tranquilizers and sedatives might seem the first logical step, these drugs may jeopardize the unborn baby because of their depressant effect on the central nervous system. An alcohol intravenous drip was the most popular drug therapy years ago, but now medications known as tocolytic agents, which inhibit contractions by relaxing the smooth muscles of the uterus, are preferred.

Ritodrine, also known by its brand name, Yutopar, is the only tocolytic agent approved by the U.S. Food and Drug Administration for halting premature labor during or after the twentieth week of pregnancy, but other drugs may be prescribed instead. Although reports of ritodrine's success are as high as 70 percent, it is not hazard-free. The U.S. Pharmacopoeia warns: "Risk-benefit must be considered since ritodrine may cause problems with the heartbeat of the mother and fetus and it may affect the mother's blood pressure. Ritodrine may also cause intestinal blockage and it may lower the amount of sugar in the blood of the fetus." No harmful long-term effects from Yutopar have been cited, but the studies have been done only on children up to the age of two years. Drug treatment takes place in the hospital by IV drip, with continuous electronic fetal monitoring, which reports how well both you and your child respond. If all goes well, you will probably be switched to an oral dose, sent home and told to rest in bed.

If labor cannot be suppressed or if drugs cannot be given, a steroid drug may be administered to the mother to stimulate production of a substance in the lining of the baby's lungs essential to efficient breathing after birth.

Efforts to reduce the 6 to 8 percent prematurity rate are being aggressively pursued by the March of Dimes and other medical organizations around the nation. Teaching pregnant women how to recognize the subtle symptoms of preterm labor can allow them to catch it in time. In the event of delivery prior to 37 weeks' gestation, intensive-care nurseries are working wonders—now about three-quarters of all premies are growing up without serious problems. (For more information, see "Premature Babies and Other Newborns Needing Intensive Care," p. 270.)

Information Sources

ADDITIONAL READING

After a Loss in Pregnancy, by Nancy Berezin (New York: Simon & Schuster, 1982).

Coping With A Miscarriage, by Hank Pizer and Christine O'Brien Palinski (New York: Dial Press, 1980).

Facts About Premature Birth, by the U.S. Department of Health and Human Services. This booklet is available free from Office of Research Reporting, NICHD, NIH, Room 2A32, Bldg. 31, 9000 Rockville Pike, Bethesda, MD 20205.

When Pregnancy Fails, by Susan Borg and Judith Lasker (Boston: Beacon Press, 1981).

ORGANIZATIONS

Compassionate Friends
PO Box 1347
Oakbrook, IL 60521
Organization with more than 200 local chapters which offers support to bereaved parents.

Local childbirth-education organizations often have groups to provide emotional support to women and men who are trying to get over this sad, sometimes frightening experience.

There are "warm" lines, where you can call and talk to parents who have gone through the grieving process after miscarriage. In Madison, Wisconsin, for example, the Childbirth and Parent Education Association offers telephone counseling, self-help discussion groups and also refers people to professionals if they wish.

Also consult "If Your Baby Dies" (p. 275).

ANEMIA, HERPES, TOXEMIA AND OTHER COMPLICATING FACTORS

Pregnancy puts great demands on your body, and sometimes the added strain causes complications. In contrast to the miraculous product of pregnancy, the maternity cycle can aggravate such chronic health conditions as high blood pressure or cause some expectant mothers to develop hypertension or diabetes for the first time.

Regular checkups improve the odds that most problems will be diagnosed early and can be treated successfully. Don't worry about sounding like a hypochondriac when you talk to your physician or midwife, because you may well be providing clues about some "silent" infection or illness. Also be sure to volunteer any information if your husband or companion is experiencing any medical problem. This is particularly important in the case of some sexually transmitted infections, where men tend to have more visible symptoms than women.

All the health conditions discussed here put you in the high-risk category, but with careful monitoring and frequent checkups, these complicating factors can be controlled. And after all, what's most important is that you and your baby are as healthy and strong as possible.

Anemia

Taken literally, anemia means "without blood," but it is not as serious as it sounds. If you are anemic, usually it is either because you have a low number of red blood cells or not enough of the hemoglobin they contain or both. Red blood cells are vital for the hemoglobin they carry. Iron-rich hemoglobin is what gives blood cells their ruby color. It is responsible for transporting oxygen from your lungs to your tissues and carbon dioxide from the tissues to your lungs. Essentially, as a team, red blood cells and hemoglobin build up your blood and make sure your tissues are kept alive.

In the first two trimesters of pregnancy there is a rapid 25 percent increase in the number of all blood cells to supply the baby and placenta. Although the volume of blood stops expanding in the final three months, you continue to need extra hemoglobin to meet your baby's increased demands for iron before birth. Except in extreme cases, your baby will get all he or she needs, but your own reserves can dip dangerously low.

Low red blood cells and/or hemoglobin usually occur if you lack iron or have lost a good deal of blood, perhaps because of a previous miscarriage. Even if you increase your intake of iron-rich foods, most medical experts believe your body will absorb only 10 to 15 percent of them, and in pregnancy twice that amount is needed to meet stepped-up demands. If iron supplements don't do the job, your physician or midwife will look for other causes, specifically infection, folic acid deficiency, abnormal red blood cells or sickle-cell or some other inherited anemia.

SYMPTOMS AND DIAGNOSIS

Without the right number of red blood cells or amount of hemoglobin, which gives them their color, you are apt to look pale. Iron-poor blood means you will also be feeling weak and more exhausted than other pregnant women. When it is severe, anemia makes you short of breath and gives you heart flutters after exercising.

Two simple blood tests will show how much hemoglobin your red blood cells contain and the overall percentage of red blood cells in your system.

TREATMENT AND MANAGEMENT

Treatment for anemia depends on its cause. For iron-deficiency anemia, iron supplements, or higher doses of them, will probably be prescribed. If it is severe and you are close to term, you may be given an injection of iron. In cases of heavy blood loss, transfusions may be necessary, followed by iron supplements.

Blood Incompatibility

Great progress has been made in combating Rh disease since the 1940s. The Rh factor is a proteinlike substance that resides in the red blood cells of most men and women. Chances are that you are Rh-positive, but about 15 percent of the population lacks this particular protein and is Rh-negative.

The potential problem arises when an Rh-negative mother carries an Rh-positive baby; her body may react to the baby's red blood cells as it would to foreign matter. At some point—after a transfusion, an abortion or the birth of her first or second child—the mother's immune system may produce antibodies to destroy the invading Rh-positive blood cells. This action is called "sensitization," and the baby may become severely anemic.

A less serious and more common incompatibility occurs if you have type O blood and your baby has inherited type A, B or AB. ABO incompatibility occurs in 20 percent of all pregnancies, but only 1 in 30 becomes sensitized, and 95 percent of the time babies remain free of the disease.

DIAGNOSIS AND TREATMENT

The initial blood work at your first prenatal checkup will tell you if you have antibodies that would attack your baby's blood cells. The best way to counteract your system's response to incompatible Rh blood is by an injection of Rhogam, short for Rh immune globulin. As an added safeguard, many doctors are now beginning to use the injection at the twenty-eighth week of pregnancy, before much of your baby's blood has entered your circulation. The combination of giving Rhogam twice, within 72 hours of possible sensitization (that is, from a previous blood loss such as occurs after a miscarriage) and at 28 weeks' gestation, can head off nearly all expected sensitizations and all but eliminate Rh disease.

If, however, you enter your pregnancy already sensitized, your baby will probably become severely anemic. The most effective treatments so far for this are intrauterine transfusion and early delivery. If nothing is done for an Rh-sensitized mother, her baby has only about a 70 percent chance of survival. Babies affected by either Rh or ABO incompatibility are born looking slightly yellow because of too much bile pigment in their blood and tissues. This may be treated by placing the baby under "bili lights" or by an exchange transfusion. (For further discussion, see "Newborn Jaundice: Common but Rarely Serious," p. 291.)

Diabetes

If you are a diabetic or develop diabetes during pregnancy, with careful management you have about a 95 percent chance of having a perfectly normal baby. That's the good news; the bad news is frequent doctor visits, lab tests and possibly a few brief hospital stays prior to delivery, all of which may add hundreds of dollars to your medical bill.

Between 2 and 4 expectant mothers in 100 develop "gestational" diabetes because their endocrine systems fail to adapt to being pregnant. Most women's metabolisms automatically regulate the amount of insulin, which is temporarily upset by hormonal changes that cause fluctuating levels of blood sugar. Nondiabetics deal with these changes by simply releasing more or less insulin as needed, something a diabetic woman cannot do without dietary controls and, oftentimes, insulin shots.

Maintenance of normal blood-sugar levels is crucial, because extremely high or low levels may be responsible for the 2 to 4 percent of malformations found in babies of diabetic women. Tight control of one's insulin and blood-sugar levels is crucial during the first trimester, when the baby's major organs are built; however, if gestational diabetes should develop, it is likely to be during the second or third trimester, so the danger to your baby is not as great as it is for women who are diabetic from the start.

Whether the diabetes is gestational or preexisting, this disease also predisposes expectant mothers to certain complications. Sometimes the placenta may cease to supply your baby with nutrients and oxygen, but since this usually happens close to term, scheduling a cesarean birth when this occurs can protect the baby from harm. Diabetic women are also more likely to develop toxemia, a condition that is believed to be brought on by a diseased placenta. Toxemia can be controlled if spotted in time.

DIAGNOSIS AND TREATMENT

A glucose-tolerance test can diagnose whether you are diabetic or have developed the disease along the way. Usually the test involves drinking a bottle of sugar water that tastes like cola concentrate, and then, after an hour or two, a blood sample is taken to measure the amount of sugar your system has used up. If the level is high, that means the insulin in your body isn't doing its job and you may be diabetic. Some physicians automatically have pregnant women take this glucose test if they are 30 or older.

Expect frequent visits to your obstetrician interspersed with checks by your internist or diabetologist, because maintaining normal blood-sugar levels demands delicate balancing of insulin with caloric intake and output. A gestational diabetic may only need to follow strict dietary guidelines. Other diabetics, who take insulin shots, may go to the hospital for periodic tests; and a severe, or "brittle," diabetic may have to spend an occasional week or two in the hospital for even finer tune-ups. Oral diabetic medicines are not advised, since they have been shown to cause serious birth defects or other damaging effects in animals.

At 36 weeks some doctors automatically hospitalize diabetic expectant mothers, just in case the placenta should fail. As a safeguard, babies used to be delivered a month prior to the due date, but now approximately two out of three of all well-managed diabetics can have a normal vaginal birth. Cesarean deliveries are not uncommon, since many diabetics tend to have very large babies. A sudden drop in one's insulin requirement, a sudden rise in blood pressure or signs of a weak placenta are some other reasons doctors will either induce labor or perform a cesarean.

Some newborns of diabetic mothers arrive with too much or too little blood sugar, with high levels of calcium or, if born prematurely, with respiratory distress syndrome. Only about 3 percent of women who develop diabetes during their pregnancy will have the disease after childbirth.

High Blood Pressure

Among expectant mothers with a history of hypertension, about one-third have no change in blood pressure at all during pregnancy, one-third have slightly elevated blood pressure but within the normal, or "normotensive," range and the remaining one-third develop toxemia (preeclampsia). The potential danger is that constricted blood vessels may limit the blood's supply of nutrients and oxygen through the placenta to the baby. By far the greatest concern in hypertension is that it can lead to toxemia, one of the most serious complications of pregnancy.

DIAGNOSIS AND TREATMENT

Women who are older or obese or who have a history of high blood pressure in their family are predisposed to hypertension. Except in extreme cases, there are no apparent symptoms. This explains why it is so important that your blood pressure be taken at every prenatal checkup, establishing a baseline normal range against which any rise can be measured (what is high for one woman may be normal for another). If you are hypertensive upon entering pregnancy, chances are that you know it and have been dealing with it. During the first two trimesters, slightly elevated blood pressure is not cause for alarm, since it is usually after 20 weeks that most cases of toxemia develop.

The controversy surrounding treatment is partly due to the fact that it is next to impossible to predict whether hypertension will run a benign course or turn into toxemia. Some tests to monitor your baby's response may be done. (See "Postdue . . . If You're Late," p. 210). If your blood pressure takes a sudden jump but remains in the safe range, you may be told to stay home and rest. A reduced-salt diet remains controversial, but diuretics, sedatives or tranquilizers are now suspected of causing further complications and possible harm to your baby. The benefits regarding the use of anti-hypertensive medications must clearly outweigh the potential risk before these drugs are prescribed.

You may be hospitalized for observation if your blood-pressure level remains high. Pregnant women with chronic hypertension who have been taking medication should make sure to discuss the importance of continuing drug therapy in the first trimester since the benevolent nature of pregnancy normally causes a drop in blood pressure, especially during the second trimester. Following childbirth, your blood pressure usually returns to its normal level.

Toxemia

Toxemia and preeclampsia are used interchangeably to describe the disease most life-threatening to both you and your baby. Toxemia, meaning "arrow poison," continues to baffle the medical community, remaining one of the most important unanswered questions in obstetrics.

Toxemia is characterized by high blood pressure, fluid retention and protein in the urine. Other symptoms include rapid weight gain, headaches and eye problems. Any one of these alone is not cause for alarm, but occurring together, they signal preeclampsia—the forerunner of eclampsia—a condition that brings on convulsions and usually death.

Although toxemia may sound grim, if treated in time it is a completely reversible condition, causing no permanent damage to you or your baby. Women not receiving prenatal care have a high rate of developing toxemia, but your own chances are only about 2 to 3 in 100. The causes remain obscure, but researchers have been able to isolate certain factors that seem to predispose certain expectant mothers to the disease:

- a first pregnancy
- 30 years old or more
- adolescent pregnancy
- twins, triplets and so on
- diabetes
- chronic hypertension

- chronic kidney disease
- poor nutrition
- particular parasite found in mother's blood

Excessive weight gain during pregnancy used to be blamed for triggering toxemia. It is recognized now, however, that the amount of fluid—not fat—accounts for the sudden weight gain.

SYMPTOMS AND DIAGNOSIS

Three of the routine checks at each office visit are for blood pressure, weight and urine. Taken together they form key detectors of the "classic triad" of symptoms indicating the sudden onset of toxemia.

Symptoms	Probable Causes
• rise in blood pressure	• your blood vessels are constricted, so you and your baby's tissues are not getting enough oxygen
• rapid weight gain (more than two pounds a week) and edema (*some* swelling is normal)	• you are retaining more salt and fluid than usual
• protein or albumin in urine	• your kidneys are not working as they should

For your baby, preeclampsia means a serious reduction in the amount of blood flow through the placenta, slowing down vital supplies. If not diagnosed, preeclampsia could escalate to eclampsia—a disease life-threatening to both of you.

TREATMENT

If you develop a mild case of preeclampsia, your obstetrician may order plenty of bed rest (lying on your left side) at home. Some physicians suggest a restricted salt intake and the use of diuretics to force the kidneys to excrete sodium and water, although the U.S. Food and Drug Administration flatly advises against the use of water pills (diuretics) during pregnancy. Dr. Tom Brewer, author of *Metabolic Toxemia in Late Pregnancy*, argues that salt retention is not a cause of toxemia but an impending sign of sodium depletion, which causes toxemia. Brewer advocates no salt restriction, a high-protein diet and vitamin injections, but this strategy is not widely accepted.

If toxemia doesn't respond to bed rest and dietary changes, you are likely to be hospitalized so the illness can be controlled until the baby is old enough to be born. One course of action consists of sedation followed by an antihypertensive drug. A less aggressive approach includes a general hospital diet with no sodium restriction or medications, and partial bed rest.

Tests may be run such as amniocentesis, nonstress and stress tests to see how the baby is doing. If conditions worsen, amniocentesis is considered unnecessary, since delivery will be necessary regardless of the baby's maturity. There is little argument that if your health continues to deteriorate, the consequences for your baby are more serious than if he or she were to be born prematurely. In that case, doctors will perform a cesarean, or induce labor if you are very near your due date.

After childbirth your baby will return to normal; if this is your first pregnancy, your chances of toxemia in future pregnancies are no greater than any other expectant mother's.

Multiple Births

The prospect of having twins clearly has the advantage of getting two for the "price" of one pregnancy. The hitch is that you have a body designed to carry one passenger. For this reason you are put in the so-called high-risk category. The most common complications involved in carrying twins, triplets or quadruplets are:

- first trimester bleeding
- miscarriage
- premature delivery
- breech or sideways position
- difficult and/or prolonged labor
- toxemia or preeclampsia.

This explains the overall 10 to 15 percent mortality rate in multiple births. The loss rate among twins is four times that for single births, for triplets it's eight times, and for sets of four, twelve times. Your babies' chances of survival do improve, however, as you move closer to term.

The older you are and the more children you've had, the more likely you are to have multiple births. They are three times more frequent, for instance, in women 35 to 40 years old with four or more children than for a 20-year-old first-time mother. Heredity is another factor, since the structure of the reproductive system is involved. In the case of fraternal twins, the ovary has released two eggs at once instead of the usual one; these are fertilized by two sperm. More uncommon are identical twins, which are actually the result of a single ovum splitting into two separate but complete ova. Both types usually grow in their own gestational sacs, but identical twins often share the same placenta.

SYMPTOMS AND DIAGNOSIS

As you might expect, pregnancy symptoms tend to be more bother-some if you are carrying extra cargo. You may suffer more from morning sickness and such pressure symptoms as swelling and varicose veins. About 50 percent of multiple births are surprises, but the routine use of sonograms now means many twins are spotted by the second trimester. Certain signs are clues to you and your medical adviser that there may be more than one child:

- rapid growth of uterus
- unusual weight gain not due to fat or fluid retention
- two fetal heartbeats
- two discernible bodies
- mild toxemia in the last trimester.

The suspicion usually will be confirmed by having a sonogram done or, to be absolutely positive, by running a fetal electrocardiogram, which would register as many waves as there are babies.

TREATMENT

Being responsible for supplying food and fuel to more than one baby is an extra drain on your own reserves. Mothers expecting twins are more likely to be anemic and hypertensive and to carry an excessive amount of amniotic fluid. Although your weight gain will be carefully monitored, 330 extra calories over the normal daily dietary guidelines for expectant mothers is often recommended.

By far the greatest risk in multiple pregnancies is preterm birth. Twins, triplets and quadruplets are born an average of four or more weeks early, making these premies more susceptible to disease. To prevent early delivery, many doctors urge women to get off their feet for at least three hours a day. Stress, in addition to chronic fatigue, is also to be avoided, since it too is believed to increase the chance of premature labor.

Most of the risks of carrying more than one child now can be controlled. Precautions, such as monitoring a mother's diet, can be taken, thanks to the early detection of twins by sonograms and other diagnostic tests. And if the babies are born too early, remember that neonatal intensive-care nurseries across the country are working miracles.

Excess Amniotic Fluid (Hydramnios)

The volume of fluid in your baby's amniotic sac reaches a little over one liter (1000 ml) by 36 weeks, then tapers off as delivery approaches.

An amount in excess of 2000 ml is considered too much, and if it climbs to two or three liters, you will have a mild, rather common form of hydramnios. This condition appears to develop more often in diabetic mothers and in women carrying more than one child.

DIAGNOSIS AND TREATMENT

Rarely does hydramnios come on quickly. It is, instead, a gradual buildup of fluid, which may cause discomfort as the expanding uterus pushes against other organs. Your medical adviser may have trouble hearing your baby's heartbeat and find it surprisingly easy to move the baby around in your womb. A definitive diagnosis is made with a sonogram.

The type of treatment will depend on how severe the case is. Mild hydramnios usually requires only careful monitoring. If you are very uncomfortable, find it hard to move around and are short of breath, some doctors may suggest you be hospitalized in order to rest prior to birth. If there is a risk that the pressure from excess fluid may cause your membranes to rupture prematurely, amniocentesis may be performed to drain some fluid (see "Amniocentesis: Risky or Not?" p. 82).

Except in rare cases where too much fluid causes damage to the placenta and other parts of your reproductive tract, hydramnios is free of aftereffects. If it is severe, however, the prognosis for your baby is less encouraging, since there is about a 50 percent chance that, owing to birth defects, the infant will not live. Eighty percent of the babies who do survive, though, have no problems.

Infections and Viruses, Including Herpes

Many germs, unfortunately, can endanger your baby either by crossing the placenta or traveling up the birth canal. Luckily, your own antibodies may be fast enough to destroy the germs that pass through the placenta. A substance has also been identified in the amniotic fluid that some researchers theorize may protect the unborn baby from bacteria entering the vagina.

To see if you have antibodies or "footprints" of past or present infections, a TORCH test may be run on the blood sample drawn at your initial prenatal visit. It checks for:

T
O > Toxoplasmosis
R   Rubella
C   Cytomegalovirus
H   Herpes

CATS or RAW MEAT = TOXOPLASMOSIS

If you have been warned not to touch cats, it is for fear that you will catch toxoplasmosis. The bacteria present in this disease are sometimes found in cat feces and raw meat. A surprisingly high number of women of childbearing age carry the bacteria without knowing it, but when symptoms do occur they are similar to those of a cold or mononucleosis.

If the TORCH test shows you are immune to this parasitic infection, you need not worry but expectant mothers may want to take the following precautions suggested by the March of Dimes:

- Meat should be cooked to at least 150°F, and watch out for undercooked pork or lamb
- Wash your hands immediately after handling raw meat
- Infection of indoor cats can be prevented by feeding them dry or canned food, which is sterilized in processing
- Cats should not be allowed to hunt mice or come into contact with other cats that may be infected
- Cat's litter box should be emptied and disinfected daily
- Disposable gloves should be worn when cleaning the litter box, and ideally someone other than you should tend to this clean-up job.

GERMAN MEASLES

If you have never had rubella, or German measles, chances are that you have been exposed, but never caught it thanks to a natural immunity. Your antibodies prevent the germ from hosting in your cells. The TORCH test will let you know. If your rubella test is negative, you lack these antibodies and will have to be checked periodically during the next nine months to make sure you have not been exposed. Vaccines against German measles should never be given during pregnancy. Even the small amount of virus that vaccines contain can damage the tiny embryo. Of course, vaccines can be safely given to you soon after birth, provided you practice effective birth control.

SEXUALLY TRANSMITTED DISEASES

Cytomegalovirus belongs to the herpes family, but its symptoms, unlike those of herpes, vary widely according to the strain involved. Although about 5 out of 100 newborns catch cytomegalovirus from their mothers, only about 3 percent of those suffer damage. The harm is most often seen in the form mental retardation, hearing loss and disorders of the central nervous system. Experimental vaccines are being tested in the hope that our daughters will be immunized before they reach childbearing age.

Chlamydia infection, another one of the most common sexually transmitted diseases, recently has been linked with such medical problems as miscarriage, prematurity, eye infections and pneumonia in newborns who become infected during vaginal birth. The signs of this infection are frequently missed in women; however, men may have a cloudy discharge, a burning during urination and other more obvious signs. Unlike cytomegalovirus, there is no routine testing for this silent condition. Antibiotics, specifically erythromycin, can clear up the infection within a week or so.

Genital herpes is a virus transmitted either by sexual intercourse or by oral-genital contact, and turns up in approximately 1 out of every 100 pregnancies. Although the virus is rarely transmitted across the placenta, a baby can still become infected if there is more than a few hours' lag-time between the rupture of the membranes and birth or if the baby is born vaginally during an active infection.

There are two broad categories of herpes, "primary" and "recurrent." In a primary infection the symptoms usually will include a low-grade fever, back pain, headache, painful urination and the appearance of what look like small blisters on the genitals. These symptoms disappear in about 10 days, but for many people, the virus does not. Instead it retreats to live in nerve tissues until the next outbreak. For reasons still unknown, herpes and pregnancy tend to aggravate each other. Not only will symptoms be a bit more uncomfortable during pregnancy, but they may recur more frequently, particularly near the due date, which is why the baby is so susceptible.

Ointments to alleviate the symptoms of herpes flare-ups are available, but so far there is no effective treatment or vaccine to cure the virus, and the prognosis for a baby who catches herpes is not good. There are, however, some safeguards to help prevent the newborn from getting infected. If you or your partner has a history of herpes, you should be monitored closely, beginning at about the thirty-second week. Many doctors take the additional precaution of biweekly tests to detect whether the infection is active. A much faster test has been developed by the government's National Institute of Neurological and Communicative Disorders and Stroke, which probably will soon replace the current one for herpes, which takes a week and does not provide the up-to-the-minute information needed for deciding whether vaginal delivery is safe. Many physicians will recommend a cesarean so as to make sure the baby is protected from infection.

DES (Diethylstilbestrol)

If your mother took a synthetic estrogen hormone known as diethylstilbestrol (DES) while carrying you, chances are that you, along with several million other women, show some signs of being exposed to the drug. Structural differences in the uterus, cervix and vagina are common, and some evidence suggests that these alterations of the reproductive tract are responsible, at least in part, for a slightly higher rate of premature birth, miscarriage and ectopic pregnancy among DES women.

A 1981 study conducted by the "father" of DES research, Dr. Arthur Herbst of the University of Chicago, found that out of 600 pregnant women exposed and not exposed to the hormone, 27 percent of the DES group versus 16 percent of the unexposed lost their babies during pregnancy, and 5.7 percent as opposed to 0.3 percent experienced ectopic pregnancies. After further investigation and follow-up, however, a higher percentage—about 80 percent—of the DES group was found to have at least one healthy, successful pregnancy.

If you suspect your mother took DES, tell your medical adviser. During an office visit, with the aid of a colposcope, positioned outside the vagina, your physician or midwife can confirm DES exposure. Your pregnancy usually will be monitored more closely, just to make sure everything is going well. In the case of an incompetent cervix, where the neck of your uterus is not strong enough to hold the weight of the baby, an obstetrician may sew up the cervix until it is time for your baby to be born.

Urinary-Tract Infections

Some of the marvelous ways your body nurtures and protects your pregnancy can also be responsible for some not-so-pleasant side effects. As it expands, your uterus puts pressure and stress on your bladder, and increased production of progesterone dilates part of your urinary tract so that urine sits there longer before being voided. Together, these changes create the ideal climate for an infection, in the bladder and perhaps the kidneys, so that 4 to 13 percent of all pregnant women have bacteria in their urine without even knowing it.

DIAGNOSIS AND TREATMENT

The only way to diagnose symptomless infection (asymptomatic bacteriuria) is by a periodic urine test. Inflammation of your lower urinary tract, mainly your bladder (cystitis), will send signals of frequent, painful or difficult urination along with a feeling of urgency, accompanied possibly by slight tenderness above the pubic bone. Warnings that the infection has traveled to the upper tract (pyelonephritis, or kidney infection) are usually rather abrupt: sudden fever, chills, lower back pain, perhaps loss of appetite and nausea. These signs can sometimes be mistaken for appendicitis, labor, premature separation of the placenta from the uterus or, after delivery, infection of your uterus.

One way to stave off urinary tract infections is to drink plenty of fluids to keep your system flushed out. Cranberry juice is believed to be particularly effective because it helps to keep the urine acidic which is not a conducive environment for bacteria. Urinating right after intercourse is also good prevention. Another way to avoid having stale urine sitting in the urethra is "double-emptying"; in other words, once you've voided, try again, to squeeze a bit more out of the bladder. Beyond this there isn't much you can do to prevent catching an infection, but prompt treatment will keep it under control. At the least sign, contact your physician or midwife, so that a urine culture can be performed. Depending on the organism that is isolated, an appropriate antibiotic will be prescribed. Erythromycin is considered one of the safer antibiotics, with no known adverse effects on the baby. Although penicillin and its derivatives appear in amniotic fluid and fetal blood and tissue, these drugs do not appear to be dangerous to the baby; the only risk would be an undetected allergy to penicillin-based drugs. Sulfa drugs or sulfonamides are other alternatives to penicillin but are not to be used after the thirty-sixth week of pregnancy since they could cause newborn jaundice. Tetracylines are often prescribed for chronic urinary-tract infections, but they are on the definite "no" list during pregnancy since they may cause permanent discoloration of the baby's teeth and affect bone development. To avoid the potential risk of premature labor, women with recurring urinary-tract infections may be advised to take a low dose of an antibiotic on a daily basis.

Information Sources

ADDITIONAL READING

"Having Children . . . A Guide For the Diabetic Women." Advice on choosing your medical team, more details on the effects of diabetes on pregnancy and what to expect in delivery and postpartum care. Available free from Juvenile Diabetes Foundation, 23 E. 26th St., New York, NY 10010.

Having Twins, by Elizabeth Noble (Boston: Houghton Mifflin, 1980). A comprehensive book focusing on the period between conception and the first weeks of life.

ORGANIZATIONS

American Diabetes Association
2 Park Ave.
New York, NY 10016
Your local chapter of ADA can provide information about and referrals to diabetologists and to different hospitals that offer special

care for diabetics. Some chapters sponsor group discussions for diabetic mothers-to-be.

Center for Study of Multiple Births
333 E. Superior #463-5
Chicago, IL 60611
Information clearinghouse that provides pamphlets and literature.

Department DES
National Cancer Institute
Office of Cancer Communications
Building 31, Room 10A19
Bethesda, MD 20205
Information for DES mothers and daughters.

Herpes Resource Center
PO Box 100
Palo Alto, CA 94306
This service of the American Social Health Association provides the latest information about treatment and management of herpes and can tell you if there is a local self-help herpes group near you.

National DES Action
Long Island Jewish Hillside Medical Center
New Hyde Park, NY 11040
Support groups for DES mothers and daughters.

National Organization of Mothers of Twins
5402 Amberwood Ln.
Rockville, MD 20853
Nine hundred local clubs across the country. Mothers of triplets, quads or more are welcome to join.

FROM TRANSFUSIONS TO OPEN-WOMB SURGERY

The inside glimpse of life in the womb provided by ultrasound and amniocentesis has set in motion experimentation with other methods of prenatal diagnosis and treatment. The fetus is fast becoming medical science's newest and smallest patient. Some exciting developments include:

- *Intrauterine transfusion.* This treats the fetus suffering from severe anemia.
- *Urinary-tract blockage.* It can be corrected with open-womb surgery on a 21-week-old fetus.

- *Drain into brain.* This is inserted to relieve severe hydrocephalus (water on the brain).
- *Operation on kidney.* Further surgery is performed after the child is born.
- *Selective abortion.* One boy twin with Down's syndrome was aborted, brother was normal and healthy.
- *Vitamin B–complex supplements.* Taken in large doses by a pregnant woman, this treated a hereditary genetic disorder in her baby.

If you think amniocentesis is mired in controversy, consider fetal medicine, which opponents refer to as "misuse of medicine," whereas advocates call it better "preventive medicine." In addition to the ethical debate over just how far doctors should "interfere" with nature is the right-to-life implication arising from treating the unborn baby as a patient and therefore considering it as a person.

The basic premise for treating a baby in utero is that the earlier the medical intervention takes place, the greater chance there will be of escaping permanent damage. Dr. Gary Hodgen, Chief of Pregnancy Research at the National Institute for Child Health and Human Development, "anticipates a rise in the number of babies diagnosed and treated in utero in the next decade." He is careful to point out, however, that not all diagnosed fetal abnormalities will be treatable; some are better treated after birth.

Two diagnostic capabilities, fetoscopy and fetal blood sampling, are seen as forerunners of more extensive fetal therapy in the not-too-distant future. With the use of a small, telescopelike instrument inserted into the amniotic sac, this fetoscope can be used to view body formations, obtain blood and tissue or administer medications directly. Principal risks of this diagnostic and treatment method are infection in the mother and premature delivery of the fetus.

One of the oldest and safest intrauterine procedures is fetal transfusion, the injection of blood into a baby's bloodstream to overcome severe anemia brought on by Rh sensitization (for more on the Rh factor, see "Blood Incompatibility," p. 172). An alternative to a transfusion is premature delivery or, in the case of Rh incompatibility, an injection of Rhogam into the mother to prevent sensitivity.

Open-womb surgery is in some ways less complicated than treatment after birth, since the fetus not only has a built-in life support system, thanks to the umbilical cord and placenta; the postoperative period may be less risky, because the fetus is in the protective and familiar environment of the womb. After fetoscopy and other therapeutic procedures, the healing process is remarkably fast, owing to the fetus's already rapid growth.

In the more distant future, scientists may develop ways to stimulate limb growth, repair skeletal defects and transplant healthy cells or even organs in utero. These potential developments seem possible because at very early stages of growth the fetal body has not yet fully developed its immune systems. This means the fetus may tolerate some tissue or organ transplants that would otherwise be rejected after birth.

Information Sources

ORGANIZATIONS

National Institute of Child Health and Human Development, University of California/San Francisco and Yale University are recognized as pioneers in the field of fetal medicine.

National Institute for Child Health and Human Development
National Institutes of Health
Building 31, Room 2A-32
Bethesda, MD 20205
Principal financial sponsor of fetal-medicine research.

BREECH POSITION: SPECIAL HANDLING

If you are in your second trimester and your passenger is riding "head up," don't worry. Ninety percent of the time babies turn around prior to delivery. The switch from rump to head-first (vertex), partly because of increased head weight and size, is nature's way of encouraging your baby to assume the best position to enter the world.

The breech position can be either legs up, with the feet near the head, called "frank"; with one or both knees flexed, "complete"; or with feet or knees lying below the rump, "footling." No one knows exactly why, but breech occurs more frequently in cases of:

- premature delivery
- multiple births
- overrelaxed uterine muscles
- excess amniotic fluid
- placenta located over the cervix instead of higher up in the uterus
- birth defects.

Because breech babies have a death rate three times higher than those in a head-first position, a breech birth requires special handling. Normally, the baby's head has time to mold itself to the birth canal and, as the first and largest part of the body to exit, stretches the birth outlet to allow the shoulders, trunk and legs to follow easily behind. The order is reversed in a breech birth. The bottom, legs and shoulders slide out quickly, especially in small babies, leaving the larger, harder head inside. In complete, or footling, breeches, the umbilical cord may be squeezed between your body and the baby's head, pinching off the oxygen supply. This is one of the chief reasons a cesarean is performed, an alternative some doctors estimate is now chosen 75 percent of the time for breech babies. Many claim the high cesarean rate is responsible for significantly lowering the chance of injury or death among breech babies, improving their chance of survival fivefold.

But breech does not automatically mean a cesarean. Depending upon certain guidelines, you may have a choice. In its 1981 *Cesarean Childbirth* study, the government's National Institute of Child Health and Human Development recommends that a vaginal delivery, often termed "trial of labor," can be attempted if:

(1) anticipated weight of the baby is less than 8 pounds
(2) mother's pelvic size and structure are normal
(3) position is "frank" breech, meaning the baby's buttocks come first, rather than the feet or legs
(4) baby's face is not tilted up (if this were the case, vaginal delivery could injure baby's spine)
(5) the physician is skilled in the art of vaginal breech delivery (having performed "several" deliveries is not adequate experience, warn many doctors).

Other breech experts believe that as long as you're not otherwise at risk, there is little difference in safety between a vaginal or cesarean delivery, provided your baby is full-term and "frank."

Since you are put in the high-risk category, even if your physician agrees to a "trial of labor," your hospital may veto the idea, particularly if other specialists and equipment are not available, including:

- an assistant who is able to support the baby's body during delivery and/or to provide steady pressure on the baby's head to make sure the face doesn't turn up
- an anesthesiologist to give emergency general anesthesia if necessary
- a neonatologist to supply the full range of resuscitative efforts and techniques
- continuous electronic fetal monitoring.

When discussing your options, be sure to ask your medical adviser about hospital policy. If you're under an obstetrician's care, don't hesitate to find out the number of breeches he or she has delivered.

How Do You Know It's Breech?

In the last three months, you may get the idea that your baby prefers the head-up position. The baby's movements may be felt low in your abdomen, and kicks against your pelvic floor or rectum might be painful. A breech presentation usually can be detected during an office visit by feeling your belly, and confirmed by a vaginal exam and, probably, a sonogram. A definitive diagnosis comes through X-ray pelvimetry in order to measure the baby's head in proportion to your pelvis and to make sure the baby's chin is tucked down against the chest. This is a controversial test that many medical professionals agree is justifiable only for a breech (for more information, see "X-Ray Pelvimetry Warning," p. 259).

Coaxing Your Baby to Turn

What can you do to encourage your baby to turn around? The best, most well-known exercise is simply to lie down for 10 minutes on a hard surface with your pelvis, raised by pillows, 9–12 inches above your head. This drill should be done twice a day on an empty stomach. If started by about the thirtieth week of pregnancy, after three weeks the baby should be turned in time for delivery.

Another method is external manipulation, in order to rotate the baby from the outside. It carries some risk and is not done often. To be successful, the external version should be done early, and only to a very relaxed uterus. If you are a first-time mother, a drug to de-tone your uterine muscles may be necessary, carrying with it possible serious side effects for the baby. The manipulation itself is not without danger, since it could cause the placenta to separate from the wall of the womb. However, if done by a pair of experienced hands early in the third trimester, this technique can prevent the baby from being born dangerously prematurely.

Information Sources

For a complete description of the breech tilt position and other techniques to help your baby turn to vertex:

Mothering Magazine
Reprint 19-2
PO Box 2046
Albuquerque, NM 87103
A one-page explanation of exercises with photographs is available for $.75.

Obstetrical Gynecological News
Volume 12, No. 1, Jan. 1, 1977
Article, "Postural Exercise Turns Fetus in Breech Position," can be found at a university medical library.

If a cesarean breech delivery is planned, see "Cesarean: What Every Expectant Mother Should Know" (p. 260).

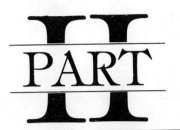

PART II

YOUR NINTH MONTH AND CHILDBIRTH

⑤

Advance

Preparation

FINAL COUNTDOWN CHECKLIST

Eight months and counting! Probably you're excited and impatient, though you may have second thoughts about becoming a parent and feel apprehensive about childbirth. Of course there is no way to predict how long labor will last and whether it will be difficult, but keep in mind what so many mothers say—any pain felt during contractions or pushing was immediately forgotten upon seeing that beautiful little baby. The sensations of childbirth are unlike anything else, and are described in "Typical Birth: Stages of Labor" (p. 215). It's also natural for you to be a bit nervous if this is your first hospital experience as an adult. If you haven't gone on a tour of your hospital, this is a good time to familiarize yourself with the physical layout and hospital policies.

During these final weeks, remember your due date is only the estimated day of delivery; best to keep friends and relatives in the dark about exactly when labor might begin. Since there is no telling if your baby will arrive early or late, it's wise to get organized well ahead of time. There's one thing you need not worry about for the time being—if you cannot choose a name in advance, you can finalize that even weeks after birth.

Questions and Answers for Your Doctor

Many mothers wish they had talked more with their doctors before-hand about labor and delivery. If you are determined to have a natural, unmedicated birth, be sure your physician knows it. The better informed you are, the more likely it is that your preferences will be respected, but don't ignore the possibility of various necessary medical procedures being done. Face up to the fact that some decisions may be taken out of your hands, on medical grounds; that is why it's in your best interest to read up on obstetrical drugs, forceps, cesareans and the like, and explore hypothetical situations with your doctor.

- Leaf through the following chapters and be sure to read about those topics you know nothing about, such as "When Is It Wise to Induce Labor?" (p. 230).
- Map out your ideal birth plan and make a list of priorities. Do you feel strongly about not being hooked up to an IV and electronic fetal monitor? Do you place great importance on the first moments with your child and want to have a Leboyer delivery?
- Discuss the feasibility and wisdom of your preferences with your medical adviser. Routine procedures may be easy to negotiate, but some decisions, such as whether or not to have an episiotomy, cannot be made beforehand. Your birth attendant may do everything possible to avoid an episiotomy, for instance, yet in the end be forced to perform one.
- Have your preferences noted on the medical chart for the hospital staff to see; this is particularly important if your personal doctor is not present when you arrive at the maternity ward.

Having done all you can to choreograph your perfect birth experience, accept the fact that it will probably not go exactly according to plan. That's why you should throw out some "what ifs" to your doctor. Scenarios you might want to work through in advance include:

- Is there a time limit on how long I can push during the second stage so long as there is no sign of fetal distress (see "Typical Birth: Stages of Labor," p. 215)?
- If I need pain relief, what drugs are commonly used by the hospital? Which regional blocks are administered, and what anesthesia is actually injected? What is known about the effects on me, my labor and my child (see "Drugs During Childbirth," p. 236)?
- If fetal distress is detected by the electronic fetal monitor, does the hospital have the capability of double-checking this diagnosis with a sample of the baby's blood (see "Electronic Fetal Monitors: Pros and Cons," p. 232)?
- If a cesarean is necessary, can my husband or companion stay

with me or does the anesthesiologist have the final word? Could I expect to have a low "bikini" abdominal incision rather than the vertical "classical cut" (see "Cesarean: What Every Expectant Mother Should Know," p. 260)?

Several checklists that run down the sequence of minor and major decisions during childbirth may enhance your prelabor dialogue with your doctor. A particularly helpful four-page pamphlet is available for $.50 from Prepared Childbirth Preference, PO Box 424, 1614 Grand Ave., North Baldwin, NY 11510.

Questions and Answers for Your Baby's Doctor

If you haven't chosen a pediatrician or family practitioner, now is a good time to select one (see "Choosing Your Baby's Doctor," p. 201). In the event that you have not selected a physician before your child is born, a doctor on the hospital staff will make the initial newborn evaluation. Sometimes these doctors expect you to bring your baby back to them for subsequent checkups, but you are in no way obligated to do so. If you plan on giving birth at home, don't delay in arranging for a physician to examine your newborn within the first 24 hours. Several questions that might be helpful to discuss now are:

- *Circumcision.* Unless you know for sure that you're going to have a girl, this decision deserves some thought. Many doctors agree with the American Academy of Pediatrics' claim that there is no convincing medical reason for this quasi-routine surgical procedure. If you opt to circumcise, you may want to explore the pros and cons of Novocain or some other local pain-killer during the five-minute procedure (see "Circumcision: Not a Medical Decision," p. 287).
- *Obstetrical drugs during labor.* Your pediatrician or family practitioner probably can help you weigh the risks and benefits to your baby of specific medications administered during childbirth. This will help you decide which anesthesia to choose should you need it.
- *Early discharge.* If you want to abbreviate your hospital stay, talk this over with your baby's doctor (see "Hospital Stay: How Soon Should You Go Home?" p. 281).

Heading Off Trouble

Here is a grab bag of suggestions to help you detect or avoid complications during the final weeks.

Preventing premature delivery prior to the thirty-seventh week. It's normal for your uterus to practice contractions as early as the twentieth week, but if you notice painless abdominal-muscle activity occurring every ten minutes, call your doctor or midwife immediately.

Flying and out-of-town travel. Get checked for any change in your cervix before you leave. The beginning of effacement and/or dilation could mean labor is imminent. If you venture away from home, be sure to take along the telephone number of your doctor or midwife as well as the name and number of a physician where you'll be. The airline may require that you obtain written permission from your obstetrical caretaker, so to avoid a last-minute snafu: Check before paying for your ticket.

Aspirin. Numerous studies have found that aspirin taken within five days of delivery can lead to excessive bleeding during childbirth and the first few days of postpartum. To be safe, stay away from it and all over-the-counter drugs that contain aspirin, such as Alka-Seltzer, especially during this final month.

Just in case... Take note of the section "Emergency Childbirth: How to Deliver Your Baby," p. 257.

Herpes and other sexually transmitted diseases. If you or your partner has herpes, a weekly vaginal exam is advisable to be sure an active infection is not present in your vagina at the time of delivery. Otherwise a cesarean may be performed, to avoid exposing your baby to it. Unlike herpes, several other sexually transmitted infections leave few clues that they are present. Often, however, men experience more visible symptoms. If your mate has any such signs, such as a burning sensation when urinating, or a mucous discharge, it's worth it to your baby's health to find out what it means. Antibiotics are effective in clearing up cytomegalovirus and chlamydia.

Mental and Physical Readiness

A few suggestions on preparing your mind and body include:

Films. Besides practicing your individual breathing and relaxation techniques, try to see a film about childbirth and also one about what it's like to be a new parent. If you are taking a Bradley, Lamaze or other childbirth-preparation class, your instructor should be able to arrange a free viewing. Otherwise, contact your local childbirth-education association, which should be listed in the telephone book.

Unspoken fears. Every expectant mother worries about whether her child will be normal. A fear that's never confronted is more terrifying than one you dare look in the face. Think through alone or, preferably, with the father how you might respond in the event that your baby is sick, is deformed or dies. Getting your unspoken fears out in the open will melt away much of the apprehension and also will lay a foundation for better communication in the unlikely event that you must deal with an upsetting or tragic situation (see "Premature Babies and Other Newborns Needing Intensive Care," p. 270, and "If Your Baby Dies," p. 275).

Prenatal breast care. La Leche League recommends that you ready your breasts for your baby's sucking by toughening up your nipples; others call this unnecessary. However, most agree that the need for preparation depends on the tenderness of your skin. One technique is to pull the nipple gently but firmly outward and roll it between the thumb and first finger, or you can rub each nipple with a dry towel.

Perineal massage. Preparing the birth outlet is suggested by many midwives and childbirth educators for those women who want to avoid episiotomies or tears during delivery. One technique is to put lubricant on your fingers and place your thumbs inside your vagina and press the perineal floor toward the rectum and to the sides. Massage not only can soften and stretch the tissues but also get you more accustomed to sensations and pressure that you'll feel during labor (see "Conditioning Exercises: What's a Kegel?" p. 68, and "Episiotomy: An Unnecessary Cut?" p. 249).

NAMING YOUR BABY

Every person reacts differently to his or her name. According to Christopher Andersen, author of *The Name Game*, "names are far more than mere identity tags. They are charged with hidden meanings and unspoken overtones that profoundly help or hinder you in your relations and your life." Many psychologists warn parents that unusual names do more harm than good; however, many children aren't bothered if they are teased about their "odd" names. Here are some questions—name checks—to help you decide.

(1) What does the name actually mean? Is there any hidden meaning, especially a slang one?
(2) Can the first name be shortened to a nickname, and, if so, do you like it?
(3) Is it one of the more popular names, and, if so, would you prefer one less frequently chosen?

(4) If the name is unusual, could it be mistaken for another word?

(5) Is the name used for either sex, and, if so, would this bother you?

(6) How does the entire name sound, and do the syllables and consonants work well together?

(7) Have you chosen a middle name or initial that may provide an alternative if your child dislikes his or her first name?

(8) Do the initials spell a word that might cause embarrassment?

(9) Have you chosen a celebrity's or public figure's name that may be a burden to your son or daughter during high school and later in life?

(10) Would you be proud if it were your name?

Take your time making this decision, and resist pressure from friends and relatives who want to decide for you. You have plenty of time to enter the full name on your child's birth certificate. If necessary, you can even change it later.

Last-Minute Checklist

Infant Car Seat. A car seat is the one piece of equipment you should be sure to rent or buy before your baby's born. Use it, awkward as it is at first, when you drive home from the hospital (see "'Car Seats, Cribs and Other Essential Equipment," p. 341).

Breast-feeding Gear. If you plan to nurse, consider buying two or three maternity bras. You can use handkerchiefs or purchase a small supply of nursing pads—you may want to experiment with different kinds. A brochure (from nursing gowns to breast pumps) is available free from Designer Series, 3015 Glendale Blvd., Suite 100 F, Los Angeles, CA 90039.

Baby Clothes and Paraphernalia. A dozen diapers, a few blankets about one yard square and several shirts are the bare essentials. Remember that you're likely to get presents after your baby arrives. A dresser drawer can serve as a bed, in a pinch (see "Baby Clothes and Supplies," p. 351).

Hospital Tour and Preadmission. A tour of the maternity floor and nurseries gives you an opportunity to question the labor- and delivery-room nurses about hospital rules. As in booking a hotel room, completing your admission form now will mean one less hassle when you arrive at the hospital once labor has begun. Pay attention to the language in any medical consent form you may be asked to sign (see "Patients' Rights and Informed consent," p. 200).

Private Hospital Room. Although your insurance plan will not cover the additional cost of a private room, the extra out-of-pocket expense may be worth it, particularly if you want your mate to spend the night with you. Of course, check first about your hospital's policy to make sure sleep-overs are allowed.

What to Pack. Here are two checklists, one for items you might want during labor and another for belongings for your hospital stay:

Labor
- talcum powder or cornstarch to reduce friction caused by massage
- Chap Stick or Vaseline for lips
- this book and your childbirth manual
- pillows to provide support for different positions (hospitals rarely have extras)
- rolling pin or tennis balls to help apply counterpressure if you experience back pain (hot water bottle also helps)
- socks in case your feet get cold
- tape recorder or radio
- camera and film
- telephone numbers of relatives and friends, along with change for the telephone

Postpartum
- nightgown and bathrobe
- slippers
- toilet articles
- hair dryer
- maternity bras if you plan to nurse
- books and magazines
- baby-name lists if you haven't decided
- eyeglasses and contact lenses
- birth announcements and address book
- blanket and other baby clothes to bring your prize home in from the hospital (avoid a bunting or papoose sack because it makes it more difficult to strap your baby in a car safety seat)

Home Birth. Necessary supplies should be collected. Be sure you've sent a map to your midwife or doctor if he or she has never been to your home (for more details, see "Home Birth: Final Arrangements," p. 204).

Food. If grocery shopping and meal planning generally fall on your shoulders, do some advance cooking and freezing for the days you'll be away or for the times when you are simply not even up to boiling an egg.

Household Help. Consider lining up a maid, relative, friend or nurse to help around the house during the first week or so, particularly if your mate cannot get away from work. If you have other children, arrange for a babysitter and/or playgroup (see "Day Care, Live-Ins and Babysitters," p. 334).

PATIENTS' RIGHTS AND INFORMED CONSENT

Presumably you have a good rapport with your doctor, so you can expect an honest dialogue about specific drugs or procedures, should the need arise during labor. Of course, the more you know, the better you can participate in any decision making, which is the primary intent of the next two chapters. Furthermore, if you feel strongly about certain issues, your preferences can be noted on your medical record for the hospital staff to see.

Probably you will not be asked to give written approval for specific medications or procedures, since informed consent means, in the words of the American College of Obstetricians and Gynecologists, "the ongoing exchange of pertinent information," unless emergency situations develop that preclude such discussion. However, should you refuse, for example, to have a cesarean even if your attending physician sees no way around it, you probably will be required to sign a nonconsent form against such medical procedures, relieving the doctor and the hospital of legal responsibilities.

Should a problem arise during childbirth, you can fall back on any of the statements spelled out next, although none of these guidelines is legally binding. If necessary, you can cite the policy statement by the American College of Obstetricians and Gynecologists, the official licensing organization, which notes:

> It is important to note the distinction between "consent" and "informed consent." Many physicians, because they do not realize there is a difference, believe they are free from liability if the patient consents to treatment. This is not true. The physician may still be liable if the patient's consent was not *informed*. In addition, the usual consent obtained by a hospital does not in any way release the physician from his legal duty to obtain an informed consent from his patient.
>
> Most courts consider that the patient is "informed" if the following information has been provided:
>
> - The processes contemplated by the physician as treatment, including whether the treatment is new or unusual.
> - The risks and hazards of the treatment.
> - The chances for recovery after treatment.
> - The necessity of the treatment.
> - The feasibility of alternative methods of treatment.

This ACOG statement should give you some leverage if you need it. The International Childbirth Education Association's "Pregnant

Patient's Bill of Rights," which is also nonbinding, pinpoints several specific questions that should be addressed:

> The Pregnant Patient has the right, prior to the administration of a drug or procedure, to be informed of the areas of uncertainty if there is *no* properly controlled follow-up research which has established the safety of the drug or procedure with regard to its direct and/or indirect effects on the physiological, mental and neurological development of the child exposed, via the mother, to the drug or procedure during pregnancy, labor, birth or lactation (this would apply to virtually all drugs and the vast majority of obstetric procedures).

Another course of action is to have your labor coach pick up the telephone and see if the hospital has a patient representative, sometimes called a patient advocate. These reps serve as intermediaries between the patient and hospital staff and try to iron out any friction or disagreement.

Information Sources

ADDITIONAL READING

"The Pregnant Patient's Bill of Rights and the Pregnant Patient's Responsibilities." This four-page report prepared by members of the International Childbirth Education Association (ICEA) is available free. Send a stamped, self-addressed envelope to ICEA, Box 1900, New York, NY 10001.

The Rights of Hospital Patients, by George J. Annas (New York: Avon Books, 1975). Discusses legal rights of patients both in emergency and nonemergency situations.

"Your Rights to Your Medical Records: Your Rights as a Hospital Patient." This report is available for $2.00 from Center for Medical Consumers, 237 Thompson St., New York, NY 10012.

CHOOSING YOUR BABY'S DOCTOR

Frequent trips to your baby's physician soon will replace your numerous prenatal appointments. The initial newborn examination, subsequent well-baby checkups and periodic immunizations make it advisable to line up a physician in advance of the baby's arrival, preferably not just a week or two before your due date.

You're bound to get the names of several doctors when you solicit recommendations from your obstetrician, friends and neighbors. Some major considerations outlined here should be evaluated in addition to your instincts and general confidence in the doctor's ability.

- *Round-the-clock availability.* Is the doctor available any hour of the day, and if he or she is out of town, who covers? Does the M.D. have a call hour on weekdays to answer questions about breast-feeding, rashes and other concerns that don't warrant an office visit? Is there a charge for telephone consultation?
- *Travel time to doctor's office and hospital.* Are the clinic, office and hospital where the doctor has admitting privileges reasonably close to where you live? Time can be critical in the event of a sudden illness or emergency.
- *Private versus group practice.* When the (solo) physician is away, is there another doctor to cover who would have access to your child's medical record? In a large group practice, can you choose the doctor you prefer or are you assigned the one who is least busy at the time?
- *Office setup.* Is the waiting room overcrowded? Is there a separate sick-child waiting area? Are lab facilities on the premises?
- *Hospital affiliation.* Are you satisfied with the reputation of the hospital(s) where the doctor has admitting privileges? Does the hospital allow you or the father to stay overnight with your child?

These questions can easily be answered over the telephone by the doctor's receptionist or nurse. Before scheduling a meeting, you may want to consider which kind of specialist you want: a pediatrician or family practitioner.

Pediatrician	Family Practitioner
Definition: Health care from birth through adolescence; some M.D.'s see children only up to 12 years of age, others through their teens.	*Definition:* Health care for entire family, with reliance on specialists such as a pediatric endocrinologist.
Training: Medical-school graduate plus 3 years' hospital-based pediatrics (or equivalent) training program; certification by American Board of Pediatrics requires passing oral and written exams; voluntary recertification.	*Training:* Medical school graduate plus 3 years' family-practice residency, which requires broad training in internal medicine, pediatrics, obstetrics, surgery and so on; recertification required every 6–7 years by American Board of Family Practice.

Pediatrician	**Family Practitioner**
Cost: Some doctors have pediatric nurse assistants on their team; these R.N.'s handle routine well-baby care, often at a lower cost than the pediatrician.	*Cost:* Fees often lower than pediatricians' but in the event your child needs to see a specialist, usually such doctor visits would cost more than pediatricians'.

For most infants, doctor visits during the first year include routine checkups and possibly diagnosis of and treatment for an ear infection or diarrhea. Both family practitioners and pediatricians are trained in well-baby care and know how to treat these common ailments. When considering a family practitioner it is wise to make sure the doctor sees a lot of very young children, not primarily adolescents. Choosing a family practitioner would mean your teenager will be less likely to switch doctors, which is sometimes a traumatic ordeal during puberty.

There are many decisions you will face hours after your baby arrives. Chapters 8, 9, and 10 discuss issues particularly relevant to that time. If you intend to schedule a meeting with a pediatrician (possibly a $25.00 fee), being prepared will enhance a two-way discussion and help you judge how much the doctor includes you in the decision-making process. In addition to the major considerations outlined earlier, the following are some questions you might want to ask the doctor:

(1) Do you have any suggestions about bonding, breast-feeding, and dimmed lights immediately after birth?
(2) Will you actually examine my baby after delivery or will some other doctor? Is it possible for both parents to be there during this newborn checkup? What's the cost? Is it covered by my insurance?
(3) What are your thoughts about circumcision? If we decide on it, how soon after birth would our baby boy be circumcised?
(4) What facilities are available in case the baby needs medical attention? Is there a newborn (neonatal) intensive-care unit in the hospital or a "baby bus" that can transfer the child to the closest one?
(5) How important is breast-feeding? How can I continue to breast-feed and resume my full-time job?
(6) What baby books can you recommend?
(7) Are infant vitamin drops necessary? I've heard that some doctors suggest them even if you breast-feed, and others claim the vitamins may interfere with the baby's ability to absorb natural vitamins contained in mother's milk.
(8) What are the charges for routine checkups? Are there standard

fees for office visits when the baby is sick? What about lab tests and shots? Which expenses will be covered by my insurance policy?

You will know if the chemistry is right after an interview. Sometimes a chat over the telephone with the doctor will give you enough confidence. If you don't feel comfortable with the doctor, neither will your child. The quality of the relationship you build during well-baby visits will stand you in good stead when and if crises occur.

Factors to Weigh

Often there is no way of knowing whether your child is okay; it is important to have a doctor who is accessible day or night and whose office is nearby. Chances are that your baby will be perfectly healthy except for ordinary growing pains or an occasional flu, which either a capable pediatrician or family practitioner can handle, but every doctor emphasizes different aspects of child care. Child care is highly individual and demands an experienced physician who is up-to-date on the latest developments in pediatrics and whose style and views match your own, so be sure to take time and shop around.

Information Sources

ADDITIONAL READING

Directory of Medical Specialists and *Fellowship List of Academy of Pediatrics.* Available at most hospital and medical libraries and some large libraries, these directories give capsule biographies about the training and experience of family practitioners and pediatricians.

HOME BIRTH: FINAL ARRANGEMENTS

The final weeks of waiting are a time of further mental preparation and practical planning. "Women who hope to deliver at home have to be very certain that this is what they want and to start arrangements for it early in pregnancies," writes Shirley Kitzinger in *Birth At Home.* Now is when you should get rid of any nagging questions by talking with your birth attendant. Speak openly about your fantasies and fears and clarify any confusion over who calls the shots in the unlikely event that problems develop during labor. This sort of dialogue will cement your agreement and partnership. Assuming you are getting pertinent information on all aspects of home birth from your midwife or physician, as well as other reading material, here is a collection of last-minute reminders you might want to consider.

(1) Collect bedding, equipment and other essential supplies about three weeks prior to your due date. Ideally, put all supplies in one place, perhaps in the bassinet or crib.

(2) Send a map of where you live to your birth attendant, particularly if he or she does not make a house visit during the last trimester.

(3) Line up a family practitioner or pediatrician to examine your newborn within 24 hours of birth.

(4) Settle the payment schedule, including any extra charges, such as an additional $150 for a "monatrice," or birth assistant.

(5) Talk with other couples who have different opinions regarding the ideal number of family members and friends to invite to the birth.

(6) Stock up on groceries so you have enough food on hand for your birth attendant and others witnessing the baby's arrival.

(7) Prepare your older child or children for the birth of a sibling (see "Older Child: Preparation for the New Arrival," p. 207).

(8) Get a copy of Gregory White's *Emergency Childbirth* or some comparable step-by-step guide if you don't have a comprehensive home-birth manual.

(9) Consider a tour and preregistration at the hospital just in case. Some midwives also suggest packing a small overnight bag. Think about filling out necessary insurance forms. (A packet of emergency backup forms plus a Bill of Rights and Birthplan Checklist is available for $3.65 from Lee Brainerd, 171 Santa Ana, Long Beach, CA 90803.)

(10) Run through backup arrangements with your birth attendant, including what local ambulance service has neonatal resuscitation equipment.

During Labor

Among the many advantages of giving birth at home is to be in your own bed. Remember that other furniture, including bean-bag chairs and rockers, may help at various stages of labor. The warmth of a shower or bath can soothe and relax you all over; in fact, it may help labor to progress. If birth at home turns out to be unadvisable, a transfer to the hospital may be a great disappointment, but it does not mean failure. As Shirley Kitzinger says, "No woman should decide that she is going to have her baby at home whatever happens. It is important to maintain flexibility and to keep the option of hospital open if needed, and impossible to know for sure in advance."

After Birth

Try to rest and stay quiet for about three hours. You might send everyone off to another room to celebrate while you and your immediate family spend some quiet time alone together. Periodic blood-pressure and temperature checks will be made, but apart from watching your vital signs, barring any problems, make an appointment for a postpartum checkup four to six weeks from now.

There are a few more reminders regarding baby care. Federal law requires that silver nitrate drops or an approved alternative ointment be put in the eyes an hour after birth. Your birth attendant will do the standard Apgar scoring (which evaluates your baby's breathing, heart rate and reflexes) at one minute and five minutes of age, but a full newborn exam should be done within the first 24 hours of life. On the third day, your child should be watched for signs of jaundice—namely, a yellowing of the skin as seen in natural light. Jaundice is normal but could become serious if color spreads below the navel, yellowing appears within the first 24 hours, yellowing shows up on the third day but does not disappear within a week or so, or the baby appears to have only a mild case but seems dopey or particularly unresponsive. Remember to schedule a follow-up well-baby visit prior to four weeks of age.

Information Sources

ORGANIZATIONS

American College of Home Obstetrics (ACHO)
c/o Dr. Gregory White
2821 Rose St.
Franklin Park, IL 60131
ACHO publishes a newsletter and provides referral service for physicians who attend home births. Dr. White wrote *Emergency Childbirth.*

The Farm
156 Drakes Ln.
Summertown, TN 38483
Midwifery journal titled *The Practicing Midwife* and other publications are available.

Home Oriented Maternity Experience (HOME)
P.O. Box 450
Germantown, MD 20874
HOME sponsors discussion groups around the country for expectant parents and publishes a newsletter and birth manual.

National Association of Parents and Professionals for Safe Alternatives in Childbirth (NAPSAC)

P.O. Box 428
Marble Hill, MO 63764
NAPSAC publishes a newsletter, books and directories relevant to couples planning a home birth.

Also refer to chapters 6 and 8, specifically "Typical Birth: Stages of Labor" (p. 215) and "Long Labor: Let the Sun Set Twice?" (p. 246).

OLDER CHILD: PREPARATION FOR THE NEW ARRIVAL

One mother tells the story of how her son "helped mommy" by brushing his baby sister's teeth . . . with a Brillo pad. To your older child, having a younger brother or sister means learning that the newest family member isn't an instant playmate, and adapting emotionally to no longer being the center of attention. No matter what you do to help your child handle the adjustment, there's bound to be some hostility, but, after all, handling jealousy is part of growing up.

Mothers expecting their second child are often troubled about the days spent at the hospital, away from the toddler. Because of fear of infection, many hospitals prohibit children under 16 from visiting parents even on the maternity floor. The current demand for family-centered births, though, has changed some policies and opened the way for siblings to see their brother or sister and, far more important, visit their mom—and sometimes in the recovery room. A handful of hospitals have gone a step further and allow an older child to witness the birth. Of course, a primary reason many parents choose an out-of-hospital delivery is to make the birth truly a family event.

There is a fair amount of planning if your son or daughter plans to be present at the birth, but first some suggestions on when to break the news about the new addition, how to make the still-invisible baby real to your child as well as ways to reduce the distress if you will be in the hospital for the better part of a week. Of course, your child's age will determine what is and is not appropriate.

- You may want to wait to break the news until the fourth or fifth month, when you begin to show, but don't delay too much longer. Otherwise, well-meaning neighbors and friends may be the ones making the announcement.
- You may want to show photographs of the developing fetus such as those in Lennart Nilsson's *A Child Is Born* or in other books geared to youngsters, which help visualize what's happening inside your tummy.
- You may want to buy a fetal stethoscope or take your child along to one prenatal checkup to hear the baby's heartbeat.

- You may want to let your child choose the baby's first gift.
- You may want to explain that you will be able to talk every day by phone while you're away at the hospital. It's also a good idea to let your child get comfortable with the sitter who will keep him or her company.
- Your husband may want to bring home instant pictures of you and the new arrival to assure the older child you're okay; you could even tape a special message on a cassette for your child.
- While in the hospital, you may want to send little things home each day along with a note, or just something from your hospital tray, such as a straw or empty medicine cup.

You probably will want to line up someone—not a stranger—to take care of your son or daughter, and to be on the safe side, get a backup sitter. A visit to grandparents may be convenient, but some children tend to feel more resentful when they return home and discover a stranger. Another option is to take advantage of sending the older child off to relatives for a few days after he or she has readjusted to your being home and at least has been introduced to the newborn.

Also check on your particular hospital's sibling-visitation policy. Owing to growing pressure from parents, more hospitals are allowing children to visit with their mothers in a lounge area and look at their new brother or sister through the nursery window. More progressive are those institutions that provide a private room, reserved for half-hour intervals, where the entire family—father, mother, sibling, grandparents—can see and touch the new addition. If the hospital has an ironclad rule of no children under 16, you may want to think about early discharge (see "Hospital Stay: How Soon Should You Go Home?" p. 281).

Additional Preparation for Birth Itself

Sensitive picture books such as *Mom and Dad and I Are Having a Baby* do an excellent job of describing to a youngster what it feels like to watch a birth. There are films, and even sibling-preparation classes, but nothing is more important than your degree of involvement in telling your daughter or son what it will be like to be with you during labor and delivery. A book recommended for parents that may help them explain the birth process is *Flight of the Stork*. Some of the other suggestions outlined next apply only to siblings who plan to witness the births.

- See a film sponsored by a local childbirth-education group or health center and explain to your child what is happening;

some parents say this is a good test run to judge how well your son or daughter responds and, equally important, how well you are able to describe what is happening.

- Have your child watch you practicing breathing and relaxation exercises so he or she gets accustomed to various positions and facial expressions; also, your child should be used to seeing you naked.
- Try "realistic" role-playing; for instance, demonstrate with your fist what it is like to push the baby out . . . it's hard work.
- See a pet giving birth if the opportunity arises. Again, talk to your child as it is happening.
- Explain certain hospital procedures, such as an IV, a shave or an episiotomy, if they apply to your situation.
- Arrange for a companion whose only job it is to look after your child and act as the child's "coach" throughout labor and delivery.
- Assemble a "quiet activity bag" that might include pipe cleaners and other knickknacks that can provide amusement in case you find your child's presence distracting or if your child wants to do something else.
- Warn your child that it isn't likely, but the chance exists that, if everything doesn't go quite right, you may stay at the hospital longer than originally expected.
- Reassure your child after the birth that you and the baby are fine.

Birth can be a frightening experience if a child is not adequately educated, which explains why many parents emphasize making sure your son or daughter is well prepared and stress choosing a companion who provides continuous attention and reassurance during labor.

Most experts say that the more your child feels he or she plays an important role as big brother or sister, the easier the adjustment will be. Don't be too afraid of physical contact between the two—newborns are remarkably sturdy, and the benefits to your first child in terms of attachment, self-esteem and confidence could be significant. Show him or her the proper way to hold the baby sister or brother, making clear it's allowed "only when Mommy or Daddy is with you." Children under about three years should never be left alone with the baby, because they may hurt it accidentally—or intentionally, out of plain jealousy. Don't be surprised if your older son or daughter starts thumb-sucking, bed-wetting or imitating the baby by asking for a bottle. Although it will be difficult at first, giving your older child your undivided attention periodically during the day, coupled with the father's actively responding to your older child's emotional needs, should help temper the rivalry. Another way of expressing your togetherness is by making your bed the family bed.

Information Sources

ADDITIONAL READING

Birth Through Children's Eyes, by Sandra Van Dam Anderson and Penny Simkin (Seattle, WA: Pennypress, 1982). Illustrated, 118-page text provides a complete discussion about children attending home birth.

A Child Is Born, by Lennart Nilsson (New York: Dell, 1975). Superb photographs of the baby in utero.

Flight of the Stork, by Ann Bernstein (New York: Dell, 1978). For parents, as an aid to understanding what young kids imagine about birth.

Mom and Dad and I Are Having a Baby, by Mary Ann Malecki (Seattle, WA: Pennypress, 1979). Picture book that describes what it feels like to watch a birth.

When the New Baby Comes, I'm Moving Out, by Martha Alexander (New York: Dutton, 1979). Cartoon book to help older children cope with their feelings toward you and the new baby.

Also see "Family Bed: Good or Bad Habit?" (p. 428).

POSTDUE...IF YOU'RE LATE

Most babies don't arrive when they are expected, and if this is your first child, you are more likely to be late than early. Yes, you are feeling frustrated, uncomfortable, tired and even angry at the thought that you will remain pregnant forever. It's not unusual to wonder if you'll have the excitement and euphoria you need to help carry you through labor; but don't worry, when contractions begin, your body calls up energy reserves to pull you through.

It is easy to forget that your due date is 40 weeks after your last menstrual period, which is the average length of gestation (give or take two weeks). In fact, you may not even be postterm, because your EDD (estimated date of delivery) may have been miscalculated. Furthermore, some embryos are late starters, making them immature for their gestational age. They simply do not get started according to the textbook, and need extra growth time in utero.

Certainly there is *less* risk with postdate babies than premature ones. If you are not having any problems yourself and all signs show that your passenger is getting along fine, there is no cause for worry. Some physicians are willing to let nature take its course and not interfere, particularly since several simple tests can be given to check on the baby's strength.

Usually, 14 days past your due date, your weekly prenatal checkups will be supplemented by a combination of tests to make sure the placenta is still functioning and your baby is in good shape. The life-supporting organ appears to have a predetermined life-span, and once it starts to go, time is limited before your baby's well-being is compromised. These tests help evaluate whether the fetus is in any danger if it is left in the womb. Other judgments play a part in the decision about whether it is safe to wait for labor to begin spontaneously. A fuller discussion is given in "When Is It Wise to Induce Labor?" (p. 230).

Estriol Levels. To make sure the placenta, the primary support system, is still functioning at 42 weeks, a simple test is usually done. Estriol is an estrogenlike hormone secreted by the placenta whose amount progressively increases as pregnancy advances. The estriol level can be measured, sometimes on a daily basis, by blood or urine specimens. A gradual or abrupt drop is interpreted as a sign that the placenta may be failing. This determination is not foolproof, and other tests are recommended to get a better profile of conditions in utero.

Nonstress Tests. The way our heart reacts to exertion tells how we will handle physiological stress. The supposition with the nonstress test is that a healthy baby's heart will speed up each time it moves in the womb. An external electronic fetal monitor is used to measure the number of fetal heartbeats per minute. For 30 minutes or so, the expectant mother indicates when she feels the baby move, by pressing a button or simply telling the doctor or nurse. If the baby is taking a nap at the time, sometimes drinking some fruit juice or changing positions will awaken it. A baby is considered "reactive" if the heart rate accelerates at least 15 beats per minute for at least 15 seconds during a period of activity, compared with the rate when the baby is still.

If the baby's heart does not react to its own movements, the test may be repeated or a doctor may recommend a stress test. The nonstress test is reasonably accurate in checking fetal well-being. And if you will be having your child at a hospital where electronic fetal monitors are routinely used, you will already be familiar with the equipment (see "Electronic Fetal Monitors: Pros and Cons," p. 232).

Stress Tests. Otherwise known as the "oxytocin challenge test," this procedure is usually more stressful to the mother-to-be because it must be done in the hospital. A mock labor is staged to find out whether the baby can adapt to the stress of being born. First, an external fetal monitor is used to determine the baseline for the baby's heart rate. Then oxytocin, a synthetic hormone that stimulates the uterus to contract, is introduced intravenously into your bloodstream until mild contractions occur three to four times within ten minutes. Your baby's heart rate is recorded to see how it responds to the "stress" of a uterine contraction. Unlike the nonstress test, where a change in fetal heart rate is a good sign, in the stress test it is not.

These predictions of the baby's ability to withstand the ordeal of labor are not always reliable, and opponents claim they often result in unnecessary cesareans.

No single measure is reliable enough by itself, so these tests are usually run in combination to cross-check the other results. There are no straightforward answers about the risks of prolonged pregnancy so long as there is no evidence of fetal distress. Many studies show the risk of waiting for labor to begin spontaneously in a truly postterm baby is higher than the potential hazard of induction or cesarean, while other research rejects the idea that an overdue baby has a special intolerance to labor.

It is more than likely that these tests will provide a reassuring profile of the placenta and the baby, and the next thing you know, you'll be feeling the first, welcome contractions.

⑥
Options
During Birth

SIGNS OF LABOR: TRUE OR FALSE?

It's not always easy to distinguish between real and false labor, even if you've given birth before. Some women dilate 5 centimeters before realizing that the premenstrual feelings and frequent tensing of the uterus were, in fact, early contractions.

If you are less than 37 weeks pregnant and notice a pattern of painless contractions or your abdomen gets hard every ten minutes or so, refer to "Premature Labor: Catching It in Time" (p. 167).

Just as many expectant mothers remain unaware that they are actually in labor, it's quite common for women to experience false labor, sometimes more than once. Each dry run is not only discouraging but emotionally and physically draining. Here are some characteristics that might help you distinguish between true and false labor:

True Contractions	False Contractions
pain centered in small of your back and extending to front of the abdomen and groin	pain concentrated in your back
contractions persist even with walking or changing positions	contractions noticeable when lying down, but walking relieves discomfort

213

True Contractions	False Contractions
contractions get stronger, occur more often and last longer	contractions may seem rhythmic but occur intermittently and don't get stronger
uterus remains hard for 30–60 seconds	uterus feels hard for 2–4 minutes

Remember that because many of the symptoms of false labor mimic the real thing, it may be necessary for you to have a vaginal exam to see where your baby's head is in relation to the bones that form the narrowest part of your pelvis (station) and to see if your cervix is thinning out (effacing) and/or dilating (dilation). For a first-time mother the signal of your baby's descent may precede effacement and dilation of your cervix. If false labor is diagnosed, you're bound to feel frustrated and possibly embarrassed, particularly if this happens after your due date.

Besides contractions, there are other signs of approaching labor, although many pregnant women will *not* experience them beforehand.

- *"Lightening."* Two to three weeks before birth, your baby may drop down into your pelvis. Breathing will seem easier, but increased pressure in the pelvic area may cause your bladder to be more impatient than ever. Lightening may not happen until labor begins.
- *"Bloody show."* As your baby pushes against the mouth of your uterus, the pressure on the cervix sometimes causes the tiny mucous plug to break loose. A small amount of mucus, tinged with blood, from the vagina is usually a sign that labor has started, but it can occur several days before anything actually happens or may not occur until labor is under way.
- *Rupture of the membranes.* A slow trickle or gush of water from your vagina indicates the amniotic sac that surrounds your baby has broken. This may occur before contractions start or not until later in labor.
- *Other signs.* These include a spurt of energy, slight weight loss, premenstrual feelings and occasional cramps.

Whether you are experiencing abdominal pain or cramps or any other signs that worry you, don't hesitate to check in with your physician or midwife. Definitely call if your water breaks or if contractions last half a minute or longer and occur ten minutes apart. Tune up for active labor by eating lightly: a few carbohydrates and liquids (Gatorade, broth, Jell-O, unsalted crackers) to prevent dehydration and provide energy.

TYPICAL BIRTH: STAGES OF LABOR

Childbirth may be the hardest work you will ever do, but it will also be one of the most exciting and memorable events of your life. Although there is no reliable way to predict how long your labor will last unless you have had a child (even then, predictions are susceptible to error), practically every woman who is prepared and educated about the physiology of labor tends to experience similar physical sensations and emotional reactions as labor progresses. An example that stands out is the final stretch, when a dozen or more intense contractions effectively force the cervix—the neck of your uterus—to open from 8 to the magic 10 centimeters. During this difficult phase, termed "transition," a laboring mother usually will not want to be touched and may be downright hostile to those around her.

Because of all the confusing terminology for the stages of labor, simply think of childbirth as a three-act play with possible variations: some women, for instance, may have contractions for hours before their bag of water breaks. The sequence of other events, such as how early in labor you go to the hospital, will depend chiefly on the recommendation of your doctor or midwife. Hospitalization prior to the onset of active labor (4 centimeters' dilation) many times promotes unnecessary intervention as care providers become anxious regarding the typical progression of normal labor.

Presumably you will arrive at the hospital during either the early or active phase of labor. A nurse will run through a list of questions including: Have your membranes ruptured? How far apart are your contractions? When did you eat last? Besides checking your blood pressure and other vital signs, an internal exam may be done to see how much your cervix is dilated. If you happen to be in the middle of a contraction, by all means ask the nurse or doctor to wait.

Depending on what you and your doctor decided or on hospital policy, you may be taken to a "prep" room or directly to a labor or birthing room, where your pubic hair will be shaved and an enema administered. Another nurse may soon arrive to put in an IV (intravenous drip), whereby a small needle is slipped into a vein in your hand or arm. This provides constant fluids and drugs, if called for. From this point until birth, most hospitals allow nothing by mouth except ice chips. Of course, every hospital and physician has its own policy.

The last part of getting set up usually includes attaching an electronic fetal monitor, which both records the pressure of your uterus during contractions and tracks your baby's heartbeat. An external monitor has belts or straps that are attached around your abdomen. If your membranes have ruptured, an internal monitor can be used, whereby a tiny electrode is attached to your baby's skin closest to the cervix. If you have qualms or questions about the routine use of a monitor or any other hospital procedures, do talk to your doctor. To learn more about prepping, equipment and other labor and delivery procedures, refer specifically to the material later in this chapter; for example, "Enema, Shave and IV: Which Ones Are for You?" (p. 222), "Episiotomy: An Unnecessary Cut?" (p. 249) or "Drugs During Childbirth" (p. 236). A birth plan outlining the individualized preferences of you and your labor coach should be discussed at about 34 to 36 weeks and updated as you become better acquainted with procedures and your wishes. If you feel adamant about certain issues, see that your doctor knows; perhaps you can have them noted on your medical record that is sent on to the hospital. It won't hurt to mention your preferences to the hospital nurses, but this is best done in a nonthreatening manner.

What follows is a blueprint for a "textbook" birth, along with specific coping tips and suggestions for your labor coach. Although you should expect to have a trouble-free birth and it's crucial to maintain a positive attitude, try to learn a little about possible complications. We don't mean to scare you, but there is a one-in-six chance that you will have a cesarean. So in addition to skimming "Cesarean: What Every Expectant Mother Should Know" (p. 260), also spend some time on other sections in the next chapter.

Act I: The First Stage of Labor

The biological guardians protecting your baby for the last nine months must now retreat. The membranes encasing the amniotic sac may break first, releasing fluid and flushing out a blood-tinged mucous plug from the cervix that isolated your baby. It's not unusual, though, for this seal sometimes to be discharged before the bag of water breaks or for contractions to start prior to both. Once labor is under way, the contractions you feel come mainly from the top outer layer of muscle in the uterus squeezing your baby down and at the same time drawing up lower uterine muscles in an effort to flatten or thin out the cervix and pull it open (effacement and dilation). The inner layer of muscles form circular bands and have been supporting your baby, keeping the cervix closed. These involuntary muscles are passive during labor.

It takes anywhere from 3 to 32 hours for the cervix to dilate to about 10 centimeters, approximately 4 inches, in diameter. The first stage has three phases: early labor, active labor and transition. Normal labor starts off slowly, then gains momentum. As you approach 8 centimeters, the last stretch, transition, stands out as the roughest yet shortest phase.

WHAT TO EXPECT

EARLY PHASE

The cervix begins to open to about 4 centimeters, roughly the width of two fingers. This is the longest phase of labor, and some women are not even aware of it. Many health professionals suggest resting comfortably at home until active labor is near; be sure to drink fluids and eat lightly to provide enough fuel for the hard work to come.

- contractions last 30–60 seconds and occur every 15–30 minutes
- menstrual-like cramps or gas-like discomfort
- feeling of warmth deep in the abdomen
- low backache
- bag of water may break, resulting in gush or slow leak (this may happen before contractions start or just prior to the second stage)
- leftover amniotic fluid may be discharged with each contraction (a clean, small, folded hand towel tucked inside your underwear will absorb this—a sanitary napkin probably won't do the job)
- mucous plug dislodged, tinged with a bit of blood
- mixed emotions, including excitement, relief, apprehension, impatience
- sociable and talkative between contractions (if early phase has not gone on too long)

ACTIVE PHASE

By now you should be at the hospital or birth center. The cervix dilates from 4 to 8 centimeters, or the width of four fingers. This phase is shorter than the previous one.

- contractions intensify, lasting 45–75 seconds, and occur every 3–5 minutes
- contractions may become painful and harder to handle
- repeated checks on baby's heart rate by stethoscope (the nurse will do this) or electronic fetal monitor
- periodic vaginal exams by doctor or nurse-midwife to check progress of dilation and baby's descent
- increasingly serious and preoccupied with labor
- occasionally doubt whether you can cope with contractions to come

TRANSITION PHASE

It takes about one hour for the cervix to expand from 8 to 10 centimeters. This is the most demanding, but relatively the shortest, part of the first stage.

- contractions every 2–3 minutes, lasting 60–90 seconds
- relaxation difficult
- "hot" pain at bottom of uterus as final tissues of cervix are pulled up over baby's head
- nauseous, may vomit as the body clears stomach prior to birth
- sleepy between contractions as uterus robs most of the blood-sugar supply
- hot and cold spells, possibly trembling
- backache worsens as baby settles into pelvis
- rectal pressure builds, but it's necessary to control the urge to push until your cervix is fully dilated (panting will help)
- loss of inhibitions (no longer modest)
- emotional reactions include panic, hostility, short temper, bewilderment

---

HYPERVENTILATION may be caused by rapid breathing when too much oxygen is inhaled and not enough carbon dioxide is exhaled. Symptoms include:

- dizziness, light-headedness
- blurred vision
- tingling sensation in hands or feet
- fainting or blacking out

If hyperventilation occurs, breathe into and out of a paper bag or cup your hands over your mouth.

Coping Tips During First Stage

(1) Eat lightly (no greasy foods) and drink fluids during early labor (there's no way of telling how long it will last, and you need food for energy and also must avoid dehydration).

(2) Rest, read and relax as much as possible between contractions.

(3) Try a warm bath or shower for relief from cramps and to help you relax (if bag of water is not broken).

(4) Consider an enema and perhaps artificial rupture of

your bag of water if you experience a prolonged first stage of labor.

(5) Move about often once contractions intensify, and change positions frequently, as it often results in spurring labor on.

(6) Urinate frequently—at least once an hour—since this helps you stay relaxed.

(7) Lie on your side and breathe slowly while rocking the pelvis gently during contractions.

(8) Experiment with different positions such as kneeling on the bed with head and arms on a pillow to relieve backache (avoid lying flat on your back).

(9) Use a hot-water bottle and counterpressure for back pain.

(10) Take one contraction at a time (don't think about how many more are coming).

(11) Control the urge to push by concentrating on breathing (puff or pant) to prevent bearing down, but don't hold your breath.

Coach's Checklist During First Stage

(1) Offer frequent verbal assurance and support throughout the first stage of labor.

(2) Help her relax, possibly give massage or back rub and apply counterpressure if backache becomes severe.

(3) Wipe her face, neck and hands with a cool, damp cloth.

(4) Offer ice chips or clear liquids every 15 minutes or more often between contractions, especially if she is not hooked up to an IV.

(5) Reiterate your preferences about specific procedures such as delayed cord cutting or waiting for an hour after birth before administering silver-nitrate eye drops.

(6) Take a break and get something to eat before the contractions intensify.

(7) Check out the ventilation in room for drafts and have an extra blanket and socks handy in the event that she gets chilled.

(8) Watch for signs of hyperventilation (see p. 218).

(9) Help by breathing with her, particularly if she has the urge to push.

(10) Stay with her even if she's hostile and does not want to be touched (if *you* need a break, be sure someone else stays with her while you are away).

(11) Provide positive guidance during transition, and remind her this phase is short and birth is near at hand.

Act II: Delivery, or the Second Stage of Labor

The hard part of coping with contractions is over. Now you get to work with them by using your stomach muscles and the forceful expulsive efforts of your uterus to help push your baby out into the world. Your cervix temporarily merges with the uterus, and your baby's way is clear to begin the journey down the birth canal. Depending on your baby's size and the resistance of your vagina, this can take anywhere from a few contractions to a few hours. After your baby's head has rotated, and inched past the bends of the birth canal—namely, your tailbone and pubic bone—the head will begin to stretch out the opening of your vagina. As the baby's body leaves your bony pelvis, the rectal pressure feels like slapping hands or a stinging sensation. Once this soft tissue of the vaginal outlet is wide enough, the head will gradually emerge; then the shoulders and body will slip out, usually from the force of a few more contractions.

WHAT TO EXPECT

- contractions last 60–90 seconds and occur every 3–5 minutes
- mixed feelings of surprise and fear caused by the pushing sensation
- backache stops as baby rotates, but if baby's face remains pointed toward the mother's abdomen ("sunny side up"), pain of back labor may increase because of the head pushing against tailbone
- urge to push down and out increases as baby gets past the birth-canal curve; similar to desire to move bowels (and it is common to expel some stool, which will precede baby's head)
- pressure in groin caused by the baby's head against your rectum and pelvic floor as baby leaves the support of the bony pelvis, which may result in a stinging, burning sensation, a feeling of being split in two
- a cut (termed episiotomy) to enlarge vaginal opening may be done
- great relief after baby is born

Coping Tips During Second Stage

(1) Wait until you feel the urge to push, and listen to your body's commands.
(2) Remind yourself it takes practice to learn how to push effectively.

(3) Rest completely between contractions.

(4) Relax thighs and pelvic floor as you push toward vaginal opening.

(5) Arrange pillows to provide a more comfortable position for pushing.

(6) Remember that every time you reinforce the work of the uterus, it brings your baby that much closer to being born.

(7) Pant to control the pushing urge if the baby is emerging too fast, to avoid tearing around the vaginal outlet.

Coach's Checklist During Second Stage

(1) Supply frequent progress reports as the baby emerges (remember, she may not be aware of how close the baby is to making its entrance—or how far away it is—the pressure of its body has numbed the skin surrounding her vagina).

(2) Remind her to take deep, full breaths and rest fully between contractions.

(3) Help support her shoulders or readjust pillows for semisitting position.

(4) Check inner thigh muscles for tension and massage to encourage relaxation.

(5) Adjust the mirror at the end of delivery table or labor bed if she wants to watch the baby being born.

(6) Offer encouragement and praise.

Act III: Finale

The strenuous work you've just accomplished leaves you shaky and cold, but leftover adrenaline and euphoria sustain your energy level. Your baby's birth soon cues the release of hormones that cause mild contractions to help your uterus shed the now-useless placenta. Once the placenta is fully detached from your uterus—which usually occurs in less than 30 minutes—it is "delivered" by slipping out the birth canal with some gentle pressure on the umbilical cord by your birth attendant. You may be encouraged to give a gentle push to aid in its expulsion from the vagina. Hormones and contractions continue their work by squeezing shut and sealing off open blood vessels the placenta has left behind. Your circulation does its part, too, by rerouting blood away from the uterus to other parts of your body. Many physicians feel that the body's natural hormonal surge needs to be supplemented by the drug pitocin which is injected or added to your IV. (For more information, refer to "Drugs During Childbirth," p. 236.)

WHAT TO EXPECT

- baby's nose and throat suctioned out, cord clamped and then cut in a matter of seconds
- baby may be given to you to hold
- baby may be breast-fed now, which helps stimulate release of hormone necessary to contract uterus, encouraging release of placenta, controlling bleeding
- local anesthetic such as Novocain (if not given prior to delivery) may be given or supplemented if episiotomy or any tears around the birth outlet need to be sewn up
- nurse performs external massage of your uterus (abdominally) and checks blood pressure, other vital signs and bleeding
- enjoy, relax, lie back and keep your son or daughter warm next to you (skin to skin if no radiant heater is available)

For more on events taking place immediately after birth, see "Eye Drops and Other Procedures Immediately After Birth" (p. 253).

Remember, the foregoing description is of a classic "textbook" labor and delivery, and, just as every pregnancy is unique, so is every birth process. Expect your baby's journey to deviate at least a bit from the norm—you might take a glance, too, at "Long Labor: Let the Sun Set Twice?" (p. 246) for an idea about what may be done in case you don't follow the average labor and delivery timetable.

ENEMA, SHAVE AND IV: WHICH ONES ARE FOR YOU?

After being admitted to the hospital, usually the next stop is the "prepping" room. The type of predelivery preparation you have often depends on hospital policy, although advance planning with your physician may allow you to forgo having an enema, shaving your pubic hair or being hooked up to an IV.

Routine prepping has come under attack on the grounds that an expectant mother suffers indignity and discomfort and, equally important, is made to feel like a sick patient. But strong arguments can be made in favor of these procedures too. An IV, for instance, prevents dehydration, and an empty bowel allows a laboring woman to push her baby out more effectively.

Enema

An enema injects fluid into your lower bowel to flush it out, making more room for your baby's journey through the birth canal and ensuring that there will be no bowel movement during delivery.

Advantages	Disadvantages
makes more room for the baby to move down the birth canal	can be dehumanizing and uncomfortable
frees you to push better during second stage of labor and eliminates fear of an "accident"	makes you feel a temporary loss of control
may help trigger stubborn labor and stimulate contractions	frightens you if contractions suddenly intensify

Claims that enemas guard against infection and contamination and tend to shorten labor have been refuted by a 1981 study published in the *British Medical Journal*. The authors concluded that enemas should only be used "for patients who have not had their bowels open in the past 24 hours and who have an obviously loaded rectum palpable at the time of initial pelvic examination."

Shave

A shave or trim of your pubic hair helps rid the area of bacteria, the argument goes, so there will be less chance of infection for you and your baby. However, many obstetricians are now reevaluating this practice in light of mounting evidence that razor nicks increase the chance of infection. Intact skin may well serve as a barrier to the entry of germs. The notion that shaving a patient does more harm than good was raised in 1982 by the government's Centers for Disease Control (CDC) in Atlanta. With regard to any surgery (in this case, cesarean), the CDC recommended *against* any razor shaving and suggested that, if there is so much hair that it interferes with delivery, shaving should be done at the time of delivery, not before.

Another reason for a shave is to avoid having hair in the way if you need a tear or episiotomy repaired after your baby is born. The counterargument is that a trim will suffice, and for most women, even this won't be necessary, because there is little or no pubic hair between the birth outlet and rectum.

From a practical point of view, the itching, as the hair grows back, can drive you crazy.

Intravenous (IV) Drip

An IV hookup consists of a hollow needle slipped into a vein in your hand or arm that allows fluid and, if necessary, drugs to drip from a bottle into your bloodstream. For the first few minutes, an IV will feel like a splinter under your skin, but soon you don't notice it.

Advantages	Disadvantages
provides energy-producing calories, essentially sugar water	limits your moving about, which may slow down labor
prevents dehydration in long labor	creates a sick-room environment
serves as a ready-and-waiting vehicle for giving pain-killers, anesthetics or labor-inducing drugs	distracts you because of fear you will dislodge it

Factors to Weigh

Prepping is often a matter of hospital policy, and many institutions are reevaluating these "old-fashioned" procedures. Check first to see what prepping entails at your hospital and how much veto power your physician has. Talk over your wishes with your doctor well before your due date, and have any special instructions included on your medical record. This is important, since your obstetrician may not arrive on the scene till much later, when labor is well on its way.

POSITIONS AND LABOR EQUIPMENT: FROM SQUATTING TO BIRTHING CHAIRS

Prior to the mid-eighteenth century, laboring women were free to assume whatever positions were most comfortable, but in 1738 that began to change, chiefly because the obstetrician to the Queen of France officially adopted the supine, or flat-on-the-back, position. Two centuries later, we are moving full circle, to rediscover some of the advantages of "natural" upright childbirth. What is commonly practiced around the world today ranges from the traditional supine position, with legs separated and raised in stirrups, to a new French style, with the mother standing but supported under her armpits. Between these two extremes are countless others, including the semiupright position in bed, with your head and back supported, lying on your side, squatting or kneeling on all fours. Sophisticated "borning" beds and ordinary bean-bag chairs offer additional support for particular positions.

It stands to reason that there are advantages and disadvantages to each one. Besides your own preference, the dynamics of labor and delivery demand changes in body position. Walking, many childbirth experts claim, is "best" during the early stage of labor, although others recommend resting in bed so as to save energy. Lying on your back or side can help you resist the urge to push before the cervix is fully dilated, yet it is next to impossible for some women to bear down during the second stage in either of these positions. Squatting can improve the effectiveness of your pushes; however, this position requires not only balance, but strong leg muscles.

Since you cannot predict what positions will be most comfortable or effective, it makes sense to move around and experiment throughout labor (although this is more easily said than done during the stretch from 8 to 10 centimeters, when the slightest movement magnifies strange and sometimes painful sensations). The chart comparing various positions is meant to be a starting point for discussion with your doctor or midwife prior to your due date. The pros and cons break down roughly into two camps, the one being physiologically better for you and your baby, the other giving both of you more efficient medical care, which is particularly important in the event of complications.

POSITION	ADVANTAGES	DISADVANTAGES
Supine, or flat on your back	allows you to rest immediately between each contraction provides best view of both abdomen and perineum for birth attendant makes it easy to keep track of baby's heartbeat with electronic fetal monitor helps you control untimely pushes, which may result in tears around birth outlet	reduces blood flow to baby because uterus is pushed against the major blood vessel, the inferior vena cava works against force of gravity to push baby out, which may necessitate medical help such as forceps increases likelihood of a tear or episiotomy, because flexed thighs tighten birth outlet, preventing gradual stretch
Left lateral, or lying on your side	allows for comfortable "sleep" position so you can catch brief catnaps reduces pressure on heart vessels and controls blood	limits view of birth works against force of gravity

POSITION	ADVANTAGES	DISADVANTAGES
	pressure during second stage of labor	restricts access to birth canal and strains your doctor's or midwife's back, but this should not influence your decision
	permits labor companion to apply counterpressure in event of severe backache	
	helps control untimely pushes during second stage and causes less tension around birth outlet, reducing likelihood of tear or episiotomy	
Upright or sitting, kneeling, squatting, etc.	may shorten labor, since body is working with gravitational pull	hinders observation and medical assistance
	ensures strong blood supply to baby because there is no pressure on lungs and heart by uterus	lessens your endurance because you may not be able to relax as frequently between contractions
	frees use of arms, chest and abdomen to help push baby out	provides no perineum support because birth attendant unable to guide baby's exit, possibly increasing likelihood of tear(s) around vaginal opening
	stretches birth canal by increasing diameter of bones of the pelvis, providing more space for baby's exit	

Fashionable birthing chairs or plain old birthing stools offer additional support for whatever positions you try. Again, your choice will largely depend on where you decide to give birth. Hospitals and birthing centers usually have setups that support particular philosophies of childbirth, but remember that some of the expensive, electronically controlled hardware such as birthing chairs are seldom used. Here's a sampler of the types of equipment, apart from the standard labor and delivery beds, in use here and abroad.

Borning or birthing bed. Found in both hospitals and maternity centers, this bed is the only piece of furniture designed to let you labor, deliver and recover in one spot. The most popular model separates into two sections: the head/chest section, angling up as far as you choose by the touch of a button, and the bottom half, either dropping into an ottoman or detaching completely, to be replaced by individual footrests, a feature that also provides quick, clear access if needed by your birth attendant.

A V shape is cut out just in front of where your hips touch, to allow space for your baby's entrance. Women like the bed because of its comfort and because it eliminates that often unspoken fear that after the final push their babies may end up on the floor! Critics of the bed argue that the soft mattress denies a woman the firmness needed to help her bear down during second-stage labor and that it requires a staff well trained in the complexities of operating all parts of the bed.

Birth stool. Before the supine position took hold in the 1700s, a stool was a standard piece of birthing equipment. Today you will see stools mainly in maternity centers, either with wide front cutouts and armrests or the plain kitchen variety, both standing not quite a foot off the ground.

Bean-bag chair. Available in many birth centers, these chairs offer firm support for your back while easily molding to whatever position you find most comfortable as labor progresses.

Tub or small plastic swimming pool. A few hospitals and some maternity centers allow a laboring woman to take a warm, relaxing bath and sometimes allow birth in the water under controlled conditions.

Birthing chair. One of the most fashionable pieces of birthing hardware, these chairs are appearing in more and more hospitals around the country. These styles and models range from primitive types, like stools with wooden backrests, in birthing centers, to space-age, fiberglass, hospital versions, costing several thousand dollars. Some hospitals use this fancy equipment to attract expectant mothers but often fail actually to use the chair. Here are some of the basic benefits and drawbacks of birthing chairs.

Advantages	Disadvantages
holds you firmly in upright position, which supports your back	may be uncomfortable (particularly models that have a rigid shell that can be adjusted only by staff); the shape may not fit all women and may cause discomfort around thighs and knees
increases oxygen-rich blood supply to your baby, since uterus is not pressing against your heart and lungs	
speeds up labor by using the force of gravity, according to some	encourages blood to pool in veins or perineum, which can cause swelling and perhaps hemorrhoids

Advantages	Disadvantages

studies, and enables mother to use more strength during the pushing phase

combines the "natural" upright position with modern medical obstetrical techniques, since it can be tilted back and angled for episiotomy repair or forceps delivery

allows mother a better view of baby as it is born

increases chance of tearing around vaginal outlet, since fixed position makes it difficult to control pushing against gravitational pull

rules out anesthetic such as an epidural regional block, since mother needs use of legs for support

makes transfer from chair to recovery bed after birth awkward

Factors to Weigh

There is growing evidence that mobility can enhance labor and delivery, and possibly speed up the entire process. Freedom of movement gives many laboring women a greater sense of control and minimizes feeling like a sick, bedridden patient. If an IV hookup and continuous electronic fetal monitoring are hospital policy where you plan to deliver, your degree of choice will probably be restricted to horizontal and semiupright positions in bed. Well in advance of your due date, check on your hospital's policy and see what you can negotiate with your doctor.

YOUR BAG OF WATER: BEST LET IT BREAK NATURALLY

Technically known as "amniotomy" (pronounced am"ne-of o-mē, cutting the amniotic sac lining) or artificial rupture of the membranes, this painless procedure simply involves reaching through your cervix to prick the amniotic sac with a small instrument resembling a crochet hook, releasing the fluid inside.

Because the breaking of the bag of water is known to bring on labor or speed up contractions, artificial rupture often serves as the first step to induce labor. Or if your obstetrician or midwife suspects your baby may be in distress, by puncturing the amniotic sac he or she is able to:

- detect any blood or traces of your baby's first stools (the latter may mean the anal muscle-ring is overrelaxed, owing to poor oxygen supply)
- attach an internal fetal monitor to track your baby's heart rate, along with a tiny catheter to measure the intensity of your contractions.

Since contractions after rupture of the membranes appear to become stronger and more efficient, some birth attendants routinely perform amniotomies even on women in normal, early labor just to speed things along. Others, including Dr. Ricardo Schwarcz, a perinatology expert with the World Health Organization, believe that nature knows best if the fluid surrounding your baby is more a hindrance than a help. The results of his comparative study of 1400 women concluded that amniotomy disturbs the important "physiological timing of the spontaneous rupture of the membranes." In his control group, the bag of water broke on its own accord for about one-third of the expectant mothers between 4 and 9 centimeters, at 10 centimeters—complete dilation—for another third, during the second stage of labor for 20 percent and at delivery for 13 percent.

The degree of risk, then, seems to center on timing, and since the membranes rupture naturally for the majority of women as they widen to 10 centimeters, the wisdom of breaking the bag of water artificially too much earlier is questionable. Artificial rupture before active labor, warns one obstetrical textbook, is "an irrevocable step—a Rubicon that, once crossed, commits the obstetrician to delivery."

Since the amniotic fluid serves as a safety measure, unless there are signs of fetal distress, removing your baby's cushion of water early in the process exposes you both to unnecessary hazards:

- your baby must bear up under the hard squeeze of contractions for a longer time without the protection of a fluid buffer
- the umbilical cord may slip into the opening of the cervix ahead of your baby (prolapsed cord) and pinch off the oxygen supply, a life-threatening situation that probably necessitates an emergency cesarean
- your baby may turn around into a less favorable position for birth
- germs from your vagina now have free entry into the womb, risking infection for you both, especially if active labor does not begin for several (six) hours after rupture.

Factors to Weigh

Barring medical indications that call for induction, the need for an internal electronic fetal monitor or the inspection of the amniotic fluid, artificial rupture of your membranes is optional. You have a right to say when and if an amniotomy is performed. To avoid a possible confrontation at the hospital, ask your obstetrician or midwife beforehand if amniotomy would be necessary so long as labor is progressing normally.

WHEN IS IT WISE TO INDUCE LABOR?

If there is reason to believe that your body is no longer the optimum environment for your baby, your medical adviser may not want to wait for labor to begin spontaneously. Prolonged pregnancy past 42 weeks ranks alongside preeclampsia, otherwise termed toxemia, as the common reasons for induction. Probably you will also be confronted with this decision if labor does not follow within 24 hours of ruptured membranes. Methods vary greatly on just how to induce labor. One physician might break your bag of water first, while a midwife might suggest herbal blue cohosh tea. Other catalysts include an intravenous (IV) oxytocin drip or another synthetic hormone called prostaglandin, available in tablet, gel or suppository form. One or all of these could be used, the sequence depending on your obstetrical caretaker's preference or the need for speed.

Before evaluating whether or not induction is a wise strategy, you need to know its possible risks:

- *Premature birth.* If your due date was incorrect, your baby may require intensive care if the lungs are not yet mature.
- *Infection.* Artificial rupture of the membranes breaks the protective seal that guards your uterus and your unborn baby from germs.
- *Fetal distress.* Long contractions with short rest periods leave less time for the baby to "catch his breath," which may lead to oxygen deprivation and consequent brain damage.
- *Cesarean birth.* If induction is not successful or there is evidence of fetal distress, surgery may be the only option left.
- *Vicious cycle.* Abrupt, intense, lengthy contractions may necessitate medication for pain relief, which in turn may slow labor, requiring more drugs to renew rhythmic uterine contractions.

For more on the risks of labor-inducing drugs and artificial rupture of the membranes, see "Drugs During Childbirth" (p. 236) and "Your Bag of Water: Best Let It Break Naturally" (p. 228).

Because every pregnancy and medical condition must be evaluated on an individual basis, often the choice is not clear-cut. Preeclampsia, for example, may necessitate immediate early delivery in one woman, while in another, induction would be ill-advised. The final decision in other than urgent cases should be a joint one, reached through discussion with your doctor. Going over the pros and cons is especially important in the gray area of postdue. Many studies show the risk of waiting for labor to begin spontaneously in a postterm baby is higher than the potential hazard of induction or cesarean, while other research points to the number of supposedly "overdue" babies whose births were induced prematurely.

In borderline cases, obstetricians often try to predict how well you would respond to induction by what is known as Bishop Scoring. Points are assigned to the condition of your cervix (soft or ripe, length and dilation), the baby's position and how far he or she is engaged in your pelvis. In addition to your readiness score, other tests probably will be run to judge whether it is best for your baby to depart from its home with some prompting from the outside.

- *Nonstress test.* An external electronic fetal monitor measures the number of heartbeats per minute to test whether the baby's heart speeds up each time it stirs in the womb (see "Post-due . . . If You're Late," p. 210).
- *Stress or oxytocin challenge test.* A mock labor is staged by giving small doses of a synthetic hormone to stimulate the uterus to contract; an electronic external fetal monitor records the baby's heartbeat to see how it responds to the stress of labor.
- *Sonogram or ultrasound scan.* This assesses whether pregnancy is at term by taking measurements of the baby, although third-trimester dimensions can be flawed, because of variations in growth rate during the final phase of development in utero.
- *Placenta's health.* A simple blood or urine test provides estriol level and other measurements to judge whether the placenta, the baby's major support organ, is no longer functioning at full strength.
- *Amniocentesis.* This is performed primarily to determine the maturity of the baby's lungs.

No single test is reliable by itself, so several of these procedures should be run to cross-check results. These diagnostic techniques, which are described in greater detail in "Postdue . . . If You're Late" (p. 210), can accurately predict whether it's wise for your baby to make its entrance.

Among nonmedical justifications for induction are a history of fast labor and excessive travel time to the hospital. However, convenience is an unspoken reason among those physicians who elect to induce simply because it fits their schedule or that of the family-to-be. The U.S. Food and Drug Administration defines unnecessary or elective induction as the "initiation of labor for convenience in an individual with a term pregnancy who is free of medical indications" and sees it as a dangerous enough practice to require warnings against it on oxytocin and other labor-inducing drugs.

Factors to Weigh

If your or your baby's well-being is clearly threatened by letting nature take its course, induction or a cesarean may be your only options. In the case of premature rupture of the membranes or prolonged pregnancy where there is no evidence of problems, often it comes down to either wait and see or play it safe and induce. The pros and cons of the various methods of induction should also be carefully considered with your medical adviser. While induction may avoid surgery, should you decide on this strategy, talk with your doctor about your specific wishes regarding cesarean childbirth in case induced labor proves unsuccessful.

For more information, see "Drugs During Childbirth" (p. 236), "Your Bag of Water: Best Let It Break Naturally" (p. 228), "Long Labor: Let the Sun Set Twice?" (p. 246), and "Cesarean: What Every Expectant Mother Should Know" (p. 260).

ELECTRONIC FETAL MONITORS: PROS AND CONS

During labor, the muscles of your uterus are contracting and relaxing in an effort to squeeze your baby down and out the birth canal. In the process, each time your uterus contracts, it momentarily reduces the flow of oxygen-rich blood supplied by the placenta. Normally your body takes care of this stress by dipping into oxygen stores in the placenta to carry your baby through each contraction. But sometimes the mechanism is faulty, depriving your baby of necessary oxygen and causing the heart rate to accelerate too much or drop too low. Electronic fetal monitors can chart contractions and the baby's heart rate to see how well he or she is "breathing" through them.

External monitors are belts or straps attached around your middle with two sensors, one to pick up the fetal heartbeat by using sound waves (a form of ultrasound), the other to "sense" muscle contractions electronically. A wireless connection to the machine called radiotelemetric monitoring, which is carried like a shoulder bag, available at some hospitals, does not hamper one's movement during labor. If the membranes have ruptured, a more sensitive device can be used internally to detect heart tones by attaching a tiny electrode to the area of your baby's skin closest to the cervix. A partner to this internal monitor is a narrow plastic tube filled with water and slipped into your uterus to measure by pressure the length, strength and timing of your muscle contractions.

Electronic monitors have made the fetal stethoscope practically obsolete at more than half of all U.S. hospitals. Many obstetricians and nurse-midwives not only feel their patients profit from "objective" reporting, but, by providing a printed record of labor progress, the machines protect the staff in the event of malpractice suits. Most importantly, in high-risk cases such as those involving toxemia or diabetes, the fetal monitor is invaluable in improving the baby's chance of survival and good health. After reviewing the use of electronic fetal monitors, the government's National Institute of Health published the following guidelines in 1979:

Monitors are strongly recommended in these situations:

(1) Expected low birth weight due to premature labor or slow growth in the womb
(2) Serious medical complications of pregnancy such as toxemia (pre-eclampsia) or diabetes
(3) Presence of the baby's first stool in the amniotic fluid
(4) Abnormal heart rate detected by listening with a fetoscope
(5) If labor is induced or contractions are artificially stimulated by a drug

Other medical conditions may make their use advisable, including:

(1) If mother has an infection
(2) Multiple birth
(3) Previous problem in pregnancy
(4) Previous unexplained stillbirth
(5) Previous delivery by cesarean
(6) If baby is in a position other than head-first

Not everyone in the medical community agrees on when and how this breakthrough technology should be used. No one questions its life-saving value in medically complicated pregnancies, but its routine use during an ordinary, healthy labor has come under attack. At issue here is not simply that electronic surveillance may unnecessarily intrude on and depersonalize the birth experience, but that it may actually be unsafe, especially in the case of internal monitors. Those opposed to routine use claim also that monitors are partly responsible for the startling increase in cesarean deliveries. Because of faulty readings or misinterpretation, they say, more babies are mistakenly diagnosed as "in distress," which results in an unnecessary C-section. A study by the National Institutes of Health, however, has failed to turn up any evidence to support this claim. Advocates of blanket use argue that benefits still outweigh any risks, since even normal labor has high-risk potential. If contractions are too strong or if the mother's blood pressure suddenly drops, both the mother's and baby's health are threatened. Arguments are strong on both sides. Here is a rundown.

Advantages of Monitoring

- listens more accurately than fetal stethoscope and picks up subtle heart irregularities
- times contractions more precisely and simultaneously compares baby's response to each uterine contraction
- focuses on the importance of the baby's ability to cope with the stress of labor
- permits long labors to take their natural course, avoiding unnecessary cesarean or forceps-assisted delivery
- tracks fetal well-being and improves a baby's chance if the mother has heart problems, pregnancy-induced hypertension, diabetes or other medical problems
- tells a mother and her coach of each oncoming contraction, since the machine's sensitivity detects muscle tightening before the mother is aware of it
- supplies printed record of progress of labor and provides reassurance to prospective parents
- predicts dangers, such as a compressed or knotted umbilical cord, faster than periodic checks with a hand-held stethoscope.

Disadvantages of Monitoring

- prevents mother from moving about, often requiring horizontal position, which reduces blood (oxygen supply) to womb and makes laboring women work against the force of gravity, possibly prolonging labor
- results in unnecessary medical intervention when machine signals fetal distress when in fact the baby is okay (estimates of the percentage of babies who are healthy yet diagnosed in distress by a monitor range from 20 to 75 percent)
- leads to inadvertent failure to detect trouble because staff tends

to rely heavily on the machine's information, ignoring other important signs (estimates of the percentage of babies who are in distress yet diagnosed by the monitor as healthy range from 7 to 20 percent)
- frightens prospective parents unnecessarily about their baby's health if machine has mechanical problems or if the printout is misread
- increases health-care costs in excess of $400 million annually—with "little evidence of benefit," claim several government experts
- might lead to yet-unknown but possibly adverse effects caused by the ultrasound device in external fetal monitors
- requires bag of water be broken artificially if membranes haven't ruptured spontaneously, in order to attach internal fetal monitor, breaking the seal that protects the unborn baby from germs, including undetected viral infections such as vaginal herpes
- increases the chance of infection in mother's uterus after birth; the internal monitor also may cause cuts on the baby's scalp

The time to explore your options with your health adviser is well before your due date approaches. Since many hospitals automatically require monitoring, if you feel adamantly opposed to the use of this equipment, you may have to decide on another birthplace and possibly switch doctors. However, there are some other options you might want to discuss with your physician. For instance, if you decide on an external monitor and find the belts around your abdomen annoying or downright uncomfortable, what about periodic checks with a hand-held fetal stethoscope? Or is radiotelemetric monitoring available, which allows you to move about more freely? Or would an internal monitor, which is more sensitive and usually more accurate, be preferred? Another scenario you might discuss in advance is, if the internal monitor picked up signs of fetal distress, does the hospital have the capability of doing a fetal scalp sampling test to double-check the monitor's reading?

If you decide on a monitor, remember to change positions frequently and don't worry about messing up the tracing. The monitor's needs are secondary to your comfort, and the belts of an external machine can be easily repositioned. *One financial footnote:* The cost of electronic fetal monitoring varies from hospital to hospital, ranging from $35 to $50 per patient, and is not always included in your labor and delivery fee. Check with the hospital beforehand to see if it is a separate charge.

Factors to Weigh

If labor begins prior to the thirty-eighth week or other medical conditions put you in the so-called high-risk category, chances are you won't have any choice about whether or not you are monitored electronically. Even if your pregnancy has been trouble-free and labor is normal, you may have little or no say, depending on hospital policy or your doctor's preference. Both the American College of Obstetricians and Gynecologists and the National Institutes of Health, however, believe the decision for or against monitors in routine cases should be reached through discussion by you with your health-care team. The NIH Task Force, looking into the role of monitors, says that they should always be used in conjunction with other tests to measure fetal well-being: "Intermittent and continuous fetal heart rate assessments are screening rather than diagnostic techniques. Failure to appreciate this limitation may lead to inappropriate clinical decisions."

DRUGS DURING CHILDBIRTH

If this if your first child, you won't know until labor is under way how well your body and mind will handle the stress of giving birth. A mother's ability to tolerate the pain of labor depends on her pelvic structure, the efficiency of her uterine contractions, her physical stamina, attitude and expectations. Some experts speculate that equally important is the amount of natural, opiatelike pain-killers, called endorphins, that are excreted by the brain.

A smorgasbord of medications can come to the rescue if one's natural defense system falters. Pain relief is the main target of most obstetrical drugs, but others are frequently used, such as those intended to start labor artificially. Although drugs can do miraculous things such as prod labor along, they can also wreak havoc with nature. By introducing a foreign agent into the childbirth process, an unwanted chain reaction of medical countermeasures may be set off. In the popular epidural block for instance, an anesthetic agent is injected into the lower portion of the back. In order for a baby to rotate naturally prior to crowning, the mother's firm pelvic floor provides the resistance that encourages the head to turn. This regional anesthetic keeps the perineal area relaxed, often necessitating forceps to position the baby properly for its grand entrance. Also, first-time mothers with an epidural often are unable to help push the baby out, resulting in a forceps-assisted delivery. But there are advantages to this type of regional anesthesia; it may arrest involuntary pushing prior to the second stage of labor, before the mother's cervix is fully dilated.

Before weighing the possible benefits and risks of many obstetrical drugs, here is a breakdown of the different categories followed by a road map of the different routes for administering the regional anesthetics.

Major Types of Medications

artificial hormones such as Pitocin to induce labor, augment contractions or arrest bleeding after delivery

tranquilizers to lower tension and anxiety during labor

sedatives containing barbiturates to calm laboring woman or help her sleep

narcoticlike analgesics such as Demerol to help increase pain threshold

regional anesthesia such as epidural block to numb some or all of the body from the waist down

general anesthesia to put mother to sleep during cesarean, although regional anesthesia is preferred for nonemergencies.

Many of the local blocks can be used to deaden pain at times other than the stages indicated in the next chart. For instance, a paracervical might be given when a laboring woman is 5 centimeters dilated and again later, during transition. Specific anesthetic agents such as Marcaine and other popular brand names used in these regional blocks are discussed in "Risks Versus Benefits" (p. 238).

PAIN SITE	POINT IN LABOR	PAIN-KILLER
Overall tension	3 cm	*Sedatives or tranquilizers may be given to stem anxiety*
Cervix (as it stretches)	4–6 cm	*Paracervical block injected into tissues surrounding cervix, eliminating pain*

PAIN SITE	POINT IN LABOR	PAIN-KILLER
		in the area and uterus, possibly causing faster dilation
Lower uterus and body of uterus as it contracts	4–8 cm	*Epidural or caudal block* injected into space surrounding fluid sac, or "dura," which houses spinal column; numbs from waist down but may not take all over
Backache	7–10 cm	*Narcoticlike analgesic* such as Demerol may reduce tension or discomfort of backache and take edge off contractions
Perineum (the area around birth outlet)	Second Stage	*Low spinal and saddle blocks* injected into spinal fluid below cord; blocks sensation from the waist down, resulting in loss of sensation and movement
Skin and tissue surrounding anus and birth outlet	Second Stage/ Pushing	*Pudendal block* injected into nerve on side of birth canal (pudendal nerve), which gives principal pain impulse at this point; deadens sensations in perineum and relaxes pelvic-floor muscles
Skin around vagina if torn or cut	Shortly after birth	*Local anesthetic* such as Novocain injected into tissue surrounding birth outlet to sew up tears or episiotomy

Risks Versus Benefits

Over 100 different drugs are administered during childbirth every day in this country, but less than half a dozen of these medications have been approved specifically for obstetrical use by the U.S. Food and

Drug Administration. One reason is the cost to pharmaceutical manufacturers of proving such safety. This partly explains the lack of follow-up studies on offspring exposed to them, although every year new research arouses more suspicion about various analgesics and anesthetics. Some experts blame these drugs for many mental or neurological problems in youngsters, but many in the medical community would agree with Dr. Phillip Goldstein of Johns Hopkins University Medical School, who suggests, "It is very likely that smoking, alcohol, and poor nutrition cause as much mischief in human development as all other drugs put together."

Many of these drugs work wonders and leave no trace of apparent adverse effect. But it is difficult to predict a drug's influence on an individual mother and her child, owing to the interplay of countless variables, including the laboring woman's size and state of health, her baby's size, the condition of the placenta, the time medication is given or taken in relation to labor or birth, the strength of the dose and its interaction with other drugs, the newborn's ability to metabolize and excrete the drug. Consequently there are inherent contradictions when discussing the pros and cons. Blood flow to the womb, for example, could be enhanced if a sedative helps you relax but hindered if you become so sedated that circulation slows and reduces oxygen supply to the baby. Artificial oxytocin may trigger abrupt and spasmodic contractions for one woman, while for another it furnishes just the extra charge needed to speed labor along.

A core issue in this debate centers on brain damage to the baby in utero. An alarming comment is articulated by Doris Haire, president of the American Foundation for Maternal and Child Health. Before a congressional committee in 1981, Haire testified,

> At no other time in an individual's life is his or her brain more vulnerable to trauma and permanent injury than during the hours which surround the individual's birth. Other major organ systems are essentially formed by the first 4 or 5 months of pregnancy. It is the nervous circuitry of the brain and the central nervous system of the fetus which is rapidly developing as labor begins, making these awesomely complex structures vulnerable to permanent damage from drugs and procedures administered to the mother during that time.

Of particular concern is that many obstetrical types of drugs depress the mother's central nervous system and, consequently, slow her breathing and lower her blood pressure. According to Haire and others, this may result in a persistently diminished level of oxygen for the baby's brain cells.

The opposing argument is that pain-killers are valuable, and perhaps essential for a laboring woman who suffers from fright or pain.

This is based on the theory that the hormonal response to fear produces too many catecholamines (essentially, high levels of adrenaline), which in turn cause the blood vessels of the uterus to constrict, possibly leading to oxygen deprivation in the unborn baby. Scientific documentation in monkeys has not been demonstrated in humans. Advocates of drug-free childbirth don't worry about catecholamines but focus instead on the high levels of endorphins, morphinelike pain-killers released by the brain, that have been detected both in newborn babies and their mothers.

Another concern is that chemicals may remain trapped in the baby's circulatory system once the umbilical cord is cut, because a newborn's liver and kidneys are not fully operational at birth and take longer to break down and excrete the drug. One study found drugs were retained in babies' systems through a six-week testing period. The U.S. Food and Drug Administration acknowledges that "all drugs used during labor and delivery may cause short-term adverse effects, such as decreased muscle tone, inability to suck, reduced responsiveness to stimulation, depressed breathing, and irregular heartbeat," but concludes that "the effects of the drugs disappeared after the first 10 days of life, and that effects beyond that period had not been proven." The timing of drugs administered can control this problem to some extent. A few medications have a longer-than-average lag time before finding their way to the baby, and if they are given late enough in labor, the infant may be born before the drug has reached him or her. However, for other drugs, the earlier they are taken in labor, the more time the mother's body has to help her baby break down and get rid of the foreign agent prior to birth.

Although you may have no intention of using any drug during childbirth, it cannot hurt to know in advance what are your doctor's "favorites" as well as what is commonly used at the hospital. Specific risks have been identified with particular groups of medications as well as individual name brands. New findings surface all the time, so the information presented here should be viewed only as a starting point in your discussion with your medical adviser. Much of the information outlined below is from the U.S. Pharmacopoeia's data base and is the foundation of this nonprofit organization's forthcoming book, *About Your Medicines During Pregnancy, Labor and Breast-feeding.*

CATEGORY AND COMMON BRAND NAMES	SIDE EFFECTS
TRANQUILIZERS used during labor to lower tension and anxiety diazepam (Valium)	Mother may have difficulty handling contractions because tranquilizer decreases awareness

CATEGORY AND COMMON BRAND NAMES	SIDE EFFECTS
hydroxyzine (Vistaril) chloropromazine (Thorazine) promazine (Sparine) meprobamate (Miltown) chlordiazepoxide (Librium)	Newborn may have trouble breathing, difficulty sucking, muscle weakness and body-temperature problems if diazepam is given in large doses within 15 hours of delivery, warns U.S. Pharmacopoeia
SEDATIVES containing barbiturates, otherwise called central nervous system depressants, may be used to sedate women or to induce sleep amobarbital (Amytal) sodium butabarbital (Butisol) phenobarbital (Luminal) pentobarbital sodium (Nembutal) secobarbital sodium (Seconal) thiamylal sodium (Surital)	Mother's labor may be prolonged since full anesthetic doses may reduce strength and frequency of contractions Mother may become disoriented, drowsy, nauseous; possible aftereffects include nightmares Newborn may have breathing problems
NARCOTICLIKE ANALGESICS may increase pain threshold; often mixed with a tranquilizer in a drug "cocktail" to boost power of the narcotic, allowing a smaller dose meridine (Demerol) morphine sulfate nalbuphine (Nubain) butorphanol (Stadol)	Mother's contractions may become overrelaxed, although this can be reversed by other drugs, called narcotic antagonists Newborn may experience breathing problems if some narcotics are taken just before birth, cautions U.S. Pharmacopoeia
LABOR STIMULANTS such as synthetic oxytocin, a hormone, may be used to induce labor or to augment contractions. Another option is use of prostaglandins including the vaginal suppositories such as Prostin E_2 which are effective in stimulating uterine contractions and also encourage cervix to dilate oxytocin (Pitocin) carboprost (Prostin) dinoprostone (Prostin E_2)	Mother may need pain relief if artificially stimulated contractions become too intense Baby may suffer oxygen deprivation because long contractions with short rest periods may reduce the oxygen-replenishing intervals Oxytocin may inhibit rather than promote expulsion of the placenta and increase the risk of maternal hemorrhage and infection, warns U.S. Pharmacopoeia

CATEGORY AND COMMON BRAND NAMES	SIDE EFFECTS

[Also refer to "When Is It Wise to Induce Labor?" p. 230.]

Oxytocin should be used with caution in mothers greater than 35 years of age, urges U.S. Pharmacopoeia

Newborn jaundice is linked by some to routine use of oxytocin but numerous studies have found no such evidence

REGIONAL PAIN BLOCKS eliminate sensations; paracervical, pudendal or other local blocks numb the pain-impulse conductors (nerves) either at the source of discomfort or at the pain-receptor center (spinal column), as with epidural, spinal or saddle blocks. The type of anesthetic agent often carries more risk than the location of where the drug is injected

    propoxycaine (Blockaine)
    mepivacaine (Carbocaine)
    prilocaine (Citanest)
    etidocaine (Duranest)
    lidocaine (Lidocaine)
    bupivacaine (Marcaine)
    procaine (Novocain)
    chloroprocaine (Nesacaine)
    dibucaine (Nupercaine)

Mother's blood pressure may drop, which may lead to inadequate oxygen to unborn baby; however, maternal hypotension usually can be corrected with IV and positioning

Mother's contractions may weaken with epidural or caudal anesthesia and forceps may be necessary, while spinal or saddle block leaves no choice but forceps or cesarean delivery, since it's not possible to push

Fetus's heartbeat may become unusually slow when chloroprocaine, lidocaine or mepivacaine are given by paracervical block, cautions U.S. Pharmacopoeia

Mother and fetus may experience adverse effects such as changes in central nervous system, heart and blood vessels if bupivacaine is administered by epidural, caudal, paracervical or pudendal block

Maternal deaths due to cardiac arrest have been reported when high dosages of bupivacaine were injected into a vein accidentally instead of into the space surrounding the spinal cord and membranes; in 1983 the FDA instructed anesthesiologists to take special precautions administering bupivacaine and to use low concentrations of this anesthetic

CATEGORY AND COMMON BRAND NAMES	SIDE EFFECTS
	Mother may suffer severe headache, constipation or inability to control bowels, with spinal or saddle blocks
	Mother more susceptible to urinary-tract infections when given many regional blocks, because clearance reflex is numb, so bladder retains germ-filled urine longer or catheter that drains inert bladder introduces more germs into urinary tract
	Newborn may have less muscle strength and tone for the first day or two of life, but the long-term consequence of this reaction is unknown, advises U.S. Pharmacopoeia
	Infant's visual skills, alertness and other cognitive development may be adversely affected by bupivacaine epidural for an undetermined amount of time, concludes one study
GENERAL ANESTHESIA is used when speed is crucial during childbirth; otherwise regional anesthesia is used, which means the mother is awake during forceps-assisted or cesarean delivery. An induction agent such as thiopental (Pentothal) may be administered first, followed by an inhalation agent such as trichloroethylene (Trilene)	Mother at risk if she has eaten within last 12 hours prior to being put to sleep and inhales vomitus, which may block airways, causing decreased oxygen to brain cells, possibly death
	Mother may suffer from reduced hemoglobin in her blood (cyanosis), which may in turn adversely affect her baby
	Baby's central nervous system depressed, since inhalation anesthesia crosses the placenta and freely enters circulatory system, possibly causing respiratory depression after birth

Ways to Avoid Problems

Well before your due date, make a point of discussing with your physician the whole range of obstetrical medicines used at the hospital.

You may want to consider having your preferences (such as no drugs during labor, epidural with an agent other than bupivacaine) noted on your medical record. You should ask about the availability of trained anesthesiologists or nurse-anesthetists on the maternity floor and inquire whether your husband or labor companion is allowed to remain with you in the event that you decide to get regional anesthesia.

After hospital admission, you may want to consider the following:

(1) Tell the labor- and delivery-room nurses of your preferences—that you intend to have an unmedicated birth or which drugs you would prefer over others.

(2) Ask about nondrug analgesics prior to deciding on drugs—if contractions are weak or irregular, consider changing positions and, if you feel up to it, walk around even if it means being followed by an IV pole and loose wires for internal electronic fetal monitoring. Although it's a long shot, ask about taking a warm bath, which helps many laboring women by reducing tension, relieving pain and promoting muscular relaxation (for more suggestions, see "Positions and Labor Equipment: From Squatting to Birthing Chairs," p. 224).

(3) Inquire about a drug's possible effects on you (nausea, vomiting, euphoria, dizziness, reduced blood pressure, headaches), on your labor (slowed or accelerated contractions, likelihood of forceps-assisted delivery) and on your baby (lower heart rate, respiratory problems, central nervous system changes). The American Academy of Pediatrics takes the position that the physician has an obligation to advise the expectant mother of the known adverse effects and potential benefits of drugs offered to her during labor and delivery.

(4) Ask the anesthesiologist specifically about your choices of anesthetic agents available for a particular regional block instead of discussing only the types of regional anesthesia.

(5) Request the anesthesiologist or nurse-anesthetist to wait before administering a drug if you are in the middle of a contraction.

(6) Weigh your need versus your ability to forgo—at 8 centimeters you may be able to stick it out, because the end of transition is near.

Factors to Weigh

Hypnosis, acupuncture and tub labor are effective in eliminating or reducing pain, but these are not acceptable options at most hospitals in the U.S. Drugs have their advantages; for instance, pain medication may give an exhausted expectant mother the rest she needs to work through the remaining contractions. Regional block can mean a woman remains awake during cesarean childbirth and suffers less post-op nausea and grogginess. On the other hand, drugs can be counterproductive in such cases where a pain-killer slows contractions, requiring artificial labor stimulants, which result in painful, sometimes terrifying contractions that call for additional pain medication or sedation.

Not even the pharmaceutical industry declares obstetrical-related drugs are positively safe. Although many doctors and anesthesiologists dismiss fears of short-term and long-term effects on exposed offspring, many unanswered questions remain. In making this decision, you owe it to yourself and your baby to weigh carefully the risks and benefits of every drug offered to you.

Information Sources

ADDITIONAL READING

Medications Used During Labor and Childbirth for Childbirth Educators, by Avis Ericson, Pharm. D. (Minneapolis: International Childbirth Education Association, 1978). Technical material but understandable to lay person.

ORGANIZATIONS

American Foundation for Maternal and Child Health
30 Beekman Pl.
New York, NY 10022
Doris Haire's eight-page report "How the FDA Determines the Safety of Drugs—Just How Safe Is Safe?" is available for $1.00.

U.S. Food and Drug Administration
Fertility and Maternal Health Drugs Advisory Committee
Anesthetic and Life Support Drug Advisory Committee
5600 Fishers La.
Rockville, MD 20857
Government agency responsible for approving drugs marketed in the U.S. and issuing guidelines for drug use.

U.S. Pharmacopoeia
Drug Information Division
12601 Twinbrook Pkwy.
Rockville, MD 20857
Data base on medications used during childbirth and soon to publish book *About Your Medicines During Pregnancy, Labor, and Breast-feeding.*

LONG LABOR: LET THE SUN SET TWICE?

Prolonged labor is not uncommon among women giving birth for the first time, in those whose membranes have ruptured before the cervix was ripe and in expectant mothers who are especially tense and fearful. The cervix may not open much or it may fail to dilate to the full 10 centimeters. Progress also may come to a standstill during the baby's journey from the cervix through the birth canal. What causes so-called dysfunctional labor often is unclear, but the reasons generally fall under the "three Ps":

- *Power*   uterine muscles too weak and cannot coordinate opening of the cervix; often happens if mother's pelvis is too small or baby is in awkward birth position, suggesting the uterus knows of the difficulty and consequently holds back

  voluntary muscles of abdomen and diaphragm are not used or used poorly because either pushing is too painful or anesthesia has disconnected nerve impulses (commands) from the brain

- *Passenger*   position of baby's body fails to provide enough of a wedge against the cervix, as in the case of a breech

  baby may be too large to pass through cervix and/or birth canal, termed feto-pelvic disproportion

- *Passageway*   stubborn cervix refuses to dilate

  pelvic outlet is too small

  soft-tissue obstruction in birth canal

Taking labor-stimulant drugs or having a cesarean or forceps-assisted delivery are some of the decisions you may have to confront if labor drags on. While some physicians and midwives patiently wait for nature to take its course as long as the baby shows no signs of distress, most obstetricians follow the adage "Don't let the sun set twice." This expression applies primarily if it takes a first-time mother more than 20 hours to reach 3 centimeters' dilation from the onset of labor or if the cervix dilates less than 1 centimeter per hour during active labor.

The average textbook timetable, based on "Friedman's curve," also puts a limit of two hours on the second stage; in other words, on the baby's travel time from the cervix through the birth canal. The major reason many doctors step in if labor deviates from the normal pattern is concern over the baby's well-being. For example, prolonged frequent, intense contractions interfere with placental circulation, jeopardizing the baby's oxygen supply; or a protracted second stage may compromise the unborn child because of pressure on his or her soft head as it pounds against the mother's pelvic floor. Others may consider exhaustion of the mother an equally important reason to intervene, though this is sometimes more a case of exhaustion of the physician. Many birth attendants who worry about hour-to-hour progression of labor prefer to coax labor along in nonmedical ways, which explains the variety of catalysts and treatments outlined in the following chart. Of course, many of the procedures are not hazard-free. The potential benefits and possible risks are discussed in detail in this chapter and the next.

STAGE OF LABOR	CATALYSTS/PROCEDURES
Prolonged Early Labor little or no cervical dilation or effacement after 20 hours; or contractions stop completely	walk around to rule out false labor rest or sleep with the help of sedatives or tranquilizers; some disagree and actually advise against resting have an enema (increased peristaltic action may irritate uterus and cause contractions) try herbs such as blue cohosh as tea or strained and diluted as an enema relax with music and massage use drugs such as artificial hormone oxytocin to stimulate or augment contractions
Prolonged Active First Stage less than 1 cm dilation/per hour; or contractions stop completely; or cervix refuses to dilate fully	empty bladder often roll nipples, which may stimulate uterine contractions experiment with different positions, and don't stay flat on your back

STAGE OF LABOR	CATALYSTS/PROCEDURES

relax in warm bath (permitted at many birth centers and a few hospitals)

avoid unnecessary sedation or anesthesia; if regional pain blocker such as an epidural was given early in labor, let it wear off, and dilation may resume

rupture membranes artificially (breaking bag of water)

use labor-stimulant drugs such as oxytocin if feto-pelvic disproportion is ruled out

perform cesarean if mother's pelvis judged too small to accommodate or baby's body is believed to be too large for vaginal delivery

Prolonged Second Stage

lasts longer than 2 hours in first-time mother

assume upright position

try artificial oxytocin or other drug to increase force of contractions

rotate baby and assist out birth canal with forceps

perform cesarean if oxytocic drug not successful, feto-pelvic disproportion diagnosed, baby in distress or beyond reach of forceps

Provided there are no signs of trouble, you have time to discuss various options with your doctor or midwife and experiment a bit. "Managing labor remains an art," writes Dr. Robert Sokol of the Ob/Gyn Department of Case Western Reserve University in Ohio. "The key to successful outcome is intensive observation and minimal intervention."

For further information, see "Drugs During Childbirth (p. 236), "When Is It Wise to Induce Labor?" (p. 230), "Your Bag of Water: Best Let It Break Naturally" (p. 228) and "Cesarean: What Every Expectant Mother Should Know" (p. 260).

EPISIOTOMY: AN UNNECESSARY CUT?

The final obstacle to your baby's arrival is the vaginal opening. Hormones have already softened you up, and the perineal muscles surrounding your vagina and rectum have a remarkable stretching capacity. But when your baby "crowns," your physician or midwife might decide to make a small cut to enlarge the opening. This incision, called episiotomy—from the Greek "epision," meaning the pubic region, and "tomy," meaning to cut—may run from your vagina toward your anus or toward your thigh.

An episiotomy (pronounced e-piz"e-ot'o-me) is often done if:

- baby's head is quite large
- baby is in an awkward position
- birth attendant thinks that you will tear and believes that tears are harder to repair and may take longer to heal than a clean surgical incision
- you are unable to control the pace and strength of your pushes, so your skin does not have the opportunity to stretch gradually
- you are not getting clear directions about when and how to push
- you have unusually tight perineal muscles (some childbirth experts caution against doing too many Kegel tightening exercises prior to birth)
- baby is in distress and needs to be born quickly, possibly with use of forceps.

Episiotomies are standard practice in the U.S., unlike elsewhere in the world, and obstetricians are trained to do them, although some hands are more skilled than others. It takes about 30 minutes to sew up the incision, and a shot of Novocain is usually given to avoid discomfort. However, don't be surprised to have trouble sitting on your derriere for the first few days. An ice pack will help reduce the swelling. (More suggestions are spelled out in "Postpartum Care: Baby Yourself," p. 307).

The episiotomy rate in the U.S. during 1980 was 62.5 percent, far higher than in any other country. A review by Drs. David Banta and Stephen Thacker, "The Risks and Benefits of Episiotomy," states that "it is the second most common surgical procedure done in the United States after cutting the umbilical cord." Most physicians justify the routine use of episiotomy for several reasons, the primary justification being that it prevents pelvic relaxation—in other words, permanent loosening of muscles in the pelvic floor. A cut enlarging the birth outlet releases the pressure on the muscles strained from the stress of pushing and pounding of the baby's head. Many doctors also believe that excessive stretching may lessen future sexual response and pleasure. But Shirley Kitzinger and other childbirth educators claim that permanent damage is often traced instead to a bad job of sewing it up, and warn that intercourse is more likely to be uncomfortable until the episiotomy has healed. They argue that a mother's perineum will regain its muscle tone naturally with the help of Kegels and other simple exercises.

By far the principal reason for routine episiotomies is the just-in-case rationale, meaning that it is better to cut than chance a tear. An episiotomy, though, is not the only preventive measure available. Birth attendants in some hospitals and birthing centers are beginning to follow the European example by coaxing a mother to go more slowly through her final pushes. By gently controlling the pace of birth, they have time to "iron out" the birth outlet and massage it back safely over the baby's head. At Minneapolis's Hennepin County Hospital in 1981, for example, the nurse-midwives report that 84 percent of their patients had no episiotomy, and only 10 percent tore.

Keep in mind that the position you assume during the pushing phase of labor has a lot to do with whether your vaginal opening is able to stretch gradually; for example, lying flat on your back with legs raised in stirrups increases the likelihood of an episiotomy or tear, because flexed thighs tighten up the birth outlet. On the other hand, lying on your left side helps control untimely pushes and causes less tension around the vagina.

Given good teamwork plus massage, you may not need an episiotomy. Whether you get one or not depends on your birth attendant's habit and clinical judgment at the time of delivery. If you would prefer to try to avoid a cut—some mothers say they would prefer to tear—let your obstetrician or midwife know well before labor.

Factors to Weigh

A shave or trim of the pubic hair is required at many hospitals just in case an episiotomy is needed (see "Enema, Shave and IV: Which Ones Are for You?" p. 222). For most obstetricians in the U.S., performing this simple procedure is an automatic reflex. Some mothers would prefer a clean cut to be on the safe side; however, others would avoid an episiotomy regardless of the consequences. Whatever you decide, try to remain flexible, since it's difficult to predict in advance just how your baby will choose to break out into the world.

FORCEPS-ASSISTED DELIVERY

The number of forceps-assisted deliveries performed in the U.S. has dropped but a 1982 *Parents* magazine poll of 64,000 mothers found steel "spoons" were used in 27 percent of all vaginal births. Certain forceps maneuvers—which are no longer used—partly explain why these surgical instruments still have a bad reputation. A mother's birth canal and cervix were often damaged and babies suffered facial injury, mental retardation and even death, but *now* forceps are never used unless the baby's head is actually engaged in the birth canal. An alternative to forceps besides cesarean delivery is a new technique, popularized in Sweden, called vacuum extraction. However, few doctors in this country are trained to use this suction-cup device, and, as one medical journal put it, older obstetricians are "reluctant to abandon hard-won skills with forceps."

The thought of clasping a baby's head with a hard metal instrument may be scary, but in experienced hands this maneuver can avoid trauma to the child and cause little or no discomfort to the mother. Two separate ends, called "blades," are angled to slip easily into the vagina and curved to fit around each side of the baby's head. When both are in place, the blades join and lock together at the arms to prevent tightening. With each contraction, the physician gently pulls on the handle, either to turn (rotation) or lift out (traction) the baby. Some doctors will combine these two maneuvers, while others will first rotate the baby's head with mid-forceps, then remove each blade, reenter the vagina, locking into a low-forceps mode, and finally slide the baby's head out.

Dozens of circumstances call for this medical intervention. Here are some of the most common reasons for using forceps:

- *Epidural, saddle block or other regional blocks.* Use of these drugs makes forceps delivery more likely, particularly among first-time mothers, who, when anesthetized by these blocks, are unable to use their abdominal muscles to help push the baby out.
- *Premature infants.* The spoons provide protection by cradling the soft head away from the mother's bony pelvis.
- *Fetal distress.* Forceps can hasten delivery; otherwise a cesarean may be performed.
- *Baby's head is posterior.* Mid-forceps can rotate the position if the crown of the head is toward the tailbone.
- *Mother exhausted or ill.* Forceps help the baby out if a woman is

too tired to push or if she is sick with toxemia or some other illness where strenuous exertion could be dangerous.

Although a positive attitude about labor is essential, no one can predict whether you might run into such problems as having your baby stuck in a posterior position. Since it is unwise to practice pushing during pregnancy, there is also no way to know how well you will be able to bear down. Some doctors watch the clock during the second stage and resort to forceps as a kind of "defense obstetrics," especially when dealing with the unproven pelvis of a first-time mother.

Often the obstetrical rationale is that forceps reduce the birth trauma to both the mother and infant by shortening this strenuous stage of labor. Although the possibility of a shorter labor is tempting, forceps still constitute a surgical procedure that is not hazard-free. There are risks to both the woman and her baby, though studies disagree about whether certain complications result from forceps or from a difficult labor itself. Keep in mind, too, that the experience and judgment of your birth attendant are the key to keeping injury to a minimum. The effects of forceps on a baby vary, but usually they are temporary. The metal tongs cause compression on the head, but overlapping skull bones provide protection. Forceps marks that look like raised bruises and abrasions heal quickly. Incorrect use of forceps can, however, cause serious eye injury, skull fracture, facial paralysis or brain damage.

One of the major advantages of vacuum extraction (using a suction cup) over forceps is that injuries to the mother are rare. Usually there is less need for pain relief, although in low-forceps delivery a local shot of Novocain will often numb the woman enough, and regional anesthesia may be used with mid-forceps for comfort as well as muscular relaxation, in order to insert the instrument. Forceps usually necessitate a generous episiotomy to enlarge the birth opening, and even with this surgical cut, tears in the vagina and cervix occur. The chance of urinary-tract infection is higher with forceps intervention, as is possible tissue damage to the bladder or urethra.

Factors to Weigh

Since it is impossible to predict the dynamics of your labor and delivery, there is no way to know whether you will be faced with this decision. However, the likelihood of a forceps-assisted delivery increases, particularly among first-time mothers who are given certain regional pain block. If you feel strongly about avoiding this type of medical intervention, talk with your doctor or midwife about specific medications and positions during labor that will reduce the chance of needing outside help.

Some obstetricians adhere to rigid one- or two-hour time limits on pushing during the second stage, while others will be patient as long as the baby's heart tones are okay. If fetal distress is detected by the internal electronic fetal monitor, ask if the hospital has the capability to confirm the diagnosis by a simple test to measure the pH or acid balance of your baby's scalp blood. In experienced hands, forceps are decidedly advantageous over a cesarean; however, if there is a medical indication that your baby needs help during this final phase of labor, it's wise to go along with whatever procedure your birth attendant knows best. Some doctors are well trained and experienced at the operating table but may not be as skilled with forceps. And, of course, forceps cannot be used if the cervix is not completely dilated or if the baby's head is not engaged.

Forceps date back to the seventeenth century and remain a basic, valuable tool in modern-day obstetrics. While for many parents a forceps delivery does not change a "perfect birth experience," for others it carries an emotional scar.

For more information, refer to "Positions and Labor Equipment: From Squatting to Birthing Chairs" (p. 224) and "Drugs During Childbirth" (p. 236).

EYE DROPS AND OTHER PROCEDURES IMMEDIATELY AFTER BIRTH

Within moments of birth, your baby must acquire an independent life-style. For the first time, your baby breathes through the lungs and reroutes the blood to travel there for its oxygen supply. At the same time your newborn is quickly learning to regulate his or her own temperature in order to keep all systems running smoothly. Not only is the infant a beginner at this, but there is less insulating fat to trap heat. That's why newborns are quickly dried off and swaddled.

Every hospital has its own policies, although obstetricians have a lot of say about what happens during the period immediately after delivery. It is becoming more common for the hospital staff to delay putting legally required silver-nitrate drops in the newborn's eyes right after birth, as well as other routine procedures that have marred the special moments of new life, often interfering with what many consider "bonding" between parents and their babies.

CONVENTIONAL APPROACH	ALTERNATIVE APPROACH
Mask covers father's nose and mouth during birth and while in delivery room	No mask worn by father or labor coach, to get fullest father-to-child contact
Immediate suctioning of baby's nose and throat to clear passageways (and to prevent inhaling fluid)	Baby allowed to take first breaths unassisted and not encouraged to cry as breathing stimulus
Umbilical cord cut right away by birth attendant	No cord clamping until pulsating stops or possibly until placenta is delivered; father may cut as part of initiation ritual
Baby cleaned to protect from infection, often weighed and measured before given to mother to hold	Skin-to-skin contact with baby immediately after birth; parents may wipe off baby themselves
Newborn placed under electronic warmer, separating mother and infant	Heat lamps positioned over mother and baby
Mother given artificial oxytocin or Pitocin by injection to expel placenta (see "Drugs During Childbirth," p. 236)	Immediate breast-feeding causes uterus to contract and expel placenta; artificial hormone may be given in addition
Silver-nitrate drops or other antibiotic ointment administered promptly	Application of drops or ointment is delayed but is required by law in most states within one hour of birth
Injection of vitamin K given to newborn to help blood clot (some say babies are born with a vitamin K deficiency)	Vitamin K not given unless baby shows a need

Some alternative approaches are further described next, and "gentle birth," with dimmed lights and a warm bath, is discussed in "Leboyer and Other Nontraditional Deliveries" (p. 114). For common procedures for treating premature infants, refer to "Premature Babies and Other Newborns Needing Intensive Care" (p. 270).

Cord Cutting

In those first moments, as your baby starts learning to adjust to the world, the placenta stands by to safeguard the infant by continuing to supply oxygen-rich blood even after the baby's first breath. Soon after the lungs are fully operational and delivering oxygen on their own, the umbilical-cord vessels shut down. In the meantime, the placenta has been draining into your baby, transfusing him or her with more blood. Debate continues on just when to cut the cord and stop this supply. The unresolved question is, how much blood does a newborn need? One school of thought argues that if the cord is cut within seconds after birth, the baby could be deprived of needed blood and become anemic. The other side believes that if cutting is delayed by three minutes or more, the additional volume may overload the baby's circulation and raise its blood pressure. Proponents of delayed cord clamping point to several studies that show late-cut newborns are alert for longer periods of time and seem to cry less. If this issue interests you, talk it over in advance with your birth attendant.

Silver-Nitrate Eye Drops

For years doctors were required by state law to place silver-nitrate drops in all babies' eyes immediately after delivery. This was to prevent a serious eye infection called gonococcal ophthalmia, caused by venereal disease in the mother's vagina but symptomless in her baby at birth. These drops not only blur infants' vision for a while but often cause eyes to redden and swell a bit. In 1980 the American Academy of Pediatrics, together with the government's Centers for Disease Control, recommended that these prophylactic drops could be delayed for up to one hour after delivery, if desired, and also approved tetracycline or erythromycin ointment instead of silver nitrate. Most state health departments now recognize this official recommendation, but check to be certain.

Mother-Child Interaction

By waiting awhile so that drops or ointment don't interfere with your baby's vision, the two of you will have a little more time to study each other. Early eye-to-eye contact is trumpeted as a crucial factor in the bonding process. Other elements include holding your baby (letting the infant lie on your abdomen, some say, helps uncoil the spine), stroking the newborn and breast-feeding. The degree of intimacy the two—or three—of you enjoy right after birth will depend on hospital policies and on whether or not either of you needs immediate medical care. (For further discussion, see "Bonding and Rooming-In: Overrated or Not?" p. 278.)

Physical and Behavorial Evaluation

Your baby takes its first "test" 60 seconds after birth, and at many hospitals and birth centers, further assessment may continue during the first few days of life. Standardized evaluations of physical and behavorial traits alert the medical staff to any life-threatening conditions. Two of the most popular methods include:

(1) *Apgar Test.* This is run twice, at one minute after delivery and again five minutes later. In the first test, the examiner (your pediatrician, delivery-room nurse or anesthesiologist) essentially checks how well your baby is breathing. The follow-up assessment can predict with some accuracy how well an infant will adjust to life outside the womb. The evaluation is based on your newborn's color, heart rate, reflex irritability (grimace, cough or sneeze), muscle tone (limp or active motion) and respiration. Each of these five categories holds a possible point value of two on the Apgar scorecard. Pink in appearance would merit a two, for example, and gray a zero. The best total score is ten, though any score from seven on up means good and healthy.

(2) *Brazelton Neonatal Behavioral Assessment Scale (BNBAS).* In many hospitals the Brazelton evaluation is begun hours or several days after birth to assess a newborn's temperament and behavior. Closely watching reactions to a 20-minute series of stimuli using light, sound and touch tracks an infant's development and gives parents an idea of areas of strength and weakness.

Factors to Weigh

These procedures happen so quickly after birth that you may not even be aware of what is being done. Experienced hands can cut the cord, administer eye drops, weigh, clean and footprint your baby in a minute or two. If you have preferences about these procedures, probably you can choreograph what you want ahead of time. Besides mapping out the sequence of events with your birth attendant, be sure to tell the labor- and delivery-room hospital staff about your desires; otherwise, quick hands may automatically go to work before you can say, "Wait!"

Unexpected Events

EMERGENCY CHILDBIRTH: HOW TO DELIVER YOUR BABY

If contractions are less than ten minutes apart and your baby can be seen in the birth canal during a contraction, it is better to stay where you are than risk giving birth en route to the hospital. Your doctor or midwife should be called, but first be sure there is someone to help you. Above all, try to *stay calm*. Most births are uncomplicated, particularly if the labor is a fast one.

Supplies

newspapers or towels and linens (if there's time, linens can be sterilized by a quick ironing)

bulb or ear syringe (boil a few minutes to sterilize)

clean white shoelaces or clean strips of linen

clean blanket

scissors (boil a few minutes to sterilize)

Directions to birth attendant:
(1) While you are scrubbing your hands and arms, get the mother to lie down or sit semiupright, with her back supported and her legs

bent and spread. Place a clean towel or newspapers under her buttocks and a clean sheet or more newspapers spread out beyond to catch the baby.

(2) The baby's head should emerge slowly, so encourage her to pant—not push—until it is out. Apply slight counterpressure to the baby's head and the skin around her vaginal opening to help avoid tearing around the birth outlet.

(3) Feel to find out if the umbilical cord is wrapped around the baby's neck. Loosen it by slipping it over the head or uncoiling it enough to let the body slip through.

(4) Baby's first breath—as soon as the head emerges, clear the passages by gentle suctioning of the nose and mouth with the bulb syringe. If no syringe is on hand, wait until the body emerges and then hold the baby's head down so the mucus drains out. If baby is not breathing, rub your hand up and down the middle of the back or try flicking your fingers on the soles of the baby's feet rather than the traditional slap on the bottom.

(5) Be patient. Do not pull the baby, but cradle its head in your hands so that the shoulders can rotate naturally.

(6) Wrap the baby in a towel or blanket and make sure its head is covered to prevent heat loss.

(7) Let the baby breast-feed, since sucking will stimulate the uterus to contract and push out the placenta.

(8) Don't pull on the umbilical cord or cut it. Wait for your doctor or midwife to arrive or get back on the telephone for directions. Many medical experts recommend clamping the cord once the blood has stopped pulsing, but another school of thought advises against cutting the cord unless the placenta is not expelled within 15 or 20 minutes or if the cord is too short to allow the baby to breast-feed. To cut the cord, take two shoelaces or strips of cloth, tie one halfway between the mother and baby and the other three inches below that, toward the baby's navel. Cut the cord between the two ties with sterile scissors.

(9) Save the placenta, because it will be examined later to make sure there are no fragments remaining inside the mother.

(10) Put one hand above the mother's pubic bone. With the other hand, feel down into the abdomen and massage the uterus gently but firmly. This helps prevent excessive bleeding; it is normal to lose approximately two cups of blood and fluid.

Information Sources

ADDITIONAL READING

Emergency Childbirth Handbook, by Barbara Anderson and Pamela Shapiro (New York: Van Nostrand Reinhold, 1982). Covers emergency procedures for unscheduled deliveries outside hospitals.

X-RAY PELVIMETRY WARNING

The verdict is that no X rays should be taken of a pregnant woman's pelvis, except perhaps to confirm that the head of a baby in breech position is tucked against the chest so the neck won't snap back during vaginal delivery. Besides the damaging effects of radiation to unborn babies, "X-ray pelvimetry is usually not necessary or helpful in making the decision to perform a cesarean," claims the American College of Obstetricians and Gynecologists, along with the American College of Radiologists and the U.S. Food and Drug Administration. "Therefore," the consensus statement continues, "pelvimetry should be performed only when the physician caring for the patient feels that pelvimetry will contribute to the decisions concerning diagnosis or treatment."

A common reason for taking an X ray is to determine whether or not a baby can pass through the mother's vagina, particularly in those cases where labor fails to progress and the mother's pelvis is suspected of being too narrow. However, this procedure cannot provide pertinent information regarding the ability of the baby's head to mold to the mother's pelvis or the capacity of her pelvis to widen in response to pressure from her child's head.

Apart from its questionable diagnostic value, the practice of X-ray pelvimetry is suspected of causing childhood leukemia. Studies conducted at an Illinois medical center found there were 4.8 deaths per 1000 in those babies who were not exposed in utero, as opposed to 7.6 deaths per 1000 in those exposed.

Factors to Weigh

Although the mounting evidence about the risk of X rays and the limited value of pelvimetry has led some health facilities to declare a moratorium on them, at some hospitals 6 out of 100 laboring women will have an X ray done. With the possible exception of the woman with a breech baby who wants to attempt a vaginal delivery, the consensus is that pelvimetry should no longer be a part of a birth attendant's diagnostic repertoire. If an X ray of your pelvis is ordered during labor or at any other time in pregnancy, be sure you know and understand why, and make sure this information is recorded on your medical chart.

CESAREAN: WHAT EVERY EXPECTANT MOTHER SHOULD KNOW

Though most new parents feel only immense relief and gratitude when a cesarean delivery has safeguarded their baby's well-being, there is no denying that many mothers who could not experience a vaginal birth sense a social stigma attached to a cesarean and feel some anger and guilt as a result. One of the criticisms leveled at Lamaze and other childbirth classes that advocate an unmedicated, natural birth is that prospective parents are told little about cesarean delivery though statistics show one in six babies is lifted out of the mother's womb by a surgeon. Skimpy information means many women simply don't know what questions to ask when their doctor recommends a cesarean. A mother's joy in having a healthy baby born by cesarean may be diminished because she wasn't adequately informed and couldn't participate fully in this decision.

In addition to advice about how to reduce your chance of having a cesarean, included here are suggestions on ways to avoid problems if abdominal delivery is necessary, as well as physical and emotional reactions you are apt to experience during childbirth and postpartum.

Cesarean section comes from the Latin "caedere" and "seco," both meaning to cut. The five most common reasons for performing a C-section in the United States are:

(1) mother's pelvis is judged to be too small for her baby to pass through, referred to as feto-cephalopelvic disproportion
(2) mother's labor fails to progress or is slow because of weak or infrequent contractions
(3) baby is in breech position rather than the normal vertex or head-first presentation
(4) baby's oxygen supply is believed to be in jeopardy, termed fetal distress; irregular heartbeat pattern may be detected by electronic fetal monitor
(5) mother has had a previous cesarean section.

Preexisting medical conditions that usually warrant abdominal delivery include pregnancy-induced hypertension, severe toxemia, placenta previa (placenta located above or near the cervix rather than higher up in the uterus, thus blocking baby's exit), active vaginal herpes infection and, possibly, maternal diabetes. An emergency cesarean is required in the unlikely event that the umbilical cord is knotted or wrapped tightly around the baby's neck or in the unusual case of a prolapsed cord (when this lifeline slips out ahead of the baby). In all three instances, the pinched supply line cuts off food and oxygen necessary to the baby. If the membranes have been ruptured for 24 hours and labor is not progressing, a cesarean is a strong possibility.

Reducing Your Chance of Having a Cesarean

In 1981, 17.9 percent of babies born were delivered by cesarean, a threefold leap over 1970. According to Selma Taffel of the government's National Center for Health Statistics, the rates in 1981 "were highest in the Northeast, among older women, among married women, and in proprietary (private) hospitals. . . C-section rates were highest in 1981 where expected principal source of payment is Blue Cross and lowest for self-pay patients." Fewer vaginal deliveries for breech babies and the trend away from using forceps, though, are not the main reasons for the steady increase. The overall rise is primarily traced to the increased frequency in the diagnosis of dystocia (pronounced dis-to′se-ah), a catch-all term. It comes from the Greek word "dys," meaning abnormal, and "tokos," childbirth or labor. This diagnosis, a *subjective* judgment, may mean that the baby's head will not fit through the mother's bony pelvis (medical jargon is cephalo- or feto-pelvic disproportion) or that labor is not progressing or a combination of both.

Routine reliance on electronic fetal monitors has given birth to the frequent diagnosis of fetal distress, another term where there is room for a lot of interpretation. Abnormal or irregular heartbeat patterns may worry one doctor but not another (see "Electronic Fetal Monitors: Pros and Cons," p. 232).

Dystocia and fetal distress are often legitimate reasons for a cesarean, but these two popular diagnoses happen to fit in well with a play-it-safe or defensive-medicine approach. The fear of malpractice—particularly those lawsuits *for failing to perform* a cesarean—prompt some obstetricians to operate at the least sign of trouble. Although surgery carries with it some risks to both the mother and baby, abdominal delivery represents the ultimate in birth-trauma protection.

Dozens of other explanations and allegations abound for the startling increase in cesareans, but cross-examining a doctor about legal, economic or personal motives won't get you very far. Regardless of how much you trust your health adviser, be sure you understand exactly why a cesarean is necessary, discuss possible options and take steps to double-check the diagnosis:

(1) If the size of your pelvis or your baby's head (cephalo- or feto-pelvic disproportion) is the reason, get a second opinion—not just a telephone consultation—by another doctor who actually examines you; hospitals that show a reversal in the cesarean trend are those with such built-in peer review. Incidentally, an

X-ray pelvimetry is ill-advised (see "X-Ray Pelvimetry Warning," p. 259).

(2) If prolonged or difficult labor is the reason, before agreeing to a cesarean birth, ask about other ways to move it along such as:
- walking around
- relaxing in a bath (if your membranes haven't ruptured)
- try an oxytocic drug such as Pitocin, to stimulate contractions
- a pain blocker such as an epidural, so you can rest for a while and regain your strength
- experimenting with squatting and other positions during the second stage of labor that may help you bear down more effectively
- a forceps delivery.

    For more suggestions, see "Long Labor: Let the Sun Set Twice?" (p. 246).

(3) If your baby is in breech position with its chin tucked down against its chest and weighs no more than about 8 pounds, discuss a trial of labor (see "Breech Position: Special Handling," p. 186).

(4) If fetal distress is detected by an internal electronic fetal monitor, ask for confirmation by a sample of your baby's scalp blood to measure acid balance (another clue that the oxygen supply may be low); pH determination is regarded by many as the most objective evaluation of fetal distress, although not all hospitals have the capability of doing fetal scalp sampling. (In order to obtain a very small blood sample, a minuscule needle is guided through the vagina and pricks the baby's skin.)

(5) If you have had a C-section before, discuss the possibility of delivering vaginally this time (see "After Cesarean: Natural Birth," p. 117).

If a cesarean is decided on, there is time, except in case of acute emergency, to question your medical team about such concerns as the timing of surgery or types of anesthesia. Before reviewing the checklist, "Ways to Avoid Problems" (p. 266), here is a rundown on the surgical procedure itself.

What to Expect

The hospital environment, particularly the operating room, can be scary even if you've had surgery before. Knowing the sequence of events and the sensations you may experience will reduce some apprehension and also help you plot out the best possible delivery. There are bound to be some deviations, especially at those hospitals where nonemergency cesareans are performed in a family-centered setting, which encourages the father's participation during childbirth and, if the mother wants, immediate bonding and breast-feeding with her newborn.

> ### Low Bikini Incision Preferred
>
> A series of separate incisions are made. The abdomen is opened first, followed by a cut in the uterus. The bikini, or transverse (horizontal), incision leaves about a 6-inch half-moon scar, and a similar crosswise incision inside opens the lower section of the uterus, which saves blood and heals with a strong scar unlikely to split if you decide to deliver vaginally in the future.
>
> A classical (vertical) incision is done in some emergency situations or if the baby is in an awkward position or very large. Another reason for a lengthwise cut in the main part of the uterus is to avoid damaging the placenta if it is positioned near the bottom of the uterus instead of the top. The classical opening means more blood loss and increases the risk of infection to the mother.
>
> In determining whether or not you can deliver vaginally next time, it's only the type of *uterine* cut that matters—a classical incision would be a bit more likely to rupture from the strain—the *abdominal* cut is unimportant.

Standard preoperative procedures vary, depending on your obstetrician's standing orders, hospital policy and whether speed is of the utmost importance to your baby. In the case of a planned cesarean, blood samples and other lab work sometimes can be done on an outpatient basis to avoid staying in the hospital the night before. Prepping usually includes an enema, a shave of the abdominal and upper pubic area, an IV hookup, which consists of a hollow needle slipped into a vein in your hand or arm, and a urinary catheter, which is essentially a tiny plastic tube inserted into your bladder. Some of these procedures may be done before you are brought to the delivery/operating room.

In nonemergency situations, your child will be born about 15 minutes after you have been given anesthesia. Regional anesthesia, such as an injection into the spinal area, may numb you from the lower rib cage to your toes. General anesthesia is reserved for acute emergencies; the risks to both the mother and unborn baby are greater with it, and postoperative recovery also takes longer. Although the thought of being awake during surgery may make you squeamish, many new mothers say that seeing the baby being born and hearing the first cry makes you forget the rest. (For more information on your choices, see "Drugs During Childbirth," p. 236.) If you choose, mirrors can be positioned so you can see your baby's birth; however, this is usually not done until after the abdominal and uterine incisions are made. Once the womb is open, the baby's head and body are gently lifted out. Slight sensations of pressure, pulling or nausea may be felt during the birth and also when the placenta is removed.

While the baby is examined and admired, the doctor will need about 30 to 45 minutes to sew up your uterus and the outermost layer of skin. With regional anesthesia, you may feel up to holding your baby until the anesthesia begins to wear off. The father or hospital staff can help position the child by your side. You may be wheeled into the recovery room or back to your own room; expect frequent routine checks on your blood pressure, pulse and bleeding. Depending on hospital policy, the baby may be taken immediately to a special-care nursery or the regular one for all newborns for observation—often for 24 hours. Complete bed rest is usually ordered for you for at least six hours, followed by taking a few steps with someone's assistance. Walking—although painful—is crucial to getting your blood to circulate properly again. Grogginess and nausea are not uncommon aftereffects if you had general anesthesia. The IV and catheter may be left in for a few days. Your recovery will depend a lot on why a cesarean was performed, how long you labored beforehand, your general physical stamina and how quickly your body repairs itself.

Physical and Mental Recovery

Parents who have a positive attitude about their cesarean or those mothers with a sense of relief that birth is over, especially if they labored hard and long first, probably won't find this necessary reading. But many women who invested much energy in planning and preparing for their childbirth experience may have a rough time adjusting to motherhood.

If you're depressed, in large part it's due to the physical pain you feel every time one stomach muscle moves. Although it hurts even to laugh, remember that tomorrow you will feel much better. There are lots of ways to speed up your post-op recovery, and the faster that happens, the sooner your attention will shift away from the operation to your new family.

Headache or shoulder pain caused by anesthesia is normal. At about the time the tender, bruised feeling subsides, your incision will start to itch as new skin forms to aid the healing process. Another discomfort that is likely to throw you is sharp gas pains, another necessary rite of passage to recovery. Here are some coping tips to help you through the first days:

- Walking around even though you hurt, because it's essential to get your blood circulating and intestinal tract moving.
- Consider pain medication when the anesthetic begins to wear off, instead of waiting until the discomfort intensifies; make sure any pain-killer is one of the preferred drugs if you are breast-feeding.
- Nursing your baby may be painful the first few times, but you will soon get used to those uterine muscles moving; cesarean recovery may be hastened by breast-feeding, and it's a great morale booster for many new mothers.
- Get out of bed the same way you did when pregnant, by rolling to your side and elevating yourself with one arm.
- Avoid carbonated beverages and ice-cold drinks, which aggravate gas pains, but be sure to drink plenty of liquids.
- Practice abdominal tightening exercises by placing a pillow over your incision, locking your hands over your stomach and taking a deep breath and inhaling.
- Rest and sleep as often as possible, to build up your stamina.
- Wiggle your toes, flex your feet, bend your knees and do other gentle exercises while lying in bed.
- Rely on the staff to make things easier, such as helping to move your baby from one breast to the other to avoid pulling those tender stomach muscles.

Playing the role of a helpless, sick patient can zap your confidence and self-esteem. Anger toward hospital staff, jealousy of other mothers, fear about subsequent deliveries, disappointment with yourself are some of the emotional repercussions that are likely to take a while to resolve. Guilt at having negative feelings when you think you are supposed to be elated over your healthy infant—one of the most common anxieties—may be further complicated if you don't feel close to your baby. Although the importance of parent-newborn attachment, or bonding, is much touted, there is no evidence that you've missed the once-in-a-lifetime opportunity for a close relationship with your son or daughter. Here are some suggestions on how to cope with the emotional baggage:

- Get out your feelings of resentment, failure, self-pity, regardless of how irrational they may seem.
- Remember, radical hormonal changes are partly to blame for your emotional upheaval. To understand more, see "Blues and Depression: It's Not All in Your Mind" (p. 313).
- Communicate with your mate and remember that he may share some of your disappointment; chances are that he too feels emotionally exhausted from the events surrounding the decision to have a cesarean.

- Try to switch rooms if you are bothered by being around mothers who had vaginal deliveries.
- Confess your need for reassurance as well as voicing such worries as "What kind of scar will I have?"
- Remember: Time heals.

If the psychological hangover continues for quite a while, you may want to consider joining or starting a support group for cesarean parents (see "Information Sources, Organizations," p. 268).

Ways to Avoid Problems

Though a cesarean ranks with an appendectomy as one of the safest operations around, it is still major surgery. You will lose more blood and be more prone to infection than if you had delivered vaginally. The chance of your baby's having minor breathing problems at first is greater, particularly if the cesarean is performed too early, when the baby's lungs may not have matured. Postpartum depression is more common and recovery time is longer.

If you have advance warning that sectioning is a strong possibility, here are a few key questions you might want to explore to keep unexpected surprises to a minimum and to ensure the quality of care to which you are entitled.

(1) Learn about your hospital's policy regarding cesarean deliveries and, if you don't want to compromise and if time permits, consider switching birth sites and perhaps doctors. Is there a built-in peer review system? Is your husband allowed to be with you in the operating room? If you are not married, does the hospital permit a friend or relative with you during delivery? If your baby appears healthy, can the child be with you in the recovery room? Can the newborn and father stay with you overnight?

(2) Check your insurance policy. A cesarean often costs about twice as much as a vaginal delivery, but probably you needn't worry, because everything will be covered.

(3) Ask for a second opinion, not just a telephone consultation between your physician and another obstetrician. As with any major surgery, it is expected that a second doctor approve a cesarean operation.

(4) Discuss the timing of a cesarean in the event of elective surgery. Inquire how the doctor has determined whether or not your baby's lungs are mature. A less conventional approach is to delay surgery until labor begins spontaneously, so as to reduce the risk of premature birth and Respiratory Distress Syndrome (RDS), although it is customary to perform a section prior to one's due

date, when the uterus is still quiet, meaning that there are no contractions.

(5) Ask for a trial of labor if cephalo-pelvic disproportion is the reason for a cesarean, in order to test whether your pelvis is pliable or flexible enough to allow your baby to descend, remembering that the child's skull has movable bones designed to mold to your birth canal.

(6) Find out whether your obstetrician regularly makes a low transverse or bikini incision both in the abdomen and uterus. The vertical or classical cut is sometimes preferred by doctors who have been doing a lengthwise incision for years.

(7) Discuss with the anesthesiologist the different regional anesthesia he or she usually gives and inquire about side effects for both yourself and the baby. Consider asking about the dosage for a regional spinal or epidural if you are small or thin to avoid being given too much anesthetic.

(8) Have specific preferences written on your medical chart, such as trial of labor, type of incision, kind of anesthesia, no X-ray pelvimetry.

(9) Ask to share a room with a mother who also had a cesarean or think about paying the extra money for a private room if you want your husband to spend the night with you.

Factors To Weigh

Even if there is no reason to suspect a cesarean will be necessary, one way to maintain control over the situation is to plot out a "just-in-case" scenario. Trust in your doctor is essential, but that does not mean you should accept his or her diagnosis on blind faith. Though you may be disappointed that your childbirth experience did not match your plans, remember that the most important thing is the final product. If you feel cheated, remember that once a cesarean no longer necessarily means always a cesarean. The chances of delivering your next baby vaginally are greater today than ever before.

Information Sources

ADDITIONAL READING

Breastfeeding after a C/Sec. Available for $.50 from La Leche League, 9616 Minneapolis Ave., Franklin Park, IL 60131.

Cesarean Birth Experience, by Bonnie Donovan (Boston: Beacon, 1977). A comprehensive guide to cesarean childbirth.

Cesarean Childbirth, by Christine Coleman Wilson and Wendy Roe Hovey (New York: Signet, 1980). About half the book is devoted to recovery and emotional responses.

Facts About Cesarean Childbirth, by National Institute of Child Health and Human Development. A handy pamphlet that is available free from the Office of Research Reporting, NICHD, NIH, Room 2A32, Bldg. 31, 9000 Rockville Pike, Bethesda, MD 20205.

Father's Fact Sheet for the Unexpected Cesarean. Available for $.50 from C/Section Experience of Northern Illinois, 1220 Gentry Rd., Hoffman Estates, IL 60195.

Silent Knife, by Nancy Wainer Cohen and Lois Estner (South Hadley, MA: J. F. Bergin Publishers, 1983). Disputes the need for most cesareans and describes success stories of women who have had vaginal births after cesarean.

Unnecessary Cesareans: Ways to Avoid Them, by Diony Young and Charles Mahan (Minneapolis: AM ICEA, 1980). This 30-page pamphlet available for $1.50 from International Childbirth Education Association, PO Box 20048, Minneapolis, MN 55420.

ORGANIZATIONS

Cesarean Connection
PO Box 11
Westmont, IL 60559
Literature, including monthly newsletter.

Childbirth Education Association (CEA)
Check your phone book for the local CEA, which probably offers cesarean preparation classes.

C/SEC, Inc.
22 Forest Rd.
Framingham, MA 01701
Information for those anticipating a cesarean and emotional support to new cesarean parents; publications and newsletters available.

You may also want to refer to "After Cesarean: Natural Birth," p. 117.

HEMORRHAGE AND POSTDELIVERY INFECTION

Moments after birth, your body shifts gears and shuts down pregnancy operations. Circulation is rerouted away from the womb, and the blood-lined uterus itself begins to shrink and expels the now-useless placenta. In a normal delivery the whole process means a blood loss of only about one or two cups, which your body anticipated by increasing your blood and fluid volume beforehand. Without the increase, there would be too little blood to keep your veins open, your circulatory system would collapse and you would go into shock. A minuscule number of mothers who do lose considerably more than one pint of blood within the first 24 hours risk not only going into shock but starving the cells of nutrient-rich blood and lowering resistance to infection as a result. Neither hemorrhage nor infection, however, is life-threatening unless undetected and left untreated, which isn't likely with periodic postpartum blood pressure, pulse and temperature checks.

Loss of too much blood can be caused by any one or a combination of malfunctions or minor tissue "accidents," including:

- *Tired or weak uterus.* Contractions usually start again soon after birth, to shorten and thicken uterine muscles. In this way the womb not only regains its normal shape and size but seals off blood vessels exposed by the detached placenta. When the uterus fails to contract, these vessels remain severed and blood flows freely. To encourage contractions, your abdomen may be massaged, artificial oxytocin may be given to stimulate contractions or your uterus may be manipulated by pressure from outside and inside the womb (termed bimanual compression).

- *Stubborn placenta.* If the placenta refuses to separate fully from the uterine wall despite a shrinking uterine surface area, either blood pools in the pocket behind it or, if only part of the organ falls away, the remaining section prevents the uterus from contracting well enough to "tie off" the now-exposed blood vessels. One approach for treating a retained placenta is to watch and wait. Other methods include using artificial oxytocin to induce even more contractions, or manually exploring the lining of the womb wall and scraping away the tissues (D and C).

- *Cuts and tears.* Some cuts and tears are common and usually heal quickly by themselves, but they do mean a little more blood loss. With an episiotomy, for example, you can expect to lose a few extra ounces. Other cuts or tears in your vagina, cervix or vulva could result from a difficult forceps delivery or from pushing too hard or too quickly when your baby crowned. Bleeding can be checked by sewing you up or, in the case of some vaginal tears, by packing, too, much the way a nose is packed with gauze if it bleeds profusely.

- *Infections.* If tissues in your reproductive tract are damaged by birth, they temporarily lose some of their infection-fighting strength, allowing germs that may have migrated up your vagina from the outside to breed and spread. If you do have an infection, the signs will be localized pain and a fever, which are easily treated with antibiotics. If you are breast-feeding, be sure to find out if the drug will "contaminate" your milk, since substitute medications probably can be used that won't require you to stop nursing.

If blood loss is significant, both the blood volume and the number of red cells will have to be replaced, usually by blood transfusions. Another, less medically acceptable treatment is to concentrate on replacing the iron, the major component of red blood cells. This is accomplished through megadoses of iron in foods and tablets along with other vitamins, minerals and protein.

PREMATURE BABIES AND OTHER NEWBORNS NEEDING INTENSIVE CARE

If your baby is born unequipped to function on its own, you will probably consider the equipment that surrounds your son or daughter an additional source of anxiety. Besides feeling frightened and confused, you are likely to wonder why it had to happen to you, to your baby. Neonatal intensive-care nurseries can be upsetting and intimidating to parents initially, but as one mother notes, "Once I got involved with my baby's treatment, that gave me courage and hope...it helped, understanding what each wire and tube was for, and which machines were monitors and which were actually for life support."

About 1 in 13 newborns in the U.S. depends on a highly controlled environment to stay alive. The greatest battle for most babies born before 37 weeks' gestation is breathing—termed Respiratory Distress Syndrome, meaning that their tiny lungs lack the lubrication needed to expand fully and adequately perform the oxygen–carbon-dioxide exchange process, often requiring the assistance of a ventilator. The breathing center in the central nervous system of a premature baby is not completely developed either, frequently causing irregular respiratory patterns, so monitors are necessary to provide a continuous read-out of respiratory and heart rates. A premie who is underweight, as most invariably are, has the added problem of maintaining proper body temperature, calling for an isolette or incubator to keep the temperature within the range required for optimal growth. Most premies do not have fully mature digestive systems or coordinated suck/swallow reflexes, and need intravenous and/or tube feedings for nutritional support. Even some babies born at or near term occasionally need special care. Some may have a transient, mild form of respiratory distress, others an excessively high bilirubin level or need the care of a pediatric cardiologist or surgeon. Also, a baby who did not receive enough oxygen during the birth process will need close observation and care, as will a newborn with pneumonia or some other infection. Until all systems—circulatory, central nervous, digestive, respiratory— are ready to perform on their own, these babies will be nurtured and monitored in a special-care nursery, a neonatal or newborn intensive-care unit (NICU).

Not every hospital is equipped to care for a high-risk infant, but there should be at least one regional "Level III" center located reasonably close to where you live. In order to prevent duplication of costly equipment, a hospital becomes a regional center and is outfitted for neonatal intensive care based on population density. Given enough notice, your doctor can arrange for you to deliver in the same center where your newborn can get special care. If not, your baby can be safely and swiftly transferred to the nearest one via ambulance, "baby bus" (specially equipped for transporting newborns), airplane or even helicopter.

Your pediatrician may not actually assume the care of your child, but ask that a neonatologist (a physician specializing in newborns or high-risk infants) take over. By virtue of the intensive-care unit's location in a large medical center, too, a talent pool, including cardiologists, neurologists, respiratory therapists and even developmental psychologists, is readily available. The nurses and doctors in the NICU consider the support of the parents an integral part of the care of their infant and will explain what is being done for your baby and make you more comfortable with understanding the function of any equipment involved.

How to Cope

Besides the usual postpartum emotional highs and lows, you face the additional strain of adapting to a situation you probably never expected. Negative reactions about yourself, your child, the intensive-care nursery and the hospital staff are common and normal. You may experience:

- depression and anxiety at the initial separation, which tends to be especially strong during the first day home
- distress, possibly revulsion, at all the high-tech equipment and the extent to which your baby is "wired"
- disappointment over your baby's scrawny, feeble appearance
- guilt that you couldn't carry your baby to term, and the feeling that you are somehow responsible
- moodiness that probably is a combination of postpartum blues and too much time to dwell on what has happened

- fear of touching or holding your baby because of all the wires and tubes
- feeling useless or helpless because the hospital staff and machines seem to be replacing you, at least temporarily
- the stress of traveling back and forth from your home to the hospital, and the financial strain
- doubts about your ability eventually to care for your baby without the help of nurses and machines
- being afraid to hope that your baby survives.

The usual steps in getting acquainted, such as touching, cuddling, feeding or nursing, though limited to some degree by your baby's condition, are still possible and strongly encouraged by the hospital staff. Human contact is vitally important, according to studies that have found preterm babies gain weight *more* readily when they are able to be cuddled, held and rocked. Focusing on your baby's individual characteristics and personality can help you feel closer to your child in the face of mechanical and physical isolation. Breast-feeding will probably not be possible until the sucking and swallowing reflex is fully coordinated or until your baby's digestive system can tolerate pure mother's milk. Meanwhile, you may still be able to hold your baby while he or she is receiving your breast milk or commercial formula via a feeding tube. NICU staffs also stress the importance of talking to your baby. No matter how tiny he or she is, your newborn needs to feel your touch and hear your voice.

Social workers at the hospital can help out if there are communication problems between you and the medical staff, and can counsel you about financial concerns. They can also put you in touch with local support groups, made up of parents whose children are in similar situations, and lend a hand in planning the homecoming.

Since it is frequently not feasible to visit as often as you'd like, daily telephone contact with your baby's nurses and doctors can help, as can having the nurses periodically take pictures for you to bring home. When your baby requires less intensive care it is sometimes possible for the regional center to make arrangements for him or her to be transferred to a hospital near your home.

Length of Hospital Stay

Your baby may need to be in the intensive-care unit anywhere from a few hours for observation to several months for more aggressive treatment. Expect daily ups and downs in the infant's condition; small setbacks, including weight loss, are normal. The first move out of intensive care can occur once your infant:

- tolerates feedings
- breathes effectively and regularly

- regulates his or her own temperature (when he or she weighs about four pounds, the baby can be "weaned" from the isolette to a crib)
- has recovered from any necessary surgery
- is free from infection.

Generally the only requirements for final graduation from the hospital are to be consistently gaining weight and to be able to take sufficient breast milk or formula by breast or bottle at each feeding. Some centers will take advantage of this final period to teach you how to respond to your baby's needs (including techniques for infant CPR, cardiopulmonary resuscitation), how to spot any signs of distress and generally to reinforce the confidence in mothering that you may have lost along the way. That you feel comfortable enough to assume your baby's care is also a prerequisite for discharge home. Premies are often ready to go home very close to the time of their mother's due date.

Translating Medical Terms

One way to feel more at ease in the special-care nursery is to learn the language. Here are some of the most common terms you may hear:

- *Apnea.* Prolonged pauses in breathing that may require tactile stimulation.
- *Bilirubin.* A normal by-product of hemoglobin (the substance that carries oxygen and gives blood its ruby color); the presence of too much bilirubin in your baby's blood causes the skin to have a yellow or jaundiced tinge. A common cause of this is simply that the baby's liver is not yet fully mature. A set of special lights over your baby's isolette may be used to help excrete the bilirubin. In this case, the infant will be unclothed, to expose the skin to the light, and the eyes will be covered with soft cotton patches for protection (see "Newborn Jaundice: Common but Rarely Serious," p. 291).
- *Blood gases.* A lab test determining the acid-base balance and amount of oxygen and carbon dioxide found in the baby's blood. This reveals how well the lungs, heart and kidneys are performing and indicates any changes needed in oxygen concentration and ventilator settings.
- *Cyanosis or duskiness.* Describes the gray-blue tinge of the baby's skin if the blood is poorly oxygenated.
- *Heel stick.* A procedure used to draw blood from your baby's heel.
- *Dextrostix.* The approximation of blood-sugar level, obtained by taking a drop of blood from a finger or toe.
- *Incubator/isolette.* Little plastic-enclosed beds that attempt to

duplicate, as much as possible, the environment of the womb by conserving body heat and moisture, and provide some isolation from germs; expandable openings along the front allow you and the medical team to touch and treat your child.

- *Intubation.* Insertion of a small tube through the mouth or nose into the airway to help your baby breathe; can be connected to a ventilating machine to provide necessary pressure and number of breaths for the lungs to function properly.
- *Monitors.* Machines that continuously detect heart action and breathing by wire "leads" taped to your baby's body; a potentially adverse change in respiration or heart rate will set off an alarm by the infant's bed.
- *Umbilical artery catheter (UAC).* A thin plastic tube inserted into a blood vessel in your baby's navel, a convenient place from which to sample blood and deliver fluids intravenously; since your baby has no nerve endings here, this is a painless procedure.

Information Sources

ADDITIONAL READING

Born Early, by Dr. Mary Ellen Avery and Georgia Litwack (Boston: Little, Brown, 1983). One premie in an intensive-care unit is followed until he goes home. Photos and text.

"Little Babies—Born Too Small, Born Too Soon." Pamphlet about preterm babies. Available free from Office of Research Reporting, National Institute of Child Health and Human Development, NIH, Bethesda, MD 20014.

Premature Babies: A Handbook for Parents, by Sherri Nance (New York: Arbor House, 1982). Practical reference guide for parents that includes advice about handling the financial load.

The Premature Infant—A Handbook for Parents. Available for $3.00 from Hospital for Sick Children, Room 1218, 555 University Ave., Toronto, Ontario, Canada MSG1X8.

ORGANIZATIONS

Hospital neonatal intensive-care nurseries have counselors and social workers to help with questions about where to stay, insurance coverage and other financial concerns.

Parents of Prematures
13613 NE 26th Pl.
Bellevue, WA 98005

Parent Support Group Packet on how to start a local group is available for $2.00; also has newsletter and provides advice on breast-feeding.

Parents of Prematures
% Houston Organization for Parent Education, Inc.
3311 Richmond, Suite 330
Houston, TX 77098
"Resource Directory," listing nationwide support groups for parents of premies, is available for $3.50.

IF YOUR BABY DIES

What you are feeling now, no one can know unless she's been through it. After the shock and disbelief, in your anger, you search for someone or something to blame, which often finds its way back to you. In the search for answers, many parents feel guilty, as though they were somehow responsible. A roller coaster of emotions is likely to plague you in the weeks and months to come—on one day you may feel overwhelmed by despair, and on another, a strange, indifferent calm.

"Push it out of your mind; pretend it never happened" is the advice that often causes delayed depression, months or even years later. It takes a long time to pull yourself together—to accept your loss—but confronting the reality of your baby's death is the first step in getting past the grief. Some hospitals have a neonatal hospice program designed to help parents—and even the hospital's own staff—better come to terms with the death of a newborn. A quiet room away from the intensive-care nursery or from other new mothers, where parents can be alone with their child, is sometimes available. Many times bereaved parents are encouraged to name the baby and to focus their feelings of grief on tangible objects, such as a photograph of their child, a lock of hair, the hospital bracelet. However, many couples find it too difficult to hold or even to look at their baby. Understanding the initial disbelief and agony, hospitals often save the baby, along with its belongings, for several days, just in case the parents change their minds.

If the cause of death is unknown, a postmortem examination may be advisable, to help assure you that you were not to blame and to help quell natural fears about whether your next baby will live. Some couples haven't the strength to discuss the autopsy results, but months later may decide they need to know, especially if they are considering another pregnancy.

A memorial service or baptism is another way parents, as well as their relatives and friends, can accept the baby's death, since it is a public acknowledgment. Social workers at the hospital can help with the arrangements, and the hospital chapel may be the best place, particularly for those couples who don't belong to a place of worship. A ceremony also has the effect of spreading the news, so you are less likely to be asked awkward and painful questions by well-meaning but unknowing friends and neighbors.

Compassionate Friends and other community support groups can help balance the lack of understanding that you find even in your closest friends. These organizations are made up of parents who not only have gone through the living hell you are experiencing but have found ways to come to terms with death. You may still feel a tremendous need four, five or six months later to talk about it; and "shadow grief"—that is, a particular sense of sadness—may surface at holidays or on what would have been your child's birthday. Rather than sharing your sorrow with friends or relatives who may, by a later date, prefer to forget, sessions with these support groups—even months later—can help you unburden yourself and let your feelings out.

Many people who urge you to forget what happened also encourage you to get pregnant soon. While it's important to look to the future, some experts caution that you first need to come to terms with your grief and allow your body to recover fully, pointing out that your next child deserves the best physical and psychological environment possible. One couple we spoke with, however, felt compelled not to wait. The mother was pregnant again within six months, and they just celebrated their daughter's first birthday.

Whether through friends, support groups, books or professional help, facing the reality of the death, of your grief and perhaps of your anger is essential in understanding your loss and keeping it from destroying you. Otherwise, the next child may have to bear all the expectations and dreams for the baby who did not survive. As one mother who lost her child years ago says, it is important "not to forget, but to remember and go on."

Information Sources

ADDITIONAL READING

After a Loss in Pregnancy: Help for Families Affected by a Miscarriage, a Stillbirth, or the Loss of a Newborn, by Nancy Berezin (New York: Simon & Schuster, 1982). Also includes good bibliography.

When Pregnancy Fails, by Susan Borg and Judith Lasker (Boston: Beacon Press, 1981). Readable and comprehensive, covering miscarriage, stillbirth and infant death.

ORGANIZATIONS

Amend
4323 Berrywich Terrace
St. Louis, MO 63128
Provides information for those parents who want to start their own group to reach out to the newly bereaved on a one-to-one basis.

Compassionate Friends
PO Box 1347
Oakbrook, IL 60521
Refers you to one of over 200 local groups in the country made up of parents who have suffered the loss of a child and are seeking support and understanding from other bereaved parents.

Infant Bereavement Group
52 Davis Avenue
White Plains, NY 10605

National Sudden Infant Death Syndrome Foundation
310 South Michigan Ave.
Chicago, IL 60604
Refers you to one of the 57 chapters in the country that offers support to bereaved parents and also advocates research into the causes of infant and child death.

Parents of Stillborn Newsletter
3509 NE 33rd St.
Tacoma, WA 98422

Resolve, Inc.
PO Box 474
Belmont, MA 02178
Support groups in 40 cities.

SHARE
St. John's Hospital
800 E. Carpenter
Springfield, IL 62702
Sister Jane Marie of St. John's Hospital will refer you to one of the 60 organizations in the SHARE network nearest to you.

Hours

After Birth

BONDING AND ROOMING-IN: OVERRATED OR NOT?

"I'm amazed, the number of hours I spend just looking at her," boasts a father about his two-day-old daughter. Eye contact, touching, nursing, talking and other expressions of affection immediately after birth are what people mean when they talk about "bonding." No separation is a main component of the bonding process; that is, your baby stays in your hospital room during the day or around the clock.

Numerous studies suggest that both the quantity and quality of interaction between you and your newborn may have such far-reaching consequences as strengthening your family unit and influencing your baby's psychological and physical development. Two leading researchers on bonding, Dr. Marshall Klaus and Dr. John Kennell, claim early parent-child attachment is "crucial to the survival and development of the infant." While you certainly have everything to gain and nothing to lose by making the most of those first minutes, hours and days with your baby, there's no real evidence that strongly supports the theories about bonding. Dr. Peter Vietze, of the government's National Institute of Child Health and Human Development, thinks the "results are equivocal. They suggest there's something there, but we don't know just what, nor how significant." Outright abuse or neglect may be a major reason for some infants' "failure to thrive," but the importance of bonding and rooming-in may be overrated. No one can argue that the first hours spent with your newborn are not some of the most memorable and intimate you'll have, but if unexpected events such as a premature delivery occur that delay your getting to know each other, don't think for a moment that you've lost out on the golden opportunity for a close relationship with your child.

Early Bonding

After the struggle and excitement of birth, your tiny baby will probably be in a quiet-alert state for about an hour, before falling asleep. Totally awake yet not crying, it is during this "sensitive period" that some experts believe babies are more keenly receptive to the new world around them. Your newborn not only is drinking in stimuli from you but is responding through clinging, gazing and sucking.

The degree of intimacy you will have depends on hospital policies as well as your and your baby's health. Many hospitals insist on adhering to their established ritual of cleaning, weighing and swaddling the infant before letting you hold her or him, but there is little or no interference with bonding during the first hour after delivery at those hospitals that encourage a family-centered birth experience. Of course, the newborn is never separated from the mother when deliveries occur at a birth center or home, unless medical complications arise.

Rooming-In

The unnatural fluorescent light in most hospital nurseries is reason enough to keep your baby in your own room; on the other hand, your son or daughter may not even be aroused by the other newborns howling in the nursery, and a solid night's sleep for you may make the most sense. Some hospitals don't allow 24-hour rooming-in and don't even honor your request to nurse "on demand" instead of at the scheduled 2:00 A.M. feeding. During the day, babies often are kept in the nurseries during pediatric rounds and visiting hours.

Perhaps the primary advantage of rooming-in is that it's a great way to get acquainted, without the distractions of home, in a secure setting where you can learn a lot about taking care of your baby from the hospital staff and other new mothers. It gives you a chance to become familiar with your baby's behavior—breathing, color change, bowel movements—so you have an idea of what is normal. Keep in mind that the sleeping patterns during the first few days will change, probably the day you go home.

Research shows that rooming-in helps develop more parental confidence, but, according to a 1980 study published in *Pediatrics*,

it must be pointed out that more than 90% of the women who did not receive rooming-in failed to demonstrate any evidence of parenting deficiency of minor or substantial degree by blind review. This indicates that, although rooming-in may enhance the mother-infant relationship to some degree, its absence usually is not associated with demonstrable harmful effects.

If you are keen on spending a lot of time with your newborn and rooming-in is discouraged or limited to certain daytime hours, you may want to abbreviate the traditional three- or four-day hospital stay so long as you and the baby are in good health (more in "Hospital Stay: How Soon Should You Go Home?" next page).

How to Cope

All of us, including obstetricians, would love to be able to predict in advance what labor will be like, but any number of minor or major complications may interfere with bonding right after birth. If you deliver by cesarean, for instance, you may feel too exhausted to reach out to your baby immediately. Or you may have weathered a 30-hour marathon labor, leaving you emotionally hung over and temporarily unable to respond. If prematurity or other neonatal health problems are the case, separation may be necessary while your baby gets stronger in the intensive-care nursery. And in the tragic situation of death, parents must decide whether or not to see and hold their baby. Some experts believe bonding with a stillborn infant enables parents to accept the death and helps them through the grieving process.

As unsettling as it may be, running a few of these possibilities through your mind ahead of time with plans on how to react might help you change gears if need be.

Factors to Weigh

Bonding with your child is a lifelong process and, say Drs. Klaus and Kennell, in no way "resembles the adhesive properties of the new, rapidly-acting glues." Your attachment only begins to set at birth, and even though immediate and close interaction with your baby will get both—or all three—of you off to a good start, a wonderful bonding session is, of course, no guarantee of faultless future rapport.

You should plan beforehand with your obstetrician or midwife what you'd like those first minutes to be like, and also find out about the hospital's rooming-in policy. Be sure to talk it over with your husband or labor coach so he or she can act as your aide-de-camp in case your instructions to the hospital staff upon admission are later forgotten.

Remember that you cannot write your labor and delivery

script, and in the event that circumstances prevent you from enjoying the initial contact with your newborn that you pictured, you have a lifetime to stimulate your child's growth and cement your emotional bond.

Information Sources

ADDITIONAL READING

Bonding: How Parents Become Attached to Their Baby, by Diony Young (Minneapolis: International Childbirth Education Association, 1977). Available from ICEA, PO Box 20048, Minneapolis, MN 55420.

Parent-Infant Bonding, by Marshall Klaus and John H. Kennell (St. Louis: C. V. Mosby, 1982). This revised edition attempts to give a more balanced view of bonding than the first book, which was titled Mother-Infant Bonding. Interaction between the father and infant is also emphasized.

Also see "Leboyer and Other Nontraditional Deliveries" (p. 114), "Eye Drops and Other Procedures Immediately After Birth" (p. 253) and "Hospital Stay: How Soon Should You Go Home?" (below).

HOSPITAL STAY: HOW SOON SHOULD YOU GO HOME?

Fifty years ago an obligatory ten days of hospital bed-rest followed childbirth. Today, barring any medical concerns, many hospitals allow you to cut short the standard three- or four-day stay and go home anywhere from two hours to two days after delivery, although the American Academy of Pediatrics recommends remaining in the hospital at least six hours after birth. Studies show that early discharge poses no greater health risk to the mother or infant provided there's adequate instruction beforehand on spotting such problems as newborn jaundice and taking proper care of such things as your stitches and your baby's umbilical cord.

You may want to escape the bland meals and dormitory environment of the hospital as quickly as possible or you may opt to have a few worry-free days at the hospital and take advantage of 24-hour nursing care, where you can pick the brains of the medical staff. Advantages and disadvantages stack up on both sides.

	EARLY DISCHARGE	STANDARD HOSPITAL STAY
Risk	Maternal infection, heavy bleeding; newborn jaundice may go undetected	Mother and newborn may run risk of infection(s) because of longer exposure to hospital bacteria
Rest	You may sleep better in your own bed, particularly if frequent checks by nurses or a blaring TV bothers you; more privacy as long as visitors are discouraged for several days	Catch up on sleep and relax by letting nurses wait on you and your baby; visiting hours protect you from getting too tired when socializing with friends and relatives
Mothering Confidence	Total responsibility for your baby may build confidence faster, particularly if hospital's rooming-in policy limits hours you can spend getting acquainted with your baby	Nursing staff can set your mind at ease about many common worries of a new parent and answer questions as they arise, making you feel more secure and confident
Breast-feeding	Your milk supply will be established sooner if your baby nurses "on demand" rather than feeding every four hours	Even if feeding on demand is hospital policy, staff may be too busy to answer your baby's cries promptly; your milk supply may take longer to come in
Convenience	A trip back to the hospital may be necessary if your baby needs blood work or if you decide to circumcise your son	People on hand to answer your questions, and hospitals often sponsor parties and classes on bathing your baby and breast-feeding, prior to discharge
Cost	Less expensive than standard hospital stay, but if you fail to receive adequate information on baby and postpartum care, the savings may be eaten up by more than the usual number of doctor visits	Each day spent in the hospital adds that much more to your bill, which, of course, is a major consideration if you are not insured or your policy doesn't provide blanket coverage for hospitalization

An overriding consideration in your decision is who will be with you at home. Equally important is that it be someone who won't get on your nerves, particularly during the first days at home, when it's only natural for you to be a nervous wreck from time to time.

Regardless of how long you plan to stay in the hospital, spend a little time reading up on how to get through the first few days (see "Help During Week One!" p. 297).

Factors to Weigh

This isn't a medical decision because early discharge will not be an option if you or your baby needs additional care. What really matters is where you will feel the most comfortable and relaxed. The hospital environment enables you to learn a lot from the staff and other mothers about handling an infant, and some women want and need the security of knowing that, every minute of the day and night, there is someone to ask. The familiarity of your own bed, food you relish and perhaps more privacy with both your partner and child make a speedy return home more appealing to others.

Regardless of when you decide to leave the hospital, jot down the phone numbers of both the maternity ward and the nursery. Don't hesitate to call for advice when your breasts are bursting and nothing works or when it's 3:30 A.M. and you know a diaper pin is not the reason your baby's been crying for two hours.

BREAST AND/OR BOTTLE?

The decision about whether or not to breast-feed is extremely personal. The evidence that mother's milk provides babies with a head start on good health is overwhelming, and even infant-formula manufacturers admit that it is a child's best possible source of nourishment. Babies also thrive, however, on commercial formula. What is most important to your baby's well-being is having a relaxed, loving and contented mother. If you intend to return to your job, several options exist. One is to nurse your child until you go back to work. Even one month is probably worthwhile just in terms of your antibodies being passed on through your milk. Some working mothers express their milk and leave it with the babysitter for the daytime feedings, which maintains the milk supply and prevents engorgement. The American Academy of Pediatrics recommends that, when possible, all infants be breast-fed for the first year, unless your doctor thinks otherwise. However, *don't* feel guilty if you bottle-feed. With the movement back to breast-feeding comes, unfortunately, a lot of psychological baggage for a working mother who cannot breast-feed her child—yet millions of babies have been raised successfully on formula.

Mothers will tell you there is nothing more rewarding than nursing a baby, but if you decide to bottle-feed, either for personal or medical reasons, don't feel guilty. If you aren't sure about nursing, the facts and comparisons outlined in the following chart may help you make up your mind. If you are still uncertain about breast-feeding, you may want to try it, since you can always change your mind later. The reverse is not true, however, as it is much more difficult, sometimes impossible, to switch from bottle to breast.

	BREAST	**BOTTLE**
Baby's Health	Colostrum, the yellowish clear fluid that precedes true milk, is rich in antibodies to fight infection until baby's own immune system is established. Mother's milk is almost always tolerated by her baby. Proteins in breast milk are easily digested and fats are easily absorbed. Baby cannot overeat; naturally limits itself to proper weight, according to recent studies; seldom becomes overweight or obese adult.	Infant formula linked to increased incidence of gastrointestinal disease, respiratory infection, allergies, overall higher hospitalization. More air is likely to be sucked into stomach, causing gas, cramps, spitting up and possibly vomiting. Baby may be allergic to certain infant formulas, so a trial-and-error period may be necessary.
Mother's Health	Nursing helps uterus shrink faster to its normal size. Hormones released by breast-feeding tend to relax the mother. Although mothers who nurse need to eat even more than the standard diet to produce nearly a	Unlike nursing mother, who must make sure to eat plenty of the right foods, with formula the mother can diet, and lose leftover pregnancy pounds. Mother is not restricted regarding drugs she can take, since the

BREAST	BOTTLE
quart of milk a day, it's estimated the energy used for lactating burns off about 500 calories a day over the normal expenditure; depending on your diet and metabolism, extra pounds may melt off.	baby will not be affected. Many lactation-suppressant drugs are suspected of posing health risks (i.e., estrogen drugs associated with higher incidence of blood clots).
Engorgement (oversupply of milk), which often occurs when milk supply is first established, several days after birth, may be painful and uncomfortable. Mother may experience discomfort caused by plugged ducts, sore nipples and other temporary breast infections.	

Nutrition

Balanced composition of carbohydrates, proteins, fats, minerals and vitamins. Higher levels of lactose, cystine and cholesterol than in formula, all necessary for development of brain and nerves.	As close as possible to mother's milk, but not a perfect nutritional match. Most formulas contain plenty of vitamins.

Purity of Milk

Mother's milk is as pure and harmless as whatever she consumes.	Infant-formula manufacturers must comply with federal guidelines on sterility, quality and recall procedures.
No sanitation worries and no spoilage unless pumped (expressed) milk is not refrigerated. Breast milk can be frozen and kept safely for at least one month.	Ready-to-drink formula has a shelf life and must be thrown out after a certain date if unopened. Once mixed, powdered formula should be drunk within 24 hours.

	BREAST	BOTTLE
Psychological Aspects	Pleasant way to nurture, and skin-to-skin contact enhances closeness. Nursing often has calming effect on infant, partly because of the familiar sound of mother's heartbeat and her scent. Mother may be embarrassed, nervous or have an aversion to breast-feeding, especially in public.	Similar degree of intimacy as with breast if mother (or father) holds baby close, smiles and snuggles during feedings. Mother may be more at ease with bottle than offering her breast.
Father's Role	Father is left out altogether if baby given breast milk exclusively for first three, possibly six months. Of course, father can participate if occasional bottle is given.	Father is on equal footing with mother in terms of having the opportunity to give his baby a bottle.
Sex and Birth Control	Hormones released by lactation usually mean little or no vaginal lubrication. Rhythm method of birth control is unreliable, since you may not menstruate, but you may continue to ovulate, i.e., produce an egg to be fertilized. The Pill or intrauterine device (IUD) is not advisable.	Business as usual once your hormones return to their prepregnancy state. You can then gauge your fertility period by keeping track of your menstrual cycle.
Convenience	Mother is equipped to feed wherever she goes, and her milk will be the perfect temperature. There is little difference between being at home and traveling.	Mother has more freedom to come and go as she pleases rather than timing her excursions away from home by the baby's feeding schedule.

BREAST	BOTTLE
If baby relies exclusively on breast milk, mother is tied down and cannot miss too many feedings or she risks decreasing her supply and/or feeling uncomfortable due to engorgement.	Frequent trips to the store to replenish your supply of infant formula unless you buy in quantity. Night feedings may mean a trip downstairs to the refrigerator. Preparation time is equivalent to making iced tea.
Certain blouses and other clothes make it difficult, if not impossible, to nurse discreetly.	

Cost

BREAST	BOTTLE
Minimal expense for 2–3 nursing bras, cloth or disposable nursing pads used for about the first six weeks, cream to prevent and/or treat sore and cracked nipples and possibly manual or electric breast pump.	Incidental expenses include bottles or nursers with disposable liners, nipples and nipple caps, heat-resistant mixing container. Major expense is formula, which can cost approximately $10.00/week once the baby begins to drink about 24 ounces, or four bottles, daily.
Breast milk is free and there's no waste, but mother must pay the price for a nutritionally sound daily diet.	

Suggestions on breast- and bottle-feeding are outlined in "Help During Week One!" (p. 297).

CIRCUMCISION: NOT A MEDICAL DECISION

Unless you know for sure it's a girl, give circumcision some thought before birth. Newborn circumcision is still a quasi-routine medical procedure in the United States, but one facing growing opposition even within the medical community. An uncircumcised male has a loose sleeve of skin, called foreskin, surrounding the tip of his penis, which slips back for urination and erection; a circumcised male—from Latin, meaning "cut around"—has had part of his foreskin surgically removed, leaving the penile tip permanently exposed.

Until recently, removal of the foreskin was thought not only to be religiously significant, particularly for Jews, but to be medically justifiable as well. In 1975 the American Academy of Pediatrics went on record saying that "there is no absolute medical indication for routine circumcision of the newborn . . . circumcision of the male neonate cannot be considered an essential component of adequate total health care." Still the debate continues, largely because a movement to forgo the procedure would mean a new generation of little boys growing up "different" from their fathers and from the rest of the locker-room crowd—a difference some fear could prove psychologically damaging. But those who favor leaving the penis alone point to the potential danger of emotional harm and risk of complications from the five-minute operation.

The United States, where 80 percent of all males are circumcised, stands alone in this dilemma, the only English-speaking country even approaching our rate being Canada, with less than 40 percent circumcised (fewer than 1 in 100 in England). Our disproportionate number may stem from the late 1800s, when the procedure was first encouraged by religious revivalists in this country as a way of discouraging masturbation, by eliminating the highly sensitive foreskin. Circumcision gained popularity for the better part of a century, building a momentum of conformity behind it. But today a deepening awareness of and concern over unnecessary hospital procedures may start to reverse the conformist tide. There are still some, though, who believe that the foreskin stands in the way of hygiene and optimal sexual performance.

	CIRCUMCISED	FORESKIN INTACT
Hygiene	prevents buildup of germs in small pocket between foreskin and tip of penis	encourages infection when germs are trapped under the skin, but build-up can be regularly cleaned simply with soap and water (similar to cleaning one's ears)
Health Risk	this surgery carries with it possible risk of excess bleeding and infection	no possible complications because no surgical procedure
	advocates claim it reduces chance of VD, penile and prostrate cancer, although there is no such evidence	tight foreskin is normal at birth unless it blocks urination; foreskin gradually retracts naturally as early as 3 years of age

	CIRCUMCISED	FORESKIN INTACT
Sexual Performance	tip of penis tends to be less sensitive than foreskin, so circumcision may prolong erection and/or alleviate premature ejaculation	nerve endings in foreskin may provide heightened sexual pleasure; sexual arousal may be more intense and rapid

If You Decide Against Circumcision

Newborn Hygiene. In most infants the foreskin has an opening only the size of a pinhole. Some doctors suggest the foreskin gently be pulled back daily to wash the head of the penis. On the other hand, some physicians and parents recommend that you leave the foreskin alone, even after your son is about 6 months old and the opening is enlarged, and just wash the genitals as you normally would.

Swelling or Infection. If there is swelling under the foreskin, gently clean with a Q-Tip and water; if swelling persists, contact your child's doctor.

If You Decide to Circumcise Your Son

Parental Permission. Though medical complications are unlikely, circumcision carries some risk, so, as with any surgical procedure, you must sign an informed-consent form.

Time Factor. The five-minute procedure will be done while you're both still at the hospital, ideally two or three days after birth. Babies who are premature, underweight or sick will have to wait until they're stronger.

Procedure/Pain-killer. Circumcision may be performed by your obstetrician or pediatrician. Because some hospitals allow medical students or interns to "practice" by performing this minor surgical operation, if your own doctor cannot do it, make sure your son is circumcised by an experienced physician. Techniques vary and include a "squeeze technique," usually done with a local anesthetic. In fact, a 1983 study published in the journal *Pediatrics* found that a simple injection of a numbing pain-killer considerably reduced the physiological stress and crying time for circumcised infants. Some hospitals permit you to watch the procedure, but most parents advise against it.

Recovery. Babies are generally sent straight off to the observation nursery. You may want to try to arrange to comfort your baby after the operation, maybe breast-feeding for a few minutes before he's whisked away.

Healing. One popular circumcision technique includes placing a plastic ring or holed cap over the tip of the penis. This protective cap falls off naturally as the wound heals, in about five to eight days. You will be given specific instructions on how to clean the penis, but don't hesitate to call your baby's doctor if you notice any unusual swelling or if you're simply concerned about the way it is healing.

Insurance. Circumcision usually costs about $100, and many health-insurance plans will reimburse only part of the physician's fee. Check your insurance policy to see if you are covered.

Factors to Weigh

Without real medical justification, the decision to circumcise becomes a personal and cultural one. Dr. Benjamin Spock says the advantages are cleanliness and practicality but advises that "parents should insist on convincing reasons for circumcision—and there are no convincing reasons that I know of." At a 1980 conference, "Benefits and Hazards of Hospital Newborn Care," Dr. John Scanlon of Georgetown University Medical School stated that "any benefit is possibly cosmetic" and cautioned that "the risks are real and include bleeding and infections."

A decision "for" is, of course, irreversible. One "against" leaves you free to change your mind later, though circumcision is probably best done while your son is very young, because the operation can be psychologically troubling when performed after infancy.

Information Sources

ADDITIONAL READING

American Academy of Pediatrics
P.O. Box 1034
Evanston, IL 60204
Single copies of two-page report on circumcision available for $.50.

"Routine Circumcision of the Newborn Infant: A Reappraisal," by David Grimes, *American Journal of Obstetrics and Gynecology*, 130 (1978), 125–129. Available at any medical library.

ORGANIZATIONS

INTACT Educational Foundation
6294 Mission Rd.
Everson, WA 98247
INTACT stands for Infants Need to Avoid Circumcision Trauma; literature available by sending self-addressed, stamped envelope.

NEWBORN JAUNDICE: COMMON BUT RARELY SERIOUS

If your baby's skin turns slightly yellow shortly after birth, it's usually no cause for alarm. In two out of three newborns, jaundice (from "jaundis," meaning yellow) is considered physiological; that is, part of an infant's normal adjustment to life outside the womb. The yellow tinge comes from a bile pigment called bilirubin, a natural waste product when red blood cells age and die, settling into your baby's tissue. Usually this yellow pigment is carried off through the blood to the liver, where an enzyme breaks it down and flushes it out the intestines. But if there is a surplus of bilirubin because of a large number of dying red blood cells and/or if the liver is unable to filter it out, the pigment backs up and colors skin, the whites of the eyes and other tissues yellow.

At birth, it is natural for babies to have an excess of red blood cells. Your baby's liver, however, may still be immature and lack the enzyme responsible for bilirubin breakdown. If jaundice (hyperbilirubinemia) results, from either one or both of these conditions, it shows up at about the third day after birth and disappears in a week to ten days, as the liver matures and the baby's red blood count levels off. If jaundice shows up sooner than this or stays around longer, the reason may be more serious, such as a blood-group incompatibility or some liver or metabolic disorder. This is reason for concern not only because of the underlying cause but also because of the possible risk associated with jaundice itself. Though bilirubin is relatively harmless in small amounts and for short periods in the body, in excess it is potentially toxic. The danger of a long bilirubin "visit" is that brain and nerve tissues will eventually host the pigment, which may irreparably damage the cells, a condition known as kernicterus.

Diagnosis and Treatment

Appearance. A baby with physiological jaundice begins to yellow at about the third day after birth, beginning at the head and working down the body. If your baby has jaundice at birth or develops it within the first 24 hours, or if the color spreads below the umbilical cord stump, a heel-stick blood test is usually done to determine the exact amount of excess bilirubin.

Blood Work. No precise threshold marks the passage from "safe" to "dangerous" levels for normal full-term babies, but there is a range:

safe = 6–7 milligrams/100 milliliters serum found in blood
acceptable = 10–12 milligrams/100 milliliters serum
unsafe = over 15 milligrams/100 milliliters serum

Bilirubin tolerance in premature or sick newborns is considerably lower.

Jaundice Meter. Recently the U.S. Food and Drug Administration approved the use of jaundice meters. By measuring light reflected from the baby's skin surface, these small, hand-held devices offer a pleasant alternative to blood-sample needle pricks and cost less than lab tests.

Jaundice usually requires no treatment other than letting nature take its course. Some experts suggest, though, that you help nature along by exposing your baby to lots of indirect bright sunlight. Others even prescribe doses of vitamin E because of its ability to preserve red blood cells. About 6 to 10 jaundiced babies in 100, however, require special medical treatment to keep excess bilirubin under control and prevent central nervous system damage. Except in extreme cases, where a baby's entire blood supply must be replaced (exchange transfusion), phototherapy is used, since certain types of light act to decompose the bile pigment. In phototherapy, babies are placed naked for 12 to 72 hours under "bili lights," with their eyes shielded. Blood samples taken periodically tell the hospital staff how well the lights are working on lowering the levels and when the "safe" range is reached. Bili lights are not without risk, however, as they have been shown sometimes to hinder brain development because of the lack of light stimulation and increased body temperature; they make parent-child attachment more difficult, owing to separation. Dr. M. Jeffrey Maisels of the Hershey Medical Center at Pennsylvania State University writes in a commentary to the International Childbirth Education Association bulletin:

Justifiable concern has been voiced regarding the potential long-term effects of phototherapy. However, in spite of the well documented effects of light on numerous organs and biological systems, no significant harmful effects of phototherapy have been noted in 20 years of use. Nevertheless, it is still the subject of intensive study and long-term complications cannot be ruled out. Thus caution is appropriate and the indiscriminate use of phototherapy is not justified, particularly in the full-term infant.

If phototherapy is to be used on your child, be sure you know that the bilirubin level is actually in the unsafe range. Some parents are disturbed by seeing their baby stretched out naked under the lights with patches covering its eyes. If this bothers you, ask about intermittent therapy, which would allow you to hold and feed your baby periodically throughout the treatment.

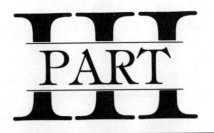

PART III

YOUR
FIRST YEAR
TOGETHER

9

The First Few Weeks

HELP DURING WEEK ONE!

Elation...exhaustion...depression...claustrophobia...these are the common, confused reactions for new parents struggling to learn how best to love and nurture their newborn. In many ways, this first week carries more emotional and physical stress than pregnancy. Your body has to heal, abrupt hormone changes trigger mood swings and blues and, to compound this adjustment process, you are on call 24 hours a day. Interrupted or sleepless nights take their toll. As one mother put it, "I was a zombie with a bad case of jet lag that lasted for weeks."

A predictable pattern will emerge eventually, but not just yet. What you need to remember now is that you and your baby will know each other that much better tomorrow, which definitely will make things easier. It also takes time for those maternal instincts to evolve. Upon leaving the hospital, many women suddenly feel overwhelmed by parental responsibility, and confidence in their ability to mother takes a dive. Decisions about how often to feed your baby or whether to offer a pacifier loom as significant and irreversible, although most often they are not.

At this juncture, simply picking up the baby is still not second nature. And you worry needlessly if his or her head drops backward accidentally, forgetting that this tiny champ survived the trauma of birth. Let's put to rest anxieties you may be harboring about the way your baby looks. Nearly all features might appear a bit peculiar—after all, the fetus-to-newborn transformation is not completed with the signing of the birth certificate.

Head. It will look enormous compared to the rest of the body, constituting about one-fourth of the total length. The egg-shaped head is the result of molding in the birth canal; it will regain its proper shape within a couple of weeks. A part of the scalp may be swollen if that area of the head tried to push its way through before the cervix was fully dilated, but this pocket of fluid, called a hematoma, takes a few weeks to disappear. The soft spots, or fontanels, at the top and back of the head prevented injury as the baby squeezed its way through the birth canal, and will grow together properly at about the time of or after your baby's first birthday.

Hair. This will be sparse for some, while other babies, particularly those born after their due date, will have lots. Either way, this hair will be replaced by new hair, probably with a color change as well. Many babies, especially premies, have delicate body hair, called lanugo, that is shed within a couple of weeks.

Skin. The skin is often wrinkled, and underdeveloped oil glands may cause tiny whiteheads around the nose and forehead. Don't fuss with them; they will go away. The skin color for Caucasians ranges from purplish to pale-pinkish gray; dark-skinned infants' coloring may be a shade or two lighter than their parents'.

Stork's Bites. Little marks on the face and neck, commonly called stork's bites or spots, usually vanish within a month or so. Your doctor can tell you whether such marks or red spots will be permanent birthmarks.

Eyes. They probably will be blue, but the color will change within the first year; a cross-eyed look and jerky movements are normal until the eye muscles learn to work in sync; a yellow discharge is nothing but a mild infection, which is very common. You may also notice crusting on the eyelids or lashes; this should clear up on its own.

Ears. Until the head assumes a more ordinary shape, the ears may look as though they stick out a bit. The only thing to be concerned about is any discharge other than wax. Q-Tips should not be used.

Dry Skin and Cradle Cap. Peeling is normal, particularly on the palms of the hands and soles of the feet. Loose skin on the scalp is also part of the shedding process. A little baby oil may help, but it's all right just to leave the cradle cap alone. The lips may peel too. "Sucking blisters," which are common on nursing infants, may also develop temporarily on the lips.

Abdomen and Umbilical Cord. A pot-bellied look is normal, and don't be alarmed if the stump of the umbilical cord looks dark and occasionally weeps a bit of blood and fluid. Try to pin your baby's diaper below the navel until the cord drops off. This usually takes a week or two. In the meantime, don't bathe the baby; simply wipe the navel with a cotton ball or Q-Tip dipped in rubbing alcohol two or more times daily.

Breasts. Even boys may have swollen breasts temporarily. This is due to an excess of hormones sponged up right before birth. A filmy discharge, playfully called witch's milk, is no cause for alarm.

Genitals. In proportion to the rest of the body, the genitals of both sexes usually look larger than normal. The scrotum or the vulva may also look red and a bit swollen, but the swelling will subside.

Vaginal Bleeding or Discharge. The vagina may ooze a blood-tinged discharge because of extra hormones absorbed in utero. This is common in girls during this first week. Also, a clear or whitish discharge does not signal trouble.

Arms and Legs. The arms also may seem out of proportion, and they actually are longer than the legs. The legs remain curled up in the fetal position, giving them a bowed appearance, and will straighten within the first year.

Hands and Feet. Until the new circulation route is established, these extremities may have less color than the rest of the body. The feet may be kinked to one side in what's called a "windblown effect," or they may be pigeon-toed or splayed outward, depending on how the baby lay in the womb. The normal position of the feet is usually established naturally within the first year.

Nails. Paper-thin nails may be long and sharp, which explains certain marks on the baby's face that will soon disappear. Do not cut nails for the first one to two weeks since the skin of the fingers adheres to the tips of the nails. It will recede after this time; in the meantime, keep hands covered with socks or closed shirt-sleeves. Then trim the baby's nails frequently with blunt-tipped scissors. One trick is to dip the nails in cornstarch so you can clearly distinguish the nail from the skin.

White Tongue. Milk tends to make an otherwise pink tongue white all over. Only be concerned if there are white patches, which may signal a mild infection such as thrush (see p. 324).

Bowel Movements. Some babies have a bowel movement at each feeding, others one a day and still others have as few as two to three a week. All are probably normal, and you will soon learn what your baby's regular pattern is. Don't be surprised at the color and consistency of stools during the first week or so. They can range from greenish-brown to bright green, from semi-fluid to mucous, and will gradually begin to change as your baby takes in more milk. Most infants grunt, strain, turn red and some even cry during a bowel movement, particularly as they grow older and solid foods are added to the diet. Diarrhea and constipation are discussed in "The Top Three Illnesses: Fever, Diarrhea, Ear Infection" (p. 385) and "Common Problems from Allergies to Rashes" (p. 391).

Hiccups, Sneezing, Coughing. These are normal, healthy ways of clearing the throat and air passages. It would be most unlikely for your week-old baby to get a cold.

Spitting Up. A moderate amount of regurgitation or vomiting is to be expected. Burping at a midpoint during feedings as well as afterward may help.

Crying

During the first few days, babies drift in and out of sleep. However, a more predictable schedule of feeding and sleeping will unfold within about three weeks. In the meantime, you have little way of knowing what the fussing or screaming is all about. Don't expect to be able to interpret what particular cries mean, and keep in mind that even if your child could talk, many times he or she would not be able to pinpoint what was wrong. The world of nipples and lights and blankets is still so new and unsettling, chances are it's just difficult for your baby to relax. When the cries sound louder and more desperate, it's easy to imagine there's a thread wrapped around the baby's toe. You check and find nothing wrong and decide to put on a clean diaper and perhaps offer your breast or a bottle, but the heart-wrenching sounds only get worse. Mysterious crying can make you a nervous wreck, and new parents' anxiety and frustration are aggravated by what we call the "nothing works twice" syndrome. You discover a particular rocking motion or a musical mobile that brings peace and quiet, but when such comforting techniques fail to work an hour later, you feel so helpless. Often, unexplained crying and overstimulation go hand in hand; some infants are just pleading to be left alone, and soon cry themselves to sleep. Remember that periods of irritability are *normal* and often have nothing to do with hunger, so don't be concerned that your baby isn't drinking enough, as long as he or she is wetting an average of six diapers a day.

After a bout of crying followed by sleep, a mother often remains too tense to close her eyes. One trick to help yourself get some badly needed sleep, whether it's midafternoon or midnight, is to try the relaxation or breathing techniques you learned in childbirth-preparation class. Remember to take the phone off the hook if you are home alone during the day, when well-meaning friends and relatives are likely to call.

A few other sanity-saving suggestions during this exhausting first week include:

- nap or at least lie down when your baby is sleeping
- relax and do as little as possible
- spread out visitors over several weeks
- forget housework, but if dishes and dust are really bothering you, hire someone if your husband, relative or friend doesn't come to the rescue
- splurge, if you can, and have groceries delivered and laundry picked up; and even order take-out dinners
- eat well, especially seeing to it that you get plenty of foods rich in vitamin B, calcium and iron to help you get your strength back
- do not fret about your weight right now; by the end of this week some of the fluid you've retained will vanish on its own
- take one day at a time and keep in mind that it *will* get easier.

Feeding

Most babies, after the first few days, take 2 to 3 ounces of milk a day for each pound of their body weight. Growth spurts often trigger bigger appetites, which may be evident during the second week and again around the fifth week or at about three months. Usually, bottle-fed babies want to have 6 to 7 feedings every 24 hours. For a seven-pound infant, this would mean somewhere between 14 to 21 ounces of formula, or 2.5 to 3.5 ounces per meal; however, many newborns' stomachs may comfortably hold only 1.5 to 2 ounces. If you are breast-feeding, don't worry about whether there is enough milk, since too little is extremely rare, and more frequent feeding automatically increases your supply.

In the past there have been suggestions that regular feeding times would be not only more convenient for the mother but also less likely to result in excessive milk intake. However, thinking on this subject has changed. It is now recommended that mothers feed their babies when they seem hungry, on the ground that "on-demand" feeding will not produce any more weight gain than a regular feeding schedule. For nursing mothers, there's the argument that on-demand feeding is less traumatic to the nipples, because a baby who is not offered the breast when hungry may suck too hard when finally fed. Several studies, however, found no significant difference in the incidence of nipple problems or breast engorgement between those who nursed on regular and on irregular schedules, and conclude that incorrect positioning may be the root of such problems as the infant's sucking too vigorously. Dr. Audrey Naylor, director of the Lactation Program at the University of California San Diego Medical Center, urges nursing mothers during the first month to feed their newborns at least every four hours, because it takes about that much time for the breasts to produce as much as they can store, and if the milk is not removed by then, the ability of milk-secreting cells may be affected, resulting in a decreased supply of milk. "Healthy weight gain for newborns and optimum milk supply in mothers occurs best with feedings of fifteen minutes at each breast eight or more times in 24 hours," advises Dr. Naylor.

Most babies will fall into a pattern of eating every three to five hours, but if your month-old child is still nursing in two-hour shifts, chances are that you are absolutely worn out. One solution is to lengthen the intervals gradually by letting your baby fuss for 15 to 30 minutes. Perhaps a bottle of water, a pacifier or a change of scenery in a Snugli may help your baby get accustomed to going a bit longer without nourishment.

There is considerable disagreement on just when the "2:00 A.M." feeding becomes unnecessary and whether or not you should break your baby's habit of waking at night to eat. Some say that if a baby is gaining well—weighing at least nine pounds—by one month the night feeding can be safely eliminated. One approach is to let the baby cry for 15–30 minutes the first night; then, if fussing persists, offer an ounce or two of warm water. Other child-care experts believe even a 6-week-old baby requires six feedings in 24 hours, and that only by the age of 3–4 months can this be reduced to five. Five feedings still mean that even with the help of expert juggling, you can count on only a six- or seven-hour stretch of sleep. The two extremes are "do whatever your baby wants" and "your baby won't starve and you need your rest." No clear answers exist as to whether, when or how night feedings should be eliminated, but talking with other parents as well as with your baby's doctor will help you decide what feels right to you.

Bottle-feeding Hints

● Homemade formula and commercial milk mixtures offer a wide choice in terms of cost and protein, fat and carbohydrate content. Soy-based and other special formulas are also available for infants who are unable to tolerate cow-protein-based food. Whole, 2 percent and skim milk contain more protein and sodium than are recommended for infants, and the prevailing opinion is that pasteurized milk should *not* be given to babies under 12 months of age.
● Sterilizing bottles and nipples is still recommended for infants under 3 months of age, although some pediatricians think thorough washing will do the trick (but don't towel-dry, as lint and bacteria will be

deposited in clean bottles). Sterilizing kits are available, but another approach is to fill clean bottles halfway with formula concentrate, add tap water until the bottle is full, invert nipples into the bottle, put caps on loosely so the steam can pass and place all bottles in several inches of water in a big pot. Simply cover and boil for 25 minutes, then let cool, tighten caps and store in the refrigerator.

• The amount of nitrosamines (a chemical added during manufacturing to give rubber products strength and resilience) in baby bottle nipples will be regulated by the U.S. Food and Drug Administration beginning in January 1985. The agency reports it has no evidence that nitrosamines have harmed babies, but that it is known to cause cancer in animals. To be extra safe, you can boil nipples for a few minutes five or six times before initial use, changing the water after each boil. The same precaution holds for rubber pacifiers.

• Nipple hole should be large enough so that milk drops slowly from the bottle when it is held upside down. The cap should be loose enough so that air bubbles can enter the bottle to allow the milk to be sucked out of it.

• Feeding position is best if the bottle sticks straight out, at a right angle to the baby's mouth. Never leave your baby with a propped bottle. Also, it is best not to let your child drink while lying flat on the back, on the theory that swallowing in a horizontal position may force milk in inner-ear canals, possibly causing an infection.

• Spitting up is to be expected, but it may occur less often if you burp midway through the bottle and again at the end of the feeding; also try giving cold formula directly from the refrigerator.

• Leftover milk should be thrown out if your baby has drunk from the bottle, and even unused formula that hasn't been touched should be discarded within 48 hours.

• Nursing-bottle syndrome or tooth decay can be prevented if you never put your baby to bed with a bottle (unless it is filled with water); see more details in "Pearly Whites: Teething and Dental Care" (p. 435).

• Overfeeding can be avoided, partly by not coaxing your baby to finish the bottle to the very last drop.

Nursing Hints

Breast-feeding soon becomes second nature, but at first there is a lot of experimenting with different positions and techniques. Besides practice, expect some adjustments during the first weeks. For instance, your breasts may seem smaller, but it means only that the swelling has gone down and the milk supply has adjusted to your baby's needs. Here are some nursing tips. Many other questions about let-down reflex, nutrition, and storing and expressing milk are discussed in detail later in this chapter in "Breast-feeding: Natural Concerns" (p. 317).

• Nipple and as much of the areola (dark area) should be in your baby's mouth to ensure the removal of milk from milk sinuses that lie directly under areola. Use a V or scissors hold with your second and third fingers to compress the areola and nipple to help your baby latch on correctly. To make more breathing space for your infant, press down on your breast next to the baby's nose.

• Different nursing positions are not only important for your comfort but also essential to prevent clogged ducts. It is wise to try the "football hold," where you sit with pillows to the side and cup your baby's head in your hands. Lying down on your side with pillows behind your head and back and a folded towel under your baby, which brings the mouth level with your nipple, is restful and takes the weight off the incision if you had a cesarean.

• Both breasts should be used for each feeding, so as to keep up the flow of milk; try to start the next feeding on the breast you used last (a safety pin on that side of your bra will help you remember).

• Burp your baby after each breast is emptied, to keep him or her awake and also to get rid of any air bubbles that may otherwise cause your baby to feel uncomfortable or full; many breast-fed babies don't need to be burped during feedings.

• Switch-nursing is a good way to build up milk supply if your baby is not nursing much on one side or tends to fall asleep. Let your baby nurse for five to eight minutes on one breast, move to the other one, and then move back to the first side and repeat.

• Break the suction with your little finger by inserting it into the corner of your baby's mouth so you can slide your nipple out easily.

• Air-dry your nipples, ideally after each feeding, and don't use soap or other drying agents on your breasts. Just wash with plain water.

• Leaking can be stopped by pressing the palm of your hand against the nipples until the tingling sensation stops (leaking will occur only occasionally after you've been nursing for about four to six weeks).

• No relief bottles—it will take approximately two to three weeks until your baby is nursing well and your milk supply is firmly established! Don't give the baby any bottles during this period in order to avoid bottle attachment, which could jeopardize successful breast-feeding.

Feeding Your Twins

It's impossible to overestimate how taxing the adjustment will be to living with and caring for two new people, both of whom depend entirely on you. Changing family living patterns to adapt to one new household member is stressful enough, but to juggle an additional person with an entirely different disposition and, perhaps, activity schedule is bound to stretch your resources to their limits. Some helpful reading material on the subject is available at libraries and bookstores, and there are about 1000 local Mothers of Twins clubs around the country, where you can meet with other parents who are in the same boat. Basic decisions—from eating and sleeping schedules to strollers and other baby equipment—will be slightly different, given your double load. But the key issue of nursing finds no consensus. Breast- versus bottle-feeding, feeding twins separately or simultaneously, have their own advocates, so you'll want to solicit advice from medical professionals as well as experienced parents of twins, in order to reach your own decision.

Because your physical reserves will be sapped in other ways such as lack of sleep and time and energy-consuming baby-care tasks, some pediatricians advise bottle-feeding twins to eliminate the additional drain on your already overtaxed system. Other experts counter that more energy is spent standing, preparing and giving the 12-plus bottles of formula necessary each day. If you decide to bottle-feed and want to have them eat at the same time, some creative gymnastics will be needed. Do whatever works, but try not to prop a bottle in your baby's mouth, as this may cause gagging and digestive upset, not to mention time without body contact with you.

Advocates of breast-feeding twins point out that you can feed both at once if you wish, whereas bottle-feeding requires both hands for each child. They also note that in the long run nursing is not only energy-saving and the most nutritious but also cost-effective. Here are some suggestions if you decide to breast-feed.

Nutrition. You will need as many calories each day as a man doing heavy manual labor; figures range anywhere from 800 to 1200 calories daily above the recommended pregnancy diet allowance, which should be distributed among the basic four food groups. To save time, cut up fresh vegetables and fruit, chunks of cheese, cooked chicken and hard-boiled eggs to keep in the refrigerator for hearty in-between-meal snacks.

Milk Volume. A balanced diet and plenty of rest will help keep up your energy level and assure a good composition to your milk, but the supply depends almost exclusively on your babies' demands: The more they suck, the more milk will be produced. This is why even night feedings are important to maintain for the first couple of months.

Separate or Simultaneous Nursing. Nursing both babies simultaneously is time-saving and may be the only way they will want to feed. On the other hand, breast-feeding each separately means giving individual care and attention. Your choice may depend both on your babies' preferences (some actually refuse to eat alone), and their waking patterns. To avoid being bound to your nursing chair all day, some mothers suggest waking one twin when the other cries to be fed. Other mothers shy away from this practice, believing it upsets their babies' natural behavior. If you choose to nurse both at once, allow a trial-and-error period and give yourself time to experiment with different positions. Some tried-and-true positions include:

- positioning both babies as you would if there were just one, overlapping their legs on your lap
- holding one in a traditional nursing position and the other with the head on its twin's lap
- positioning both babies as you would a football: their bodies under each arm, babies' faces looking at you, heads supported by pillow(s) in your lap
- one in the traditional, the other in the football hold (see p. 304)
- lie on your abdomen on the bed, supporting your weight on your elbows, with the babies underneath.

Alternating Breasts. Although La Leche League says to give in to your babies' preferences for one breast over the other, others caution against letting the same baby nurse on the same breast for too long. For one thing, the harder sucker of the two will stimulate more milk, making your breasts lopsided. Most importantly, sticking to one side allows only one of your baby's eyes to focus on you, depriving the other eye of needed stimulus and exercise. One suggestion is that you offer each baby both breasts at each feeding or offer the same breast on alternate days so that the "barracuda" nurser will stimulate a larger supply for the slower twin.

The first few days and nights at home together tend to be demanding—often stressful—for the entire family. Remember to give yourself time to adjust. Before you know it, a fairly predictable routine will develop, and you'll have plenty of energy and good humor.

Information Sources

ADDITIONAL READING

The Care of Twin Children available for $6.95 from Mothers of Twins Clubs, 5402 Amberwood La., Rockville, MD 20853 or the Center for Study of Multiple Birth, 333 E. Superior, #463-5, Chicago, IL 60611.

Double Talk: For Parents of Multiples. Quarterly newsletter, subscription available for $5.00 a year from PO Box 412, Amelia, OH 45102.

The First Three Years of Life, by Dr. Burton L. White (New York: Avon, 1978).

Having Twins, by Elizabeth Noble (Boston: Houghton Mifflin, 1980).

"Mothering Multiples." A 52-page booklet on nursing twins, available for $2.50 from the La Leche League International, 9616 Minneapolis Ave., Franklin Park, IL 60131.

Twins and Supertwins, by Amram Scheinfeld (New York: Pelican Books, 1973).

ORGANIZATIONS

Center for Study of Multiple Birth
333 E. Superior, #463-5
Chicago, IL 60611
Information clearinghouse and publisher of books about multiple births; send stamped, self-addressed envelope for their booklet "The Care of Twin Children" and a list of books.

National Organization of Mothers of Twins Clubs, Inc. (NOMOTC)
5402 Amberwood La.
Rockville, MD 20853
Publishes newsletter and will refer you to the local NOMOTC chapter near where you live.

You may also want to refer to "Crying and Sleeping" (p. 423) and "Breast-feeding: Natural Concerns" (p. 317), "Postpartum Care: Baby Yourself" (see below) as well as "Blues and Depression: It's Not All in Your Mind" (p. 313).

POSTPARTUM CARE: BABY YOURSELF

Looking six months pregnant after you've just given birth probably is not what you expected. Don't despair—that beach-ball belly will deflate considerably during the first week. Many of those essential pounds you gained will disappear, but don't count on losing the final ten pounds so soon. Regaining your prepregnancy shape is a gradual process, unlike the speed with which your body recovers.

The pregnancy equipment which was built over a period of nine months now will be dismantled in the space of a few weeks. Because of the magnitude and speed of all these changes, the first six weeks postpartum is described by one medical textbook as "a period of physiological tumult." Your uterus shrinks back to the size of a pear, blood volume decreases by a third, approximately four pounds of excess fluid disappear and hormones shift gears. Your system must also repair any damage—wounds in the womb where the placenta was attached, tears or stitches around the birth outlet, strained muscles and stretched tissues—and normalize other body functions, such as your urinary and intestinal tracts. Hair loss, heavy perspiration and skin problems are other temporary symptoms of the internal upheaval.

The most dramatic steps in reversal and recovery occur during the first ten days after birth, with more gradual adjustments during the next four to six weeks.

TYPICAL TIMETABLE: BIRTH TO RECOVERY

	First Ten Days	Second to Sixth Week
Moods	Exhilaration and emotional "high"; hormonal activity, seeking prepregnancy levels, may play havoc with emotions; blues could hit around second or third day; weakened physical state keeps you feeling dependent and vulnerable; blues will probably subside by end of the first week.	About 1 in 10 women experience some degree of depression, possibly occurring months rather than weeks after delivery (see "Blues and Depression: It's Not All in Your Mind," p. 313); you may long to get some free time from your mothering responsibilities; fewer fears and anxieties as you grow more confident as a parent.
Bleeding	Blood loss totals at least 1 cup at birth; sudden large gushes, sometimes containing clots, continue during the first 3 days; discharge (lochia) from healing cells becomes brown, then pinkish brown toward end of week and turns yellow around the tenth day.	Discharge continues for about 6 weeks; if bleeding starts again, you are probably overdoing; if bottle-feeding, menstrual periods will return in 4 to 10 weeks; if nursing, within 2 to 18 months—you *can* get pregnant even though periods have not resumed.
Breasts	Soft and supple at birth but become firm and tender second to fourth day; yellowish fluid, colostrum, is replaced by milk several days after childbirth; if bottle-feeding, milk engorgement of breasts begins to subside by sixth or seventh day, but any real discomfort disappears in 48 hours.	Milk supply established if your baby nurses regularly (see "Breast-feeding: Natural Concerns," p. 317).
Pelvic Floor	Muscles are stretched and sagging; swelling of veins (hem-	Around 4 weeks postpartum, pelvic-floor muscles have toned

TYPICAL TIMETABLE: BIRTH TO RECOVERY

	First Ten Days	Second to Sixth Week
	orrhoids) and skin surrounding episiotomy or repaired tears may be particularly painful around the third day; by week's end, tenderness and redness should begin to disappear.	up; episiotomy usually healed well enough for intercourse by one month, though some doctors suggest waiting until sixth week (see "Sex: Intimate Questions," p. 330).
Uterus	Womb continues to contract (termed after-birth cramps) during the first 3 days, especially if you're nursing; uterus shrinks about 1 cm daily.	Uterus will measure slightly larger than before pregnancy and will weigh only about 3 oz. within 5 to 6 weeks.
Urinary Tract	Normal pattern of urination will return by end of a week; anesthetic given during childbirth may distend bladder; soreness may cause you to be afraid to urinate.	Within 2 weeks your body's prepregnant fluid levels return; regular kidney function resumes by fourth week.
Intestines	Sluggish due to lack of tone, anesthetic or poor diet; you may get constipated if you delay having a bowel movement because of episiotomy discomfort.	Normal bowel pattern usually returns in about 4 weeks.

A major source of discomfort during the first week tends to be the skin and tissues surrounding the vagina, especially if you have stitches and/or hemorrhoids. As blood circulates more freely, the episiotomy or tear repair begins to heal, and clogged blood vessels loosen up. Meanwhile, you can speed up the process and ease the pain by keeping the stitches clean and dry. Some helpful remedies you might want to try include:

- placing an ice pack on the area soon after delivery
- moving around and starting Kegel exercises, which tighten and relax perineum (see "Conditioning Exercises: What's a Kegel?" p. 68) to increase circulation
- soaking in a shallow Sitz bath—essentially bathing in warm water—three times a day

- sitting in tepid water and adding ice cubes will extend the anesthetic effect after you get out of the tub or Sitz bath
- standing under a warm shower
- using a heat lamp or ordinary reading light several times a day
- resting on your side, with knees up, to relieve pressure
- reducing hemorrhoid discomfort by consuming lots of liquids and bulk foods to keep stools soft; applying cold witch hazel and compresses such as Tucks or other hemorrhoid preparations; lightly massaging the area.

When to Call Your Doctor or Midwife

Discharge or "lochia" has peculiar color or odor (foul, not like that at the end of a period)

Bright red bleeding resumes; if small amount, you're overdoing and not resting enough; if flow is brisk, you may be hemorrhaging

Unusual increase in frequency of urination or burning sensation

Abdominal pain other than slight tenderness

Severe pains in chest, legs or lower abdomen

Bleeding nipples

Tender, inflamed lumps in breasts, flulike symptoms (do not confuse plugged milk ducts with breast infection; if problem is milk ducts, there will be no miserable, under-the-weather feeling)

Chills or fever of 100°F or more

Regardless of how you've chosen to feed your newborn, your breasts need special attention. If you're nursing, nipples may redden, crack or become exceptionally painful. Smooth on lanolin-rich breast cream and air-dry your nipples, ideally once or twice a day (see "Breast-feeding: Natural Concerns," p. 317). If your baby is formula-fed, your breasts will feel heavy and sore the first few days, until the milk buildup subsides. Some doctors will prescribe drugs to stop milk production, while others prefer to let nature take its course, and suggest you ease the discomfort by applying ice packs for the first 24 hours, wearing a snug bra and taking aspirin or some other mild pain reliever. Of course, don't pump your breasts or express milk from them, as this only stimulates more milk to come in.

In order to restore itself fully, your body requires rest, so that energy can be spent on repair. If you are tempted in these first weeks to use your baby's nap time for unfinished projects or reorganizing your household, think again. Nighttime feedings rob you of a solid night's sleep for many weeks, so the only thing to catch up on in your "free time" is rest.

A balanced intake of the right foods, too, will renew your energy:

- a diet low in fats, high in protein, to heal tissues, plus extra servings of protein if you are breast-feeding
- lots of liquids, about 6 to 8 glasses a day, to make up for approximately 8 to 10 pounds of fluid and tissue lost at birth.

Postpartum Exercises

Launching into an all-out recovery workout should probably be held off for about four to six weeks, but doing several easy exercises within hours of delivery is recommended.

(1) Lie on your tummy, with pillows supporting your abdomen, hips and breasts for comfort; resting this way for about 20 minutes coaxes your uterus forward, back into position.
(2) Make circles with each foot, lying or sitting down, to improve circulation.
(3) Squeeze the muscle that controls the flow of urine and hold it for several seconds; the Kegel exercise strengthens many stretched tissues.
(4) Breathe deeply, expanding your stomach; hiss as you slowly exhale, then forcibly draw in your abdominal muscles.
(5) Lift your chin to your chest and hold it there for five seconds. Start by doing just a few and work up to 15 a day.

Somewhat more strenuous exercises may be started once the red bleeding has stopped. If any of the exercises don't feel quite right, listen to your body and quit. After all, you really can be lazy for a while, since your stomach will deflate considerably on its own. A sampling of some of the early recovery exercises include the following:

(1) lie on your back with your knees flexed, tilt your pelvis inward and tightly contract the buttocks as you lift your head
(2) lie on your back with legs straight, raise your head and lift left knee slightly, then reach for—but do not touch—the left knee with the right hand; repeat, using right knee, left hand
(3) lie on your back with your knees bent and draw one knee toward the abdomen, then stretch it out, as if bicycling; repeat with other leg

(4) lean on your elbows and knees, keeping forearms and lower legs together. Hump your back upward, strongly contracting buttocks and drawing in abdomen; relax and breathe deeply

(5) stand with your back straight, arms hanging loosely; stretch the right arm down toward the floor, bending sideways at the waist, and simultaneously offer counter-resistance from the left side, to make movement harder; repeat, bending sideways to the left and offering counter-resistance from the right.

There are any number of exercises with which you can experiment, but during the early postpartum weeks and months, concentrate on those, besides Kegels, that help tone up muscles and tissues, particularly around the vagina. Strengthening weakened abdominal muscles is also important, not only to regain control over your tummy but to prevent backache, as your center of gravity adapts to its old state.

In addition to your baby's body weight, you've lost a whopping 12 pounds at delivery—4 pounds each of blood, tissue fluid, uterus and breast tissue—and the scales will continue to show a loss over the next few weeks as fluid retention drops. The rate at which you shed the final pounds will depend on your metabolism, the number of calories you consume and the number burned off (in breast-feeding and activities). Aim at three to six months for reaching your prepregnancy weight. A concerted effort to cut down on the quantity—not quality—of food, coupled with a regular fitness program when your body's strong enough, should do the trick. (If you're nursing, factor in the number of calories expended in breast-feeding.) Ask yourself, too, if dipping into the cookie jar might be the result of stress and tension rather than hunger pains.

General Advice

Dos	Don'ts
Do rest, try to nap.	Don't lift anything heavier than your baby.
Do take your temperature twice a day if you suspect you have an infection.	Don't stand for long periods.
	Don't bend from the waist without bending at the knees.
	Don't overdo, particularly until your body has recovered.
	Don't douche without checking first with your health adviser.
	Don't lose your sense of humor!

Information Sources

ADDITIONAL READING

Essential Exercises for the Childbearing Years, by Elizabeth Noble (Boston: Houghton Mifflin, 1976).

Jane Fonda's Workout Book for Pregnancy, Birth and Recovery, by Femmy DeLyser (New York: Simon and Schuster, 1982). Cassette or double album also available.

The Post Partum Book: How to Cope with and Enjoy the First Year of Parenting, by Hank Pizer and Christine Garfink (New York: Grove Press, 1979).

"Special Diet Section for New Mothers," *American Baby*, February 1982. Weight Watchers sample day's menu; a week's menu plan along with recipes.

For more about recovery from a cesarean birth, see p. 264 as well as "Blues and Depression: It's Not All in Your Mind" (below) and "Sex: Intimate Questions" (p. 330).

BLUES AND DEPRESSION: IT'S NOT ALL IN YOUR MIND

"It hit me the seventh day after my daughter was born," one mother recalls. "All of a sudden I felt I was on a roller coaster that went down and didn't go up—the drop from euphoria to depression was so dramatic, so acute." You may be lucky and sail through the days and weeks after birth without a tear, but if you are plagued instead by unexpected crying bouts or twinges of despair, don't worry. Varying degrees of postpartum depression are now recognized as normal and temporary. Although the causes remain obscure, most experts agree these mood swings result from the interplay of biochemical changes taking place in your system, stress of new parenthood and less emotional resilience, owing to chronic fatigue. If hormones have never thrown off your emotions before, this temporary loss of control can be particularly disturbing and frustrating to both you and your mate. Just knowing it is natural and short-lived can lift some of the gloom and help you ride out the storm.

Roughly four to six mothers in ten will come down with the "baby blues," usually between the second and sixth day after birth, often peaking either just before hospital discharge or right after the return home. If it hits, you may experience any number of the following:

weepiness for no particular reason; spirits rising, then plummeting unpredictably; poor concentration; forgetfulness or occasional confusion; anxiety, unusual sensitivity and hypercritical attitude toward yourself and others; vulnerability or overdependence. The emotional tempests usually start to blow over in a few days, though they may last as long as two weeks.

For one woman in ten, the blues persist or resurface within the month. This type of postpartum depression varies widely in intensity and length. Along with low spirits and mood swings, you may find yourself short-tempered, easily irritated, self-critical, feeling "everything's hopeless," indecisive, unable to concentrate. The few whose depression lasts up to a year may also feel upset, apathetic, listless and often negative about motherhood.

Researchers have yet to zero in on exactly why you can be intensely proud and exhilarated one moment and in the depths of despair the next, or why depression may be delayed or linger on. As Dr. David Rubinow of the government's National Institute of Mental Health's biological psychiatry branch describes it, in terms of research, postpartum depression is still "virgin territory." Studies remain inconclusive, and most theories are speculative, though some explanations are more popular than others. Hormones could play a central role, but "the state of the art is such," says Dr. Rubinow, "that a one-to-one correlation between a single hormone and mood change has not been established."

Possible Causes

Your body abruptly shifts gears after the nine months of pregnancy and hours of strenuous childbirth. Some of your mood swings are probably related to physiological factors.

Depression may be caused by overall physical weakness due to:

- diminished blood volume; your body works overtime to make up the loss stressing your system and lowering its resistance to physical and emotional assaults
- "combat fatigue" from the trauma of labor and delivery and, possibly, from drugs, forceps, episiotomy or cesarean
- chronic fatigue—you may never enjoy a full night's sleep in the first days and weeks after your baby's birth, yet your body demands rest to gather its forces and repair itself.

Mood swings may also result from massive hormonal changes in your endocrine system ("hormone," incidentally, means to set in motion or stir up):

- progesterone and estrogen hormones, previously busy sustaining your pregnancy, drop dramatically

- the pituitary gland releases prolactin, the milk delivery hormone, the third day after childbirth; some scientists suspect rising levels of prolactin may make imbalances in other hormones more pronounced
- the thyroid, which regulates your metabolism, reduces its hormone production; some new mothers suffering from depression also show unusually slow thyroid activity
- endorphins, your natural opiatelike pain-killers, which were activated during childbirth, also may be associated with emotional highs and lows; some experts theorize that as endorphin levels dip after birth, their retreat is followed by a similar drop in spirits.

The adjustments to a new role and to the added responsibility of motherhood are stressful, too, and can contribute to depression. There are other psychological factors that may increase emotional vulnerability.

(1) Feelings of anticlimax are not unusual after your baby is born; they are a normal reaction following any major achievement.
(2) Your self-esteem may be low if you are disappointed for not "handling labor better," feel you can't measure up to a self-imposed standard of supermom or see the temporary, leftover pads of pregnancy fat as unattractive.
(3) Insecurity and isolation are common feelings, particularly during the first days home, when you are really alone with your baby for the first time.
(4) The father's attention may be centered on the baby, leaving you on the sidelines, or his degree of involvement in actually helping out may fall short of your expectations.
(5) Other stressful situations unrelated to your baby—job change, new home, serious illness in the family—may drain emotional resources and wear away your usual resiliency.

PREVENTION/REMEDIES FOR POSTPARTUM DEPRESSION

Medical	Nonmedical
Many physicians flatly oppose drug therapy; others would like to see it combined with counseling sessions.	recognize you are going through a natural phase and that it will pass
	warn your mate and relatives that you may be depressed and not yourself
progesterone injections at delivery and in suppository form for one week following as preventive measure; thought to compensate for abrupt fall in hormone level after birth	plan to have help once you get home (relatives, domestic help); arrange in advance for sitters

PREVENTION/REMEDIES FOR POSTPARTUM DEPRESSION

Medical	Nonmedical
gradual reduction in use of estrogen, progesterone and/or thyroid hormones for several weeks postpartum to ease natural leveling out	get as much rest and sleep as possible; steal naps during the day
antidepressant drugs, tranquilizers; some psychotropic drugs turn up in breast milk; if these medications are necessary, they should be taken under medical supervision	eat well-balanced meals low in sugar and high in whole grains; some nutritionists link moodiness with vitamin B deficiencies and/or an overload of unrefined carbohydrates (sugar, white flour and so on)
counseling sessions with a medical professional, ideally one trained in dealing with postpartum blues	spend time with other couples who have young children
	save your energy; don't be concerned with how tidy your home is; letting tasks slide is for your own good and your baby's
	try to maintain outside interests to avoid feeling isolated, but don't load yourself with fresh responsibilities
	be sure to express your feelings and communicate honestly with your spouse, particularly about parenting concerns and responsibilities
	laugh at yourself; a sense of humor often diffuses anger and self-pity

Information Sources

ADDITIONAL READING

Mother Care, by Lyn Delli Quadri and Kati Breckenridge (Los Angeles: J. P. Tarcher, 1978). Full of advice and specific suggestions to new mothers and those experiencing postpartum depression.

ORGANIZATIONS

Local groups for new parents; some have support sessions designed specifically to help mothers through difficult periods. Also, postnatal exercise classes may offer mothers an opportunity to meet others experiencing similar mood swings. To learn if there is a "parent connection" or similar group where you live, ask other mothers, women's groups, your pediatrician or the local chapter of the La Leche League.

If you had a cesarean birth, see section about Physical and Mental Recovery in "Cesarean: What Every Expectant Mother Should Know" (p. 264).

BREAST-FEEDING: NATURAL CONCERNS

Highlighted here are some common concerns about breast-feeding, ranging from sore nipples to the use of prescription drugs during lactation. Basic questions such as different nursing positions are discussed earlier in this chapter (see "Help During Week One!" p. 297).

Let-Down Reflex

At your baby's first suck and pull on your nipple, the stimulated nerve endings in your breast send a message to your brain that signals the pituitary gland to release the hormone prolactin for making milk and another hormone, oxytocin, for making the alveoli (milk sinuses) contract to squeeze the milk out. At the outset, the full interplay of hormones, nerves and glands takes a few moments to complete, but after nursing is established, the reflex can be triggered simply by hearing your baby cry. Though a few mothers are unaware that the let-down reflex has been set off, most feel a tingling or tightening in their breasts and notice some milk dripping even before their baby starts to suck.

Because it is a complex physiological chain reaction greatly influenced by fatigue, cold, pain and emotional stress, any kind of real distraction can inhibit the reflex—a barking dog, a blast of cold air, sharp words with your husband—so, in order to achieve optimal milk flow during nursing sessions, get as comfortable as you can, and try to be in a quiet place. Some lactation experts suggest sipping a little beer or wine just before and during feeding times, for relaxation.

Milk Supply

As long as your baby is sucking well and you are getting enough nutrients and rest, don't worry about not producing enough milk. You know you are supplying adequate nourishment if your baby:

- wets about six or more diapers each day while being breast-fed exclusively (disposable diapers will feel drier than cloth ones)

- gains an average of four to seven ounces a week, or one pound a month; remember, though, babies put on weight at different rates
- nurses irregularly but is gaining some weight
- looks healthy, with good color and firm muscle tone; appears alert and is active.

If you are not producing enough milk, it could be because your baby is a weak sucker, you are not eating and/or drinking enough, you are taking certain medications (particularly hormones, which dry up the milk supply), your breasts are too sore to nurse or you are under considerable stress.

La Leche League and other experts recommend the following to increase your supply:

- nurse frequently; plan to spend a day or so building up milk volume
- make sure you offer both breasts at each feeding
- stay away from pacifiers or a relief bottle; your baby's sucking is the best milk-production stimulus and needs full play on your breasts
- drink six to eight glasses of liquids daily, about four of which should be milk, but don't force them if you are not thirsty. You'll know if you are drinking enough by checking your urine; it will turn dark and be scanty before the milk volume is affected
- get plenty of rest and do anything you can to relax before nursing; for instance, play soft music, take a warm bath, sip some wine or beer, since tension interferes with the let-down reflex
- try the herbal tea Blessed Thistle, which some mothers claim increases their milk flow
- consider taking oxytocin, sometimes prescribed to stimulate milk release.

Milk Production of Well-Nourished Mother

First month: 600 ml or less/day

Third month: 700–750 ml or less/day

Sixth month: 750–800 ml or less/day

After the sixth month, there is usually a slow decline in volume.

Nutrition

Additional calories carefully selected from among each of the basic food groups will not only meet your milk production needs but protect against depletion of your own nutrient stores as well. Although an inadequate diet will affect the volume of milk, the composition will remain relatively stable, because your breasts draw any missing protein, calcium and fat from your own body supply. The amount of other nutrients passed on, however, such as amino acids, certain fatty acids and water-soluble vitamins, will vary according to your intake.

After water, the principal components of human milk are protein, milk sugar (lactose) and fat, which constitutes the bulk of its calories. To maintain a nutritional balance, it is widely believed that you need major increases in calories and nutrients:

- 300 to 500 extra calories/day beyond a normal diet
- a total of three or four 2–3-ounce servings of protein each day
- 20 percent increase in all vitamins and minerals (prenatal vitamin pills normally do the job, although vegetarians are advised to take daily B_{12} supplements); see RDAs, in "Nutrition and Essential Extra Pounds" (p. 26)
- about 50 percent increase in folic acid (good sources include liver, broccoli, mushrooms, spinach, orange juice, lemons, bananas, strawberries, cantaloupe, brewer's yeast)
- about 50 percent more calcium, phosphorus, magnesium (there is some evidence that magnesium and calcium affect the production of oxytocin, the milk-release hormone).

A food combination that supplies nearly all of the foregoing nutritional requirements is a peanut butter sandwich and an eight-ounce glass of milk. Be sure to consume six to eight glasses of liquid daily.

Food to Avoid: Fact or Fiction?

Apart from large quantities of caffeine, which may make your baby restless or fussy, and foods that tend to trigger allergic reactions, such as chocolate and strawberries, experts are divided about whether or not your baby can actually have the same response to foods when they are passed on through your milk as you do. Particularly suspect are gas-producing and spicy foods, such as raw fruits and vegetables, including garlic and onions. Some mothers swear their infants suffer from diarrhea, colic and other gastrointestinal problems after they themselves have eaten some of these foods. There is no scientific evidence to back up these claims, but there is also no reason to believe some of these "upsetting" foods are not transmitted through human milk. In other words, infants will react variably to foods; what may be a problem with one may not be for another. If a breast-fed baby is colicky, some nutritionists recommend eliminating cow's milk from the mother's diet. (More on colic in "Common Problems from Allergies to Rashes," p. 391.)

Dieting

It is estimated that the energy used for milk production burns off approximately 500 calories a day, so it's possible to maintain your prenatal diet and still lose pounds; however, this is probably unwise unless you are ten pounds over your prepregnancy weight. If you do choose to diet, a good rule of thumb is to check to be sure you're getting the maximum amount of nourishment from a minimum of calories. Substitute skim milk for whole milk, for example, and lean meats and fish in place of pork and fatty beef, and avoid foods that provide only "empty" calories, such as candy and high carbohydrates, like pastry and alcohol.

Expressing and Storing Milk

Express milk for storage any time except just before a feeding, the ideal time being in the morning after a long sleep. If it's done during a feeding, your baby stimulates the flow while nursing from the other breast, so you can simply collect the overflow in a sterile container or put a hand or electric pump to the breast to further milk production. If it's done between feedings, you'll need to massage your breasts first, from back to nipple, without touching the nipple, then squeeze gently, cupping the breast by placing your thumb above and forefinger below the edge of the areola. Supporting the breast with your other hand while in this squeezing position, push back toward your chest wall until milk comes through. The process is sometimes frustratingly slow, yielding just a few drops at first, then a thin stream. Pumps usually work faster, but if you are dissatisfied with the job yours is doing or find the instructions confusing, talk to other mothers who've had experience expressing their milk, or call your local chapter of La Leche League.

When you store breast milk it's important that anything that comes in contact with the milk—from your hands to containers—be clean, and it is essential that it be chilled to prevent spoilage. Here are some steps for storing and some specific tips:

- express milk into a clean or sterilized glass or plastic jar; La Leche League advises using plastic, since immunological properties in human milk tend to stick to the sides of glass containers, although recent scientific research casts doubt on this

- chill milk promptly in the refrigerator, where it can be kept for 24 hours, although some lactation specialists say 48 hours is safe; as it cools the bluish tinge will become white and cream will look curdled on top
- freeze milk by pouring it into container, leaving enough room at the top for expansion; ideally, freeze in proper amounts for each feeding (4 ounces or 8 ounces) so none is wasted
- keep milk in freezer compartment of refrigerator for no more than two weeks, but in a separate deep freezer it can be stored safely for several months
- add newly expressed milk to that already frozen, but first chill for 20–30 minutes in the refrigerator before adding; otherwise part of the frozen milk will defrost
- defrost milk by putting container under tepid tap water—too much heat will kill the good properties in human milk; don't let it thaw at room temperature, since slow defrosting allows for bacterial growth
- throw out whatever the baby doesn't drink—never refreeze milk
- have formula ready as backup just in case of an accidental spill; also, it's easy to think you have more frozen milk on hand than you actually do.

Your choice of equipment will depend on how often and regularly you need to stockpile milk. Some hand pumps come with parts that convert into storage containers, eliminating another step in preparation. Some regulate the amount of suction you need. Check hospitals for rental information on electric pumps if you need faster action because you work, have a premature infant or are trying to get over some breast-feeding complication, such as mastitis or cracked and bleeding nipples. Take a glance, too, at the classified ads or call a local childbirth-education group, which might help you locate mothers who have pumps to sell.

Engorgement, Plugged Ducts or Breast Infection

By backing up milk and clogging ducts, inadequate emptying of one or both of your breasts can cause painful swelling (engorgement) and set the stage for a possible breast infection. Engorgement is common when milk first comes in, a few days after delivery, as the stepped-up circulation of blood swells tissues and pressure increases from newly produced milk. Relief from the tenderness and tightness will come as soon as your baby nurses more. If engorgement continues, fluid may back up into the ducts, swelling the tissues and making it even harder for milk to pass through. These clogged ducts—also called "caked" breasts—are small, painful red lumps in your breast. If left untreated, they could become infected, since the weakened tissues will have a lower resistance to bacteria. You'll know if your breasts have become infected (called mastitis) if, in addition to painful swelling and redness, you have symptoms similar to the flu.

The way to relieve all these problems is to empty your breasts fully at each feeding, even in the case of mastitis, when nursing may be especially painful. Continuing to breast-feed is important, since weaning will produce more engorgement and aggravate the infection. Antibiotics are usually used to combat an infection. Here are some ways to prevent or reduce swelling and plugged ducts:

- change nursing positions so pressure will be exerted on all ducts to varying degrees (for example, use the "football hold")
- choose a bra that offers good support but is not tight
- nurse more often and for longer periods, offering the sore breast first to be sure it's emptied
- apply extremes in temperature, either very cold or hot; use ice packs or some form of moist heat. For instance, soak in a hot tub, shower or use hot, damp towels
- express a little milk manually before putting your baby to the breast in order to start the flow, and then let your baby empty the rest
- gently and patiently massage the blocked area with your fingers
- soak your breasts in hot comfrey tea
- wash off dried secretions with sterile water, to prevent further blockage

SORE AND CRACKED NIPPLES

Possible Causes	Possible Remedies
nipples are unused to constant irritation, so they become sore, and wetness adds to softening of skin	expose nipples to air as much as possible; wear milk cups or breast shields; other techniques include shining a sun lamp or 60-watt bulb on sore nipples a few minutes a day or using a hair dryer after each feeding
	smooth on pure lanolin or vitamin E oil after washing and drying, following each nursing session; this lubrication also prevents cracked skin from reopening, but don't slather on too much, as it may block pores

SORE AND CRACKED NIPPLES

Possible Causes	Possible Remedies
	dip breasts in ice water or apply ice packs to them
	offer less sore breast to baby first
	try Dr. Naylor's Udder Balm, sold in feed stores, recommends one nurse-midwife
baby is nursing too long initially	limit length of each feeding to 5 minutes on each side but increase frequency (at least every 2 hours); if baby craves to suck, consider a pacifier
milk is slow to come in, which makes baby strain and suck too hard	sit in warm tub or stand in shower before you nurse; sip some wine or beer to help you relax while breast-feeding
	express a little milk manually before putting baby to breast, to get flow started
baby is sucking improperly	be sure baby is latched on to most or all of the areola (darker part around nipple), not just the nipple
	experiment with holding the baby in different positions so baby is not pulling downward on nipple (try nursing lying down, with baby on top, or sitting down, with baby propped by pillows on your lap)
nipples are sensitive to skin irritants, possibly nursing bra, detergent residue; pulling baby off nipple	avoid synthetics and use cotton fabrics; use only warm water for cleaning, and double-rinse your underwear after washing
	break baby's suction on your breast before pulling away by inserting a finger gently into the mouth

SORE AND CRACKED NIPPLES

Possible Causes	Possible Remedies
yeast infection (thrush)	look inside baby's mouth for white spots signaling a fungal infection (refer to "Common Problems from Allergies to Rashes," p. 391)

If your nipples become cracked and/or bleed:

- no nursing on bleeding nipple for 24 to 48 hours; switch to formula
- then manually express or nurse every two hours around the clock to stave off plugged ducts or mastitis
- wake baby if you are not too tired for night feedings
- after bleeding stops or crack no longer looks red, resume nursing, but for *no longer* than five minutes; use nipple shield (available at drugstores) to protect cracked areas during healing period
- expect one to two weeks before completely eliminating the formula you have been substituting

Drugs During Lactation

Just as drugs in your bloodstream crossed the placenta to your baby in utero, many medications you might take now can be passed on to your baby through breast milk. Although they are partially metabolized, detoxified and excreted by you, your baby, with a still-immature enzyme system and as yet not fully functioning kidneys, is responsible for breaking down the rest. This is why, despite the relatively small amounts that slip through, toxic levels of the drug may build up over time if traces of previous doses remain unmetabolized in your baby's bloodstream. At issue here is not whether a drug is excreted into your milk, since most drugs are, but how or whether it affects your baby and whether drug therapy will mean giving up breast-feeding, if only temporarily.

Apart from a few drugs that are known to harm infants, little is known about the possible adverse effects of others. Animal studies are often unreliable, variables in epidemiological studies are difficult to control and experiments on humans are obviously not desirable. While you cannot rely on scientific data to determine safety, there are a few steps you can take to try to protect your nursing baby. Before a drug is prescribed:

(1) be sure your doctor knows you are breast-feeding
(2) ask about any known adverse effects on you and your baby
(3) find out if there are substitutes available, which, though perhaps less effective for you, would be safer for your infant
(4) ask if there is a risk of sensitization. Some babies whose mothers have taken penicillin during lactation later develop an allergy to the antibiotic
(5) double-check the advisability of the medication with your baby's doctor.

The degree of adverse reaction—if any—will vary from drug to drug, but not necessarily in proportion to the strength of the medication. A prescription pain-killer, for instance, may actually carry less risk to your baby through breast-milk transfer than an over-the-counter pain-relief preparation, so always read labels, and to be safe, clear any nonprescription or over-the-counter drug with your baby's doctor.

Your baby should be closely watched for side effects if you are taking barbiturates or sedatives, and nursing is absolutely out of the question if you are undergoing anticancer, radioactive or hormone therapy. Antibiotics, in part because treatment is generally short-term, are not known to be beneficial or harmful, except for the possibility of your baby's developing an allergic reaction to them later on.

The amount of the drug your baby receives depends chiefly on the physical and chemical properties of the medication, the dosage and the lag time between taking it and nursing. Here are a few suggestions that should help keep the amount passed on to your baby to a minimum:

- schedule doses for times when your baby is least likely to nurse; plan for the maximum time span between when you take the drug and the next feeding
- watch for side effects in your baby, excessive sleepiness or lethargy, weight loss, refusal to nurse, loss of muscle tone, lowered body temperature, change in color (that is, becoming grayish blue), vomiting and diarrhea; catching them early will help keep toxic levels down
- opt for the short-acting form of the drug to avoid accumulation (for example, take medication that works for only 4 hours rather than 12 hours)
- if given a choice, choose a water-soluble drug rather than a fat-soluble one, which would settle in the fat of your breast milk.

In the event that your health demands that you take a medication harmful or toxic to your child, some options to consider include:

- pumping, expressing and discarding milk while on medication, to keep up your milk supply; use formula until you are off the drug and can resume nursing
- considering the use of a wet nurse
- weaning and controlling engorgement (rapid weaning is going to be initially unpleasant for both of you); instead of wearing a tight-fitting bra, fold a turkish towel in thirds and pin it firmly around your breasts and keep it on for 48 hours, retightening it from time to time; also try putting Baggies full of ice cubes on each breast with a towel in between; take Tylenol and remember the discomfort will pass.

If you have a question about a specific medication, you can write or call the La Leche League International between 9:00 A.M. and 3:00 P.M. (central time zone) at 312-455-7730. Consult *Physicians' Desk Reference* and *USP DI: Advice for the Patient*, which are available at many public libraries and at most hospital or medical libraries.

Back on the Job and Breast-feeding

It is indeed possible to combine breast-feeding and employment outside the home even if your employer doesn't provide on-site day care or if arrangements cannot be made to nurse your baby once or twice during the day. More practical advice is available as more women succeed in pumping milk between 9:00 and 5:00.

Stockpile milk. If you don't want to introduce infant formula at all, you need to build up a supply of frozen milk before returning to work, generally by expressing small amounts of milk (0.5 to 1 ounce) before or after your baby's feedings for several weeks before your routine changes.

Early introduction of the bottle. Don't wait until you return to work to introduce the bottle, because your baby may well reject it. With early introduction of the bottle after several weeks of exclusive breast-feeding but before 5 weeks of age, you are likely to avoid such problems. After it is introduced, a bottle of expressed breast milk or formula should be used once a day to maintain the baby's acceptance of it. Babies several months old who absolutely refuse to have anything to do with a bottle may have less resistance to atypical bottle nipples such as Playtex or Nuk.

Missed feedings. One solution is to replace one or more breast-feedings with formula feedings. If you prefer to maintain an all-breast-milk diet, it will be necessary—for your own comfort and for the maintenance of your milk production—to express milk once or perhaps twice during your workday. This expressed milk can be used for your baby's lunch the next day. It takes practice and patience to learn how to pump milk, and consider having someone, even nurses at the hospital maternity ward, help you master the technique. Some mothers rely on a pump to initiate the let-down reflex and then switch to manual expression, which involves compressing the areola (dark area around the nipple) in a repetitive fashion, either pressing it back against the rib cage or not, depending on what works better for you.

Sterilization and storage of expressed milk. Clean rather than sterile techniques will do; the instructions about expressing milk you read about elsewhere are often intended for the donation of milk to sick infants, and such sterility requirements are neither necessary nor practical for working mothers, according to several pediatricians who themselves breast-fed their babies successfully while on the job. Milk must be stored in a refrigerator until you leave for home.

Weekends. As your baby grows, your milk supply needs to keep pace with your baby's demand. This occurs naturally if you nurse full-time, but some provision must be made if you combine formula and breast milk. One suggestion is to maintain the weekday bottle-feeding schedule during the weekends, except for one additional breast-feeding. This may lead to discomfort on Monday, but it reduces the likelihood of inadequate milk supply.

Travel. If you travel on business, there are basically two options, as you well know. You can take your baby with you (and perhaps a babysitter) or arrange for bottle-feeding (breast milk or formula) while you are away, pumping milk in the meantime for your own comfort and to maintain milk production. Unfortunately, however, a public rest room in a hotel or on an airplane is not well suited for expressing milk, so other arrangements should be made. Remember to build in enough time in your schedule so you aren't too rushed when you empty your breasts.

Encouragement is crucial for full-time working mothers who want to breast-feed. Find a pediatrician or family practitioner who is pronursing and can offer practical advice. Although the La Leche League's focus is on full-time mothers, the local chapter may be able to put you in touch with women in your situation.

Environmental Toxins in Breast Milk

Today, traces of herbicides and pesticides can be found in body fluids of most Americans and, consequently, in nursing mothers' milk. The unanswered question for these mothers is, "At what level does the threat of these contaminants become greater than the many nutritional and immunological benefits of human milk?" No one knows. Thus far there is no information that would correlate contaminants with adverse effects on a nursing infant, yet that is not to say categorically that every woman should breast-feed regardless of environmental contaminants in her system. It must be a decision based in part on the degree of exposure not only in the home but also in the workplace. Unless you use bottled water, even a switch to bottle feeding will make little difference since, if contaminants are present in your breast milk, they are inevitably present in your water supply and will find their way into your baby's system. If you are concerned, some sophisticated labs can test your milk for environmental toxins, but at this time there are no guidelines for determining what is a safe level. This may be something to discuss with your baby's doctor.

Weaning Process

There is no consensus on the ideal time to begin taking your baby off the breast. Timing and method will depend on your personal and professional circumstances and your child's developmental and emotional needs. A move directly from breast to cup, for instance, in order to avoid a second "weaning," from the bottle, won't be possible until your baby has the strength and coordination to manage it. Then again, your child may take the decision out of your hands by weaning himself or herself between 8 and 18 months, as interest in the world "outside" broadens. La Leche League would encourage you not to put an artificial stop to breast-feeding, but to continue well into toddlerhood, so that a feeling of security is established that will allow your child to feel "safe" enough to be truly independent. Others agree with child-rearing expert Dr. T. Berry Brazelton, who believes that nursing after the baby's first birthday tends to do just the opposite, and encourages excessive dependence.

How to Wean. Here again, the physical and psychological needs of the two of you will dictate your weaning method. Expect to experiment first to see what suits both of you, be flexible and try not to commit yourself to an ironclad timetable. Some suggestions are:

- Very gradually cut back, eliminating one feeding daily over a number of days, preferably beginning with your baby's least favorite, usually the midday one.
- Substitute either a bottle, a cup or solids (remember, pureed foods contain a lot of liquids) for the breast-milk feeding you skip; a cup won't be possible until your child is about 4 or 5 months old, and you must be sure you offer enough milk throughout the day—12 to 16 ounces—to be certain the baby is getting enough.

● Once you work down to just one feeding daily for a few days, begin dropping days of nursing altogether until your supply dwindles away or your baby loses interest.

The more gradual the weaning, the more comfortable for you physically, so if you opt to go cold turkey, expect a few days of painful, engorged breasts and maybe a stiff neck or back from their weight. (Suggestions for controlling discomfort if you must wean rapidly are discussed on p. 326.) Another possible by-product of abrupt weaning is milk fever—flulike symptoms, possibly accompanied by a fever—which is believed to come from quick reabsorption of milk into your system. Another withdrawal symptom could be depression at the reality of finally cutting this special closeness, an emotion aggravated by a drop in the milk-producing hormone prolactin, high levels of which are associated with feelings of well-being.

Objections are bound to be voiced at first by your baby, yet many infants make the break or transition without too much fussiness. You may find it helps to have another person offer the bottle, since the baby is less likely to refuse it from someone other than you. Because your child's gastrointestinal tract has been used to easily digestible mother's milk, a switch to formula and/or solids could show up at first in loose bowels, but the change is more likely to be in firmer and darker stools.

There is no "right" way to wean, and what works for another mother won't necessarily be the best approach for you and your son or daughter. Regardless of how you do it, don't forget to throw in lots of extra loving attention to make up for the body contact your baby will miss initially.

Information Sources

ADDITIONAL READING

Breastfeeding: A Guide for the Medical Profession, by Ruth A. Lawrence (St. Louis: C. V. Mosby, 1980). Useful reference guide, available at many medical libraries.

Breastfeeding Basics, by Cecilia Worth (New York: McGraw-Hill, 1983). Suggestions for on-the-spot help.

The Breastfeeding Book, by Maire Messenger (New York: Van Nostrand Reinhold, 1983). Techniques of breast-feeding, as well as its many advantages.

The Complete Book of Breastfeeding, by Marvin Eiger and Sally Wendkos Olds (New York: Bantam, 1973). Answers questions frequently raised by mothers.

Tender Gift: Breastfeeding, by Dana Raphael (New York: Schocken, 1979). Emphasis on support system for nursing mother.

You Can Breastfeed Your Baby. . . Even in Special Situations, by Dorothy Patricia Brewster (Emmaus, PA: Rodale, 1979). Reassuring and specific advice.

ORGANIZATIONS

Human Lactation Center Ltd.
666 Sturges Hwy.
Westport, CT 06880
Research organization that is not staffed to handle questions; however, its publications and studies are available to nonmembers.

Lactation Associates
123 Aldrich St.
Boston, MA 02131
Group of health-care professionals work principally with other health-care providers but have literature available to mothers.

La Leche League International (LLLI)
9615 Minneapolis Ave.
Franklin Park, IL 60131
Information clearinghouse with local chapters nationwide; LLLI will send free brochure listing its many pamphlets and books on nursing.

SEX: INTIMATE QUESTIONS

The same basic guideline applies for sex postpartum as for sex during pregnancy: Anything is fine, as long as it feels comfortable. Though that usually means waiting to resume intercourse until soreness disappears and stitches have healed (the standard is six weeks after birth), your body and psyche may dictate a different schedule altogether. As long as bleeding has stopped and you can easily insert a finger or tampon into your vagina, you've got the green light to resume making love. The initial discomfort of intercourse is just one of the several factors that may call for temporary adjustment in your sex life. These adjustments aren't all negative, though, as many couples claim some of these same factors are also responsible for improving their intimate relationship. Described below is a composite of what commonly influences a couple's sexual rapport during the first several weeks postpartum, some suggestions on how to smooth the adjustment and, finally, a rundown on contraception.

Physiological Changes. While many women become multi-orgasmic or orgasmic for the first time, owing to a temporarily fuller blood supply in the pelvis and genitals, others experience a drop in sex drive. A lower level of estrogen is largely responsible for this drop, as well as for drying the vaginal tissues and diminishing secretions, and may be particularly pronounced in lactating mothers, since the milk-producing hormone, prolactin, further inhibits estrogen production. The pleasure of making love may be lessened for a while, until loose tissues and temporarily dulled nerve endings in and around your vagina return to their prebirth condition.

Fear or Anxiety. Even if labor wasn't especially painful, you may tense up for fear that intercourse will hurt, and be especially guarded because of episiotomy stitches, which may prickle and pull still-tender sore skin. Apart from the discomfort, you may worry about opening up wounds and introducing infection; yet the risk of this is slight. Anxiety-provoking, too, may be the possibility of getting pregnant again soon, which is in direct contrast to the last nine months of worry-free intercourse.

Emotional Changes. Though the two of you may sometimes feel like strangers in bed if good communication has been impossible during the day, many couples feel more intimate than ever now, partly because of the man's involvement in the birth process or perhaps because the baby seems to have cemented their commitment to each other.

Overall Tension. Besides the underlying stress of round-the-clock baby care, with one ear always cocked to hear if your newborn is all right, you may sense resentment building toward your mate if he hasn't shouldered as many of the responsibilities as you'd like. Or your mate may feel excluded if you don't allow or encourage him to diaper, cuddle, bathe or feed your baby. The two of you may worry that lovemaking won't be as good as before, that it may hurt or that your vagina will be too stretched to please your mate. Trying an unfamiliar birth-control method during postpartum may also inhibit you.

Breast-feeding. About as many women report heightened sexual desire because they are nursing as do the number who complain about a lowered sex drive during this period. Some feel sexier because of larger, more sensitive breasts that receive repeated stimulation, whereas others perceive their breasts as sexless, functioning only as milk machines and the sole property of their babies. Don't be surprised if during intercourse your breasts leak, since sexual arousal releases oxytocin, which in turn triggers the milk let-down reflex.

Fatigue or Postpartum Blues. Constant baby care and middle-of-the-night feedings may leave little energy for sex play. You may crave nothing but sleep. A hallmark of depression is a loss of interest in sex, and depression is often aggravated by exhaustion.

Self-Esteem. Having had a baby may make you feel all the more womanly and sensual, proud of your body and what it can do. However, it may undermine your confidence and belief in your desirability not only because of a doughy tummy but because of skin problems and temporary hair loss as well. Give yourself time to regain completely your prepregnancy state.

Sex Suggestions

The opportunities for spontaneous sex dwindle rapidly after your baby comes home. Like many couples, however, you may find that, with planning, what is lost in quantity is made up for by the quality of time you do get to spend alone together. In addition to finding a new schedule for lovemaking here are some other suggestions for adapting during the postpartum period.

- *New and different positions.* The man-on-top position will mean penile thrusting is directed against your episiotomy stitches, so you may want to try a female-superior position, so that pressure is off this sore spot and you can better control the speed and depth of penetration. Another suggestion is side-by-side or rear entry, and bearing down during entry rather than pulling back.
- *Additional lubrication.* Unless you are using a birth-control method that already calls for it, try applying a water-based lubricant, such as K-Y jelly, and make its application part of sexual foreplay.
- *Exercises.* Kegels are highly recommended to tone up the figure-eight muscles that surround the vagina and anus; the beauty of them here is that they can be done during intercourse and heighten the pleasure at the same time (see "Conditioning Exercises: What's a Kegel?" p. 68).
- *Dispelling the fear.* If you hesitate to make love for fear of pain or disappointment, one way to reassure yourselves is to predict what penetration will probably feel like by inserting two fingers into your vagina and rotating them.
- *Communication.* Covering up or shutting in feelings, whether good or bad, gradually builds a wall between you and your mate. Trusting enough to share emotions—grievances, worries, jealousies—will enable you to feel closer and more relaxed about sharing your bodies as well.

Sex and Contraception

Your choice of contraception is somewhat limited if you are nursing. Getting pregnant, though less likely because ovulation may not be as regular, is still possible. Breast-feeding as a form of child spacing is unreliable because, as an American Academy of Pediatrics report points out, "between five and ten percent of women with lactational amenorrhea [no menstrual periods] become pregnant and an even greater proportion of nursing mothers who have reinitiated menstruation become pregnant." One nurse-midwife recalls seeing two nursing mothers who conceived again before their sixth-week-postpartum checkup. If avoiding another pregnancy soon is important to you, contraception should be begun by at least the fourth or fifth week postpartum.

Of the contraceptive techniques available, the safest and most reliable for nursing mothers are the barrier methods: sponge, diaphragm with jelly and condom. If you use a diaphragm, you need to be refitted after birth, because of your changed internal dimensions. Some health professionals recommend rechecking the new one, too, once you stop breast-feeding. Steroidal contraceptives such as the Pill are not recommended for lactating women, since the hormones they contain tend to reduce milk production and are passed on to the baby through the breast milk. IUDs (intrauterine devices) should definitely not be inserted until after six weeks postpartum, and mothers should carefully monitor the latest research findings. Preliminary evidence links IUD use and breast-feeding to uterine perforation on the theory that the walls of the uterus remain thin because lactation keeps estrogen levels low. Relying on the rhythm method (Fertility Awareness Method)—counting days, charting basal temperature, evaluating cervical mucus—is risky, since your cycle is bound to be irregular and the amount and the nature of secretions will be misleading. If this is the method you prefer, however, seek a professional who is a "believer," in order to get specific guidelines on what to watch out for and special precautions to take.

Mothers who are not nursing can use just about any form of contraception. If you want to continue using a diaphragm, be sure to get refitted, since you may well have changed size. The IUD should not be inserted prior to the sixth-week checkup and is ill-advised if you have a history of ectopic pregnancy, pelvic inflammatory disease or severe anemia. Oral contraceptives are not recommended if you have a medical history of high blood pressure or if you experienced toxemia. Another warning about the fertility awareness method: It is a bit risky during the first few weeks after birth, since the presence of lochia makes it nearly impossible to judge your cervical mucus.

If you decide to get vaccinated against rubella now, be meticulous and thorough about contraception for at least three months afterward, since a baby conceived while you are exposed to the German measles vaccine could suffer birth defects.

DAY CARE, LIVE-INS AND BABYSITTERS

If you plan to return to work, unless you are one of the lucky few whose employers offer on-site day care, you will need to research options available in your community. Begin at least a month or two before you expect to need child care. Home care is the most popular choice among parents with children under three years old—whether it means having someone come into your own home or taking your baby to someone else's—not only because very few private or commercial day-care centers will accept children before that age but also in view of an infant's or toddler's special need for individual care and attention. Once your child has developed adequate communication skills and socializing becomes more important, center-based care is ideal, especially when coupled with educational, cultural or religious programs. Many parents end up mixing and matching day-care options. A friend or relative may watch a child in the morning, for instance, then drop him or her off in a home-care program for the afternoon hours.

As a parent, you are bound to wonder if treating your child like a hot potato and having him or her spend so much time with a surrogate parent might not have some negative psychological impact, especially if begun early in life. Should day care wait until your baby reaches a certain age? Is it a good idea at all? "There is no conclusive research on the subject, just formal opinions of people," answers Dr. Stanley Greenspan, Director of the Clinical Infant Development Program at the government's National Institute of Mental Health.

> The basic issue is not day care versus no day care but the quality of mothering when available. Though there is no best time to put a baby in another's care there is a best way. First, a mother needs to solidify her new emotional relationship with her child and establish a high quality of interaction with him or her. Secondly, she must be satisfied with the quality of her child's care-giver, making sure that that person offers the same experiential nutriments not only in love and affection but in helping the baby master an array of developmental tasks.

The following are brief descriptions of the three basic child-care options along with some suggestions, primarily from the U.S. Department of Health and Human Services, on how to evaluate the one you choose.

Care in Your Own Home

In-home care provided by a babysitter or live-in such as a "nanny" may be an excellent choice for infants and young toddlers or for babies needing special care. In the case of a live-in, though, it is not a simple employer-employee relationship. "It's almost like a marriage," says one mother, "in which the partners must continually communicate about their needs and their expectations and what's going on with the development of the child."

Once you have located a candidate, a phone interview is the first step in the selection process, followed by a visit in your home if the prospective sitter or live-in seems promising. In the interview, throw out questions such as:

- Have you worked with children before? What were their ages?
- What kinds of things do you like to do with children?
- What other kinds of work experience have you had?
- Why did you leave your last job?
- Are you considering other types of work?
- May I have the names of the people for whom you have worked before?

Besides checking out references and before signing someone on, it is a good idea to get a written agreement regarding responsibilities and policies. Be sure you both agree about the following:

- days and hours care-giver is to work
- terms of payment
- policies concerning visitors, phone calls, television and radio while care-giver is working
- other tasks (housework, shopping, preparing meals, and so on)
- amount of notice and pay necessary to end arrangement.

INFORMATION CHECKLIST FOR SITTER

(1) List 911 or number for emergency

(2) Number of police, fire and poison-control center

(3) Phone number of where you can be reached

(4) Name and number of baby's doctor

(5) Name and number of nearby friend or relative

(6) Special instructions about feeding (such as prepar-

ing and handling breast milk, when you expect
the baby to be hungry, how to burp)

(7) Ways to calm a crying baby: favorite positions,
toys, books and so on

(8) Specific don'ts such as no bottle in bed; no
chocolate, peanuts or other foods baby may be
allergic to; no smoking

(9) Estimated time of return.

Care in Another Person's Home

"Family day care" is care given by a friend, parent, relative, neighbor
or someone you haven't known previously. Family-day-care mothers
usually watch no more than 6 children; if there are between 6 and 12,
the setup is referred to as a group home and required by state law to be
staffed by at least one additional care-giver. This option is especially
attractive if you are a single parent who wishes her child to have
contact with another adult or if your toddler still needs extra attention
yet is eager to play with other youngsters. Family-day-care homes may
be licensed, certified, registered or approved, according to individual
state laws, whereas all child-care centers must be licensed. The ideal
time to evaluate a day-care home is while child care is in progress;
when there are a few free moments for discussion, find out:

- how she got started as a family-day-care-giver
- how long she has been doing it
- how many children she cares for each day and their ages
- what types of things she likes to do with children
- how she cares for sick children.

If the family-day-care mother has no contract, you may want to draw
up your own, stipulating:

- care-giver services
- terms of payment
- your responsibilities (times for arrival and pickup, phone numbers,
  instruction for feeding and giving medication)
- specific policies (care for sick child, taking trips and so on)
- written notice and pay needed to end the arrangement.

Day-Care Centers

So-called centered-base care usually will not take children younger
than 2½ or 3 years old. Nursery schools or preschools fall into this

category. All such centers must meet specific safety and hygiene standards in order to be licensed by the county or state. Many have an educational, cultural or religious focus. When you check out the ones you are interested in, go while the children are there, ask to speak with the director and be sure the child-adult ratio is appropriate for the age group. For children under 3 years there should be one adult to four to five children, and for 3- to 5-year-olds, one care-giver for seven to nine children. Most centers provide their own contracts and information forms.

General Evaluation Checklist

Does your child's care-giver

- have the right materials and equipment on hand to help children learn and grow mentally and physically?
- patiently help children solve their problems?
- encourage good health habits, such as washing hands before eating?
- talk to children and encourage them to express themselves through words?
- seem to have enough time to look after all the children in her care?
- take time to discuss your child with you regularly?
- child-proof the setting so your toddler can crawl or walk safely and freely and will not be confined to a crib or play-pen?
- help your child learn to speak by talking with him or her, naming things, reading aloud, describing what she is doing and responding to your child's words?

Does the child-care home or center have

- an up-to-date license, if one is required? Was theirs ever revoked? If so, why?
- a clean and comfortable appearance?
- enough space indoors and out so all the children can move freely and safely?
- equipment that is safe and in good repair?
- an outdoor play area that is safe, fenced and free of litter or debris?
- nutritious meals and snacks made with the kinds of food you prefer for your child?
- gates at the tops and bottoms of stairs?
- a potty chair or special toilet seat in the bathroom?
- separate crib sheets for each baby in care?

Are there opportunities

- to play quietly and actively, indoors and out?
- to crawl and explore safely?
- to play with objects and toys that help infants develop their senses of touch, sight and hearing? These would include mirrors, mobiles, cradle gyms, crib toys, rattles, things to squeeze and roll, pots and pans, nesting cups, different-sized boxes.
- to rest and take naps?

Checking References

No one likes to give a bad reference, so to avoid yes-or-no or evasive answers to your inquiries, try asking:

(1) Would you choose this person or center again?

(2) What did you like most about this person or center?

(3) Did you have any problems?

Even if the answers are vague and noncommittal, you can get an idea of the person's true feelings just by the tone of voice or readiness to respond.

Adjustments to Separation

Except for infants, the younger the child, the more stressful separation is going to be. Dr. Bryna Siegel-Gorelick, child psychologist at Stanford University Medical Center, writes in her *Working Parents' Guide to Child Care* that feelings of security and "strength of attachment [are] determined in part by the parents' behavior and partially by the innate character of the child." Some children appear to have inborn feelings of insecurity despite the love and attention their parents lavish on them, yet even the most secure will show some reaction to separation from the familiar and to change in routine. One key to smooth transition from your care to another's is to make it gradual. Try to spend a day or at least a few hours for a couple of days with your child and the care-giver, to ease him or her into this new world of strange people and objects. Important, too, is reinforcing feelings of love and constancy by spending a little extra "special" time with your child in the morning before dropping him or her off. Expect the first time you part with him or her to be somewhat emotional on both sides. If your child is aged 9 to 14 months, the period of greatest "separation anxiety," it will be particularly difficult. Reunion at the end of the day may be either joyous and clinging or indifferent and resentful as your child unconsciously tries to make you feel guilty for having left. Other initial reactions of small children include tantrums, eating constantly or not at all, and waking at night or having nightmares. If the child is placed in a good day-care center, these negative responses will gradually fade away, particularly once your child has learned that you will always return and as he or she grows in attachment to the care-giver and other children under her care.

If, on the other hand, after two weeks or so, things do not improve, reevaluate the day-care setup. From her clinical experience, Dr. Siegel-Gorelick finds that any lasting difficulty in adjustment is generally due to an inappropriate child-care arrangement, not to a child's inability to adapt. Don't hesitate to make other arrangements but, again, try as much as possible to make the transition gradual.

Backup Arrangements and Finances

In case your child's sitter or care-giver gets sick, be sure you or the care-giver has an "on call" substitute. In the event that your child becomes ill while you are at work, the care-giver should have written instructions about whom to contact—you, the father, a relative, the doctor, the health center—and to check with you before giving any medication, such as baby aspirin.

The cost of child care varies not only from one type to another but from one location to the next. Just keep in mind that expensive care does not necessarily guarantee that it is the best. Be conscientious about keeping good records of costs, for use on next year's taxes, as you may qualify for a federal income tax credit of up to 20 percent of your child-care expenses. Driving up the cost of child care in your own home is your obligation to contribute to the sitter's or live-in's Social Security tax (FICA), to federal unemployment tax and to withhold state and federal taxes from her salary. A woman caring for children in her own home, however, is responsible for paying her own FICA and state and federal taxes. Check with your local Internal Revenue Service office for current regulations.

Information Sources

ADDITIONAL READING

Day Care Services Through the Workplace, prepared by The Women's Bureau, U.S. Department of Labor, to provide information on industrial-based day care. Available free by writing the Bureau at 3rd and Constitution Aves., Room S3005, Washington, D.C. 20210.

First Feelings: The Emotional Care of the Infant and Young Child, by Dr. Stanley Greenspan and Nancy T. Greenspan (New York: McGraw-Hill, 1984).

A Parent's Guide to Day Care, prepared by the U.S. Department of Health and Human Services. Available for $4.75 from The Superintendent of Documents, U.S. Government Printing Office, Washington, D.C. 20402. Ask for stock number 017-091-00231-2.

The Pocket Guide to Babysitting, prepared by the U.S. Department of Health and Human Services. Available for $4.50 from The Superintendent of Documents, U.S. Government Printing Office, Washington, D.C. 20402. Ask for stock number 017-091-00236-3.

Pointers for Participating Parents. Manual on how to set up your own day-care coop. Available for $5.50 from California Council of Parent Participation Nursery Schools, Inc., 682 E. 67th St., Long Beach, CA 90805.

The Working Parents' Guide to Child Care: How to Find the Best Care For Your Child, by Bryna Siegel-Gorelick, Ph.D. (Boston: Little, Brown, 1983). Covers the pros and cons of three types of care available, addresses issues such as the psychological impact of day care, adjustments, locating and assessing the center and/or care-giver.

ORGANIZATIONS (local resources)

For a list of licensed day-care centers in your area:
- contact local, county or state public welfare agencies, the Community Coordinated Child Care Program if there is one, the United Way of America or the Community Chest
- contact churches, synagogues, other places of worship
- contact colleges and universities, which may have their own centers
- look at bulletin boards in shopping malls, grocery stores and so on
- read the classified section of the newspaper under the headings "situations wanted," "domestic services," "babysitting services," "child care"
- look in the Yellow Pages under "Day Nurseries" and "Child Care," as well as under local chapters of women's organizations, parents' groups, child-care associations
- find out by word of mouth—from other mothers in the area, neighbors, coworkers; also try retired people in the community or local retirement homes or senior-citizen clubs.

⑩

Baby Supplies

CAR SEATS, CRIBS AND OTHER ESSENTIAL EQUIPMENT

Unlike an infant car seat, where having one can be a matter of life or death, most of the baby equipment and nursery furniture doesn't fall into the category of essential. Your expense can be negligible or you can spend hundreds of dollars if you want the top-of-the-line stroller or even accessories for the crib. This shopping guide provides you with a quick checklist designed to help you decide what to buy—for example, a high chair or portable seat—and also what to look for when comparing different models.

Car Seats

Buying a car safety seat should be at the top of your list of things your newborn will need. Remember to bring it to the hospital so the first ride is a safe one. Many models represent a four-year investment, because they can be used through the toddler and preschool years. Not even a full-size crib is used for this length of time by any one child.

Grim statistics are the reason that buying a child-restraint system is *your most important purchase.* Car accidents are the leading cause of death to infants and children. And thousands more are seriously injured. Studies by the government's National Highway Traffic Safety Administration show that:

- if you hold your child in the same lap belt with you, the weight of your body can crush the child in a crash
- an infant held in your arms can weigh as much as 300 pounds in just a 30-mile-an-hour crash
- a baby held in the arms of an unbelted adult can be crushed between the adult and the dashboard
- children behave better in car seats, according to numerous studies
- child-restraint systems have been shown to reduce the probability of a fatal injury in automobile crashes by 80 percent.

All but a few states have laws requiring that youngsters under five years of age ride in safety seats that meet federal regulations.

There are over 30 different models of child-restraint systems on the market that meet dynamic government crash-testing standards. Most car seats cost between $25 and $75 and are sold by discount, retail and juvenile-products stores as well as catalog outlets and car dealerships. There are three basic types of safety seats available from which to choose:

(1) *Infants only:* Safety seats are designed for use only in the rear-facing position for infants up to 17–20 pounds which means you will have to make a second purchase when your baby outgrows this type of restraint. By and large, infant car seats fit almost all cars and are secured to the vehicle by the car safety belt. Another advantage is that they are lightweight and can double as an infant carrier and a feeder seat. Several models include Questor Dyn-O-Mite, Chrysler Infant Love Seat, Ford Infant Love Seat and Cosco/Peterson First Ride.

(2) *Infants and Toddlers/Convertible type:* Convertible seats are the most cost-efficient choice since they can be used from birth through 40 pounds. Convertible seats can be adjusted to carry infants in the rear-facing position and in a forward-facing mode for toddlers. Before you buy a convertible model, make sure the seat can be anchored properly in both the infant and toddler position in your car by the safety belt. The majority of seats are elevated and let your child see more out the window. Some models must be secured by both a vehicle seat belt and a tether strap. The tether strap which offers extra protection must be installed by drilling a hole in the rear window shelf or cargo area.

(3) *Toddlers only:* Some seats can be used for children weighing from 20 to 50 pounds. There are models that resemble shields which are very easy to use but provide no side protection so it is best to install them in the center of the back seat. Toddler restraints with a harness provide more protection and it's harder for children to climb out. Booster seats such as Century Safe-T-Rider Deluxe and

Strolee Wee Care 602 are designed for toddlers who have out-grown their safety seats but are too short to use adult lap and shoulder belts. These seats provide the child with upper body protection and allow them to see out the car windows.

The National Traffic Highway Safety Administration operates a toll-free hot line (800-424-9394; in Washington, D.C., call 202-426-0123) providing consumers with literature about buying a car seat. For advice on choosing a model that is compatible with your car or for other safety seat information, you can call the American Academy of Pediatrics at 800-323-0797 or contact the National Child Passenger Safety Association at 215-525-4610 (PO Box 841, Ardmore, PA 19003). For more help, contact your Governor's Highway Safety office. Here are some of their suggestions:

- Any seat you consider buying should have a label on the back that reads, "meets or exceeds Federal Motor Vehicle Safety Standard 213."
- Consider both the size of your child and your car. Some seats in the rear-facing position for infants may not fit some small cars. Many Japanese-made vehicles have rear seat belts with oversized buckles that are too large to be threaded through some safety seat frames and even when threading is possible, they sometimes cannot be adequately tightened.
- Figure out how many straps and buckles need to be fastened each time the seat is used. Also, before making a purchase, check to see if your child can move his/her arms freely and also can see out the window. If the seat has an armrest or shield, make sure the ceiling of your car is high enough to raise the armrest or shield completely and when it's unfastened—in an upright position—it does not block the driver's view out the back window.
- Be wary of secondhand car seats. Some older models, which merely hook over or under the passenger seat, do not protect and should not be used. The organizations listed earlier can tell you whether or not a particular seat meets minimum safety standards.
- Shop carefully for the best deal, since the same car seat may sell at a wide range of prices in various stores in your area. Ask about rental or wholesale programs being run by community service groups or your state health agency.

If you travel a lot, you may want to consider buying a car seat that has been approved by the Federal Aviation Administration for use on commercial flights. One catch, though, is that children under 2 years, who usually fly free, may be charged 75 percent or full fare because they occupy a seat. When you are away from home, either take your own car seat or make arrangements to rent or borrow one. Some car-rental companies have child-safety restraints but be sure to reserve one. In Orlando, Florida, the home of Walt Disney, the demand for car seats is fierce, so don't wait until you arrive at the airport to make arrangements.

Here are some practical tips along with a few other safety measures for you to keep in mind:

(1) Remember that the center of the back seat is the safest place in the car.

(2) Try using blankets or rolled diapers to support newborn baby's head and body until he/she is big enough to be supported by the safety seat frame.

(3) Make sure the harness is snug and the car seat belt is tight around the restraint system. Double-check the instructions regarding proper installation. If your seat requires a tether strap, be sure to use it.

(4) To keep your baby comfortable in the seat and to ensure a snug fit of the buckles, use outfits with legs and save papoose buntings and sack sleepers for those times when you aren't on the road.

(5) Many toddlers go through a stage of wanting to climb out of their car seats, often between 12 to 18 months. Pediatricians describe this as a developmental stage that is temporary, but do not allow your child to ride in the car in any place but the safety seat. Be consistent and hold your position—it will pay off when your child is older.

Changing Tables

A changing table is relatively inexpensive and avoids back strain every time you diaper or dress your baby. Many parents, however, find their double bed or a wide, sturdy table works just as well. If you decide to purchase a changing table, there are several shopping checkpoints to consider:

- security rim surrounding all four sides, ideally about three inches high
- sturdy frame and legs
- easy-to-use buckle.

One word of caution: Never turn your back while your baby is on the changing table. It takes only a split second for a 4-month-old infant to roll over or a year-old child to fall. Another precaution is to keep talcum powder (cornstarch is preferred), ointments, creams and other bath products out of your child's reach. Such substances are easily ingested or inhaled and may cause potentially serious respiratory problems.

Cribs

Standard-size cribs must meet certain federal standards, although manufacturers no longer have to put a label on this furniture indicating compliance with government regulations. If you are buying a new crib, the U.S. Consumer Product Safety Commission offers the following suggestions:

- Crib slats should be close together, so babies' heads and feet cannot slip through the slats and get caught. Buy a crib with as narrow a space as possible between the slats, which should be no more than 2⅜ inches apart.
- The mattress you use should fit the crib very snugly. If you can fit more than two fingers between the mattress and the crib frame, the mattress is too small.
- Locks and latches on the drop side must be safe from accidental release.
- Buy a crib with as large a distance as possible between the top of the side rail and the mattress support. This will discourage your baby from trying to climb out.
- Bumper guards are recommended, but they can be risky once your baby is able to stand up, since they could be used for climbing and lead to a fall; straps on bumper pads should be trimmed so they aren't long enough to wrap around an infant's neck.

If you already have a crib or are fixing up an antique, make sure it is safe.

- Check for any missing bolts, slats and other fasteners, and get the necessary replacement parts from the manufacturer.
- Replace the mattress if it does not fit the crib snugly (the width of two fingers between the crib and mattress means it is too small and the baby could suffocate if wedged in that space), although you can roll towels to provide a safe fit.
- Use only nontoxic paints or finishes.
- Bumper pads are even more important on older cribs because they have far too much space between the slats; these guards should run around the entire crib, tie or snap into place and have at least six short straps to hold them in place.

NO MATTER WHAT THE AGE OF YOUR CHILD:

(1) Set the mattress at its lowest position as soon as your child can pull up to a standing position.

(2) Don't leave any toys or other large articles in the crib that your child can use as help in climbing out.

(3) Don't keep your child in the crib once the height of the side rail is less than three-fourths of your child's height.

(4) Replace any damaged teething rails. They can cut your baby's mouth.

(5) The crib should not be used as a playpen.

(6) If you put crib extenders on the side rails of your crib, they should not make the side rails taller than the end panels of the crib. The extenders should have no easily removable nuts or bolts, and their slats should be narrowly spaced.

Many imported cribs convert to beds, which can be used for a child up until the age of 4 or 5 years. This avoids another purchase when your son or daughter is about 24 months old and climbing out of the crib. All foreign manufacturers must comply with the government regulation that crib slats be no more than 2⅜ inches apart, but you will need to check for other safety features.

Bedding

In addition to the furniture, suggestions on a minimum of bedding include:

- 2–4 fitted crib sheets
- 2–3 waterproof sheets or pads (to protect mattress)
- 2–3 area pads such as small flannelized rubber pads (to protect mattress or your lap)
- 1–2 crib blankets
- 3–4 receiving blankets
- 1   crib bumper guard
- *No* pillow

Infant Carrier Seats

These plastic shells or hammocklike infant seats serve many purposes. Often they are convenient for feeding and carrying very young infants. Some seats fit safely in grocery carts, and others can be placed in the sink or tub when bathing an infant. Buy a seat with a wide, sturdy base. There are several precautions to keep in mind when using such equipment:

- Don't use it as a car restraint unless you have a seat that is designed for such a purpose and has a label indicating that it meets government auto safety standards.
- Use the seat and crotch belts.
- Certain seats with a springlike frame are best used only on the floor or on areas low to the ground.
- Lightweight models can tip over easily; also be careful about infant seats' sliding off slippery surfaces.
- Attach rough adhesive strips to provide a nonskid bottom surface.
- Check supporting devices that snap on the back of the carrier. They can pop out, causing the seat to collapse.

Plastic infant carriers are easy to clean and often adjust to several positions. The benefit of such models as the Bouncinette and other cloth seats is that babies often love the motion provided by the springlike frame. Usually infant seats can be used until your baby is 4 or 5 months old.

Front Carriers and Backpacks

Front carriers such as Andrea's Baby Pack and Snugli are well suited for babies from birth to 6 months, whereas Gerri Kiddie Packs and other back carriers are good once a baby's neck is strong enough to withstand jolts, usually by about 4 or 5 months of age. Most front carriers, many of which convert to backpacks, provide close body contact and often calm fussy or colicky infants. Lightweight, metal-frame backpacks allow a parent's arms to be free, which can be an advantage over a stroller, particularly in crowds. Even well-padded shoulder straps cannot altogether eliminate the shoulder strain, but many parents find they adapt quickly to the extra weight on their shoulders.

In selecting an all-fabric carrier, check for adequate support for your baby's wobbly neck and also consider whether you want a lightweight or heavier material, depending on the time of year you are most likely to use it. One other suggestion is either to try it on with your baby in it first or wait to clip off the price tags until you test it once or twice, because not all babies like being confined in front carriers.

The U.S. Consumer Product Safety Commission suggests checking for the following when buying a framed back carrier:

- enough depth to support baby's back
- leg openings small enough to prevent baby from slipping out but large enough to avoid chafing little legs
- soft, padded covering over the metal frame near the baby's head or face
- hinge mechanism on the movable stand (which supports certain backpacks when they are placed on a surface) should not be able to close accidentally, pinching or cutting baby's fingers.

It's important to choose a carrier to match your baby's size. Be sure to check the carrier periodically for ripped seams, missing or loose straps, frayed seats or safety straps, and repair promptly.

Playpens

Not long ago mothers were convinced of the importance of babies' learning to amuse themselves in a playpen. Now, however, many early-childhood-development experts claim the use of the playpen for more than an hour or so a day does not allow enough varied stimulation, which they believe is essential for maximum intellectual growth, particularly during the first year. Certainly the mesh netting on many playpens blurs a baby's view and restricts his or her attention only to the toys within reach. Some parents who believe in letting their babies be physically free to roam in a child-proofed home use the playpen as safe temporary confinement, perhaps while the parent is on the telephone or downstairs in the laundry room, or to discipline when "no" is not heeded.

If you shop for a new playpen, the U.S. Consumer Product Safety Commission suggests you check for the following features:

- mesh netting with a very small weave—smaller than tiny buttons and snaps on infant clothing
- wooden slats no more than 2⅜ inches apart (otherwise, interweave sheeting between the slats and fasten securely)
- on folding models, hinges and latches that lock tightly to prevent scissoring action when the playpen is being used
- foam pads that don't mildew and are long-lasting.

Here are several precautions to take when using the playpen:

(1) When your toddler can climb over the side, it is time to put the playpen away.

(2) Accidents do happen; for instance, a child may fall when trying to climb out. Mesh playpens with large, open-weave netting provide an easy toehold, and buttons on the baby's clothing may catch on the netting, so keep an eye on your child if you have this type of playpen.

(3) Never leave an infant in a mesh playpen when the side is down. A baby may roll into the space between the mattress pad and loose mesh side, possibly causing suffocation.

(4) Remove large toys, bumper pads and boxes from inside the playpen, since they can be used for climbing.

(5) Avoid tying decorative toys across the top of the playpen, since they can also be used for climbing; if toys are hung from the sides, excess cord should be trimmed short enough that it can't be wrapped around your baby's neck.

Strollers and Carriages

Many strollers come with canopies, wind screens and other accessories that offer carriagelike protection from the elements. Other reasons that carriages are nearly extinct include their expense and the room it takes to store them. Compact, lightweight strollers with a semireclining feature such as the Maclaren or Silver Cross fold easily and can be tucked away in a closet.

When shopping for a stroller, consider safety and comfort features:

- backrest not sharply erect but nearly vertical for firm support
- waist and crotch safety belts (some strollers have a padded guard rail that serves for safety and child restraint)
- a two-wheel brake, which provides an extra measure of safety
- wide base and wheels that are large in diameter
- when child is far to the rear of the stroller, it doesn't tip backward
- no sharp edges or scissorlike mechanism that can trap baby's fingers
- handles are long enough (without handle extenders) that you aren't forced to lean far over the stroller
- adequate headroom for growth when the canopy is down, and a canopy that locks in forward horizontal position but rotates to downward position at rear of stroller
- shopping basket sits low on the back and is located so that its center is directly over or in front of the axle of the rear wheels.

As in buying other types of equipment, you may find that talking with other parents about their strollers will help you decide on the model best suited for your purposes.

High Chair Versus Portable Seat

Before you buy a high chair, consider the other options, such as a portable table-side perch. Kari-Chair, Sassy Seat and other models are less expensive than a high chair, easily transportable and actually allow the baby to sit at the table with the rest of the family. However, unlike those high chairs that have a rim around the tray, there is nothing to catch an overturned cup except fast reactions. Most high chairs can support up to 100 pounds, whereas portable seats are good for between 25 and 40 pounds. Some seats are better for babies under 12 months, while other models have more leg room, to accommodate a toddler.

You have many choices when shopping for a high chair. There is even one that converts into a chair and table with a removable eating tray, leaving the chair freely accessible. Here are some essential safety features to check before buying a high chair:

- choose one that has a wide base, for stability
- check the tray (some have a high, splash guard rim) to be sure it stays in position once it is locked
- try the straps to see if they are sturdy and are easy to use (both waist and thigh belts are best for sitting and should not be attached to the tray).

The U.S. Consumer Product Safety Commission recommends taking certain precautions when your baby is in a high chair.

(1) Attach rough-surfaced adhesive strips to the seat of the high chair if it seems slippery.
(2) Always use all restraining straps provided. The belt around the waist should be fastened as soon as the child is placed in the chair and unfastened only when the child is to be removed.
(3) Never allow your child to stand up in the high chair (there have been thousands of falls because safety belts weren't fastened).
(4) Buy a safety harness if the high chair lacks adequate safety straps.
(5) Use the high chair in an area free of traffic—away from doorways, refrigerators, stoves and other kitchen equipment.

Safety Gates

Unfortunately, safety gates are not totally safe or effective. The traditional, accordion type of gate can pinch hands and fingers; the latticework also provides a foothold for a climbing toddler. If you buy this type for your stairs, get the longest one that will fit into the opening; and when you install it, leave as little space as possible between the floor and gate. Portable mesh gates pose problems and have their limitations. They are more expensive than accordion models, and are available only for openings about four feet wide. Also, the plastic or rubber bumpers that help hold the gate in place give way if pushed hard enough. Another way to seal off dangerous areas or stairs is to build a locking plywood gate yourself. Of course, once babies start crawling, they can be taught how to negotiate the stairs by backing down them, but a watchful eye is still needed.

Information Sources

ADDITIONAL READING

The Complete Baby Book, by the editors of *Consumer Guide* (New York: Simon & Schuster, 1979). Compares different products and offers helpful buying suggestions.

ORGANIZATIONS

Auto Safety Hotline
U.S. Department of Transportation
National Highway Traffic Safety Administration
Washington, DC 20590
Toll-free hot line on buying infant seats is 800-424-9393 (in District of Columbia: 202-426-0123).

Consumer Product Safety Commission
Washington, DC 20207
Toll-free safety hot line is 800-638-CPSC for more information on cribs, high chairs and so on.
Report a product hazard or a product-related injury by writing this government agency or calling the toll-free number.

BABY CLOTHES AND SUPPLIES

You need to buy surprisingly little for dressing your baby the first few months, and it is wise to shop for only a few basics in the beginning until you've worked with what you have and recognize just what is and is not necessary. Besides, you will be given gifts of baby clothes, which usually take care of the more expensive garments. Unless your baby needs special tiny newborn or premie clothes, consider buying the 6-month size, which will offer room to grow; many styles run small anyway. Here are suggestions for an adequate layette—taken from the French word "laie," meaning packing box or drawer, and referring to the complete outfit for a newborn baby, including clothes, bedding, accessories.

Clothes for the First Few Months

Besides the time of year, which has a lot to do with what your baby needs, another important consideration is how often laundry gets done. Obviously you will need far less if you do a wash every day.

This shopping list will get you started:

- 80 diapers (if you don't plan to wash cloth ones yourself)
- 2–4 knit undershirts, 6 cotton shirts or 6–8 undershirts
- 2–4 stretch suits
- 1–2 nightgowns or 3 kimonos or 3 sleeping bags
- 1–3 sweaters or jackets
- 4 waterproof panties (if you use cloth diapers)
- 1 hat or knitted "helmet" for winter, hat for summer
- 1–2 outdoor outfits (snowsuit)
- several pairs of socks or booties

When buying clothes, you may want to make sure garments have:

- no buttons, long string(s) or ribbons
- no zippers that lock tightly at throat
- metal zippers that are covered at the top with cloth tabs
- easy access to diaper area
- no loose threads that could get twisted around a toe or finger
- a tight knit, especially in sweaters, so as not to catch fingers
- snap or Velcro closing, particularly on hats; they are easier and more comfortable than tie closings
- room to grow, with raglan sleeves, sturdy seams, loose elastic.

Imported garments cannot be sold as sleepwear in the United States, because they do not meet the U.S. Consumer Product Safety Commission's requirement for treatment with a flame retardant; stores will instead sell them as "daytime wear" (some parents prefer clothes untreated by any such chemicals because of the 1977 cancer scare involving the flame-retardant TRIS).

Laundry Tips

buy only washable fabrics

wash clothes before baby wears them, to remove chemical sizings used to give them a stiff shape

freshen clothes further by adding baking soda to water

soak fresh stains immediately in cold water (especially important once your baby is eating solids)

check garments periodically for unraveled threads, which might twist around or catch on fingers or toes

Diapers: Cloth Versus Disposable

Your choice boils down to either cloth or disposable diapers, although some parents opt for washable diapers at night for greater absorption and switch to throwaways during the day, when the baby can be changed frequently. Advocates of cloth diapers point to the softness of the natural fabric against the baby's skin and the fact that nondisposable diapers are ecologically desirable. Those favoring disposables emphasize their convenience in terms of time and trouble, as well as the elimination of plastic pants and diaper pins. A 1982 study of 200 infants, published in the *Journal of Pediatrics*, compared the incidence of diaper rash found in babies wearing home-laundered diapers with those using disposables. The cloth-diaper group had diaper rash significantly more often than the babies using three different types of throwaways. This study, unlike previous ones, checked infants' diaper areas weekly for nine months. A similar comparison between disposables and diaper-service-laundered cloth ones has not been done.

	CLOTH	DISPOSABLE
Cleanliness	Messy clean-up, but if properly washed, they are just as clean as disposables. Less for you to do if you use a diaper service	Sterile from the package, and clean-up is easy, although toilets will clog if you dispose of them that way
Convenience	Time-consuming if you rinse, soak, wash and disinfect diapers yourself; takes a bit longer to attach pins and put on plastic pants	No folding or pinning is necessary; easy to fasten, with self-adhesive straps
Cost	Initial outlay for diapers, liners, pants, pail, pins, and cost of detergent and hot water. Diaper service brings price closer to cost of disposable diapers	Ongoing expense, since you use only once. One estimate puts the cost at four times that of cloth

Diaper rash is discussed in detail in "Common Problems from Allergies to Rashes," (p. 391).

Toilet Training

There's no need even to think much about giving up diapers before your son or daughter's second birthday. Nowadays, most experts say your child must be ready to be toilet trained both emotionally and physically—able to control the muscles around the anus—or your efforts will be in vain. Basically, training involves several elements:

Readiness, which usually comes between 18 and 24 months for girls and as late as 2 or 3 years for boys. One important sign of psychological readiness is baby's displeasure with a soiled diaper (when he or she comes to you asking to be changed immediately).

A potty chair placed beside your toilet early on is a good idea just in case your baby is ready early or wants to imitate Daddy or Mommy—an excellent way to learn.

A parent's impatience or stress can interfere with training, so don't begin or push it if your household is going through a change or a tense time.

Be consistent in giving and withholding praise, and use the same words each time to describe what you want your child to do or to ask if "it's time."

Pacifiers

Since babies have greater sucking needs when very young than can be met by nursing or bottle-feeding and because others who are chronically fussy, jumpy or colicky are easily soothed when given the opportunity to suck, pacifiers are a godsend to these babies and their parents. Most experts agree that using an artificial sucking device to "plug up" the cries of a demanding or irritable baby is to misuse it and, more importantly, is harmful to the child in the long run. However, child-care professionals do disagree on what the short-term use of pacifiers should be. Some say they should be phased out at about four months of age as the bona fide desire for surplus sucking fades, while others think a two-year-old has just as much right to be pacified by extra sucking when under stress or during moments of insecurity. As far as possible orthodontic trouble is concerned, pacifiers threaten the position of your child's teeth only beginning at about age 5 or 6 years. There is, in addition, no evidence linking pacifiers to future thumb-sucking, and there may be some proof that it actually discourages it if sucking needs are met early.

Advantages	Disadvantages
satisfies extra sucking needs	baby may not want to give it up
soothes to sleep and relaxes baby after an upset	you may be tempted to use it just for some "peace and quiet"
may mean baby won't suck thumb later on (although this is not proven)	unhygienic unless you rinse it off constantly, especially if there are household pets
if baby awakens at night, may suck his/her way back to sleep if paci-fier is in place*	if it falls out during sleep, it may cause baby to awaken*

*Some pediatricians advise removing pacifiers before bedtime, since extra sucking is not important during that time.

Other Paraphernalia

The list of essential supplies is short, but once your baby is mobile, you might want to stock up on Band-Aids and other first aid. Remember to keep thermometers, which contain poisonous mercury, and all medicinal products out of reach.

Basic Supplies

petroleum jelly

rectal thermometer

rubber bulb syringe for nose

rubbing alcohol

fever-reducing medication such as Infant Tylenol Drops

Syrup of Ipecac

zinc oxide ointment such as Desitin, for diaper rash

sterile absorbent cotton

hot water bottle

blunt-tipped scissors for trimming nails

Shoes

As your baby's feet grow, the fat pads under his or her arches will disappear, revealing the true arch as bones harden and muscles strengthen around the instep. Though you should let this happen without any unnatural support the first year, you still need to protect your baby's feet from extremes in temperature and injury. Foot specialists suggest using lightweight flexible shoes with soft leather sides and soles, which allow lots of room for wiggling toes. Another reason for a thin, pliable sole is to have less interference between the baby's foot and the ground, thereby helping his or her balance. Once your baby is standing and walking, switch to shoes that offer support without restricting movement too much—sneakers are a good choice, since they provide traction, are flexible and are easy on your budget.

Some tips on buying footwear for you to bear in mind:

- Ask other parents about good shoe stores; usually the old-fashioned family store offers more personal attention, and their aim is to cultivate you as a continuing customer. They may not only be more responsive to complaints than larger stores but keep records as well and send you reminder notices advising you it's time for a size check.
- Be sure you rely on a qualified fitter. Both feet should be measured while your baby stands up. When your child tries out the new fit and lifts his or her heel to take a step, there should be easy creasing across the toes in a lace-up shoe and moderate creasing at the sides.
- New shoes should have about one-half to three-quarters of an inch to spare in front of the longest toe, for growth and freedom of toe movement (again, important for balance).
- Don't buy secondhand shoes, since your baby's foot could easily be molded into the shape of the original owner's.
- Look for signs of a bad fit—complaints, crying, constantly pulling off shoes; redness around the big toe; tips of sole worn on outside; and wear marks on inside of shoes extending to the front.

Socks that are too tight can also pose problems. To help prevent rashes or foot infections such as athlete's foot, particularly during the hot weather, use pure cotton socks; they serve as excellent moisture absorbers.

There is no way to predict when your baby will need a new pair of shoes, as feet grow in spurts, but usually every two to three months is a safe bet. Your child probably will outgrow the shoes before outwearing them.

POUNDING TOYS, PUZZLES, PICTURE BOOKS

Toys are more than just baby entertainment. When chosen with a specific age group in mind, they can be learning tools that will promote physical, intellectual and emotional growth. Owing to the fast pace of your baby's development, the appropriateness of the toys should be periodically evaluated, some put away and new ones added to keep up with changing interests and developmental needs. Outlined below are suggestions for suitable toys according to the activities your baby enjoys at certain stages during the first 18 months. Of course, pots and pans, along with many other odds and ends, prove to be safe, enjoyable, no-cost toys.

Birth to 3 months
- mobiles placed above crib, playpen, changing table, where baby can enjoy color, movement and sometimes sound; remove as soon as your baby is able to touch them (usually at about 4 or 5 months)
- stuffed toys
- automatic swing (not before about 6 weeks)
- mirror toys

4 to 6 months
- clutch balls help baby practice grasp-and-release reflex
- rattles and teethers
- activity toys such as Busy Box or Activity Center, where baby can develop gross- and fine-motor skills and satisfy desire to bang and hit, open and close; some toys can be attached to sides of crib, playpen or wall
- jumpers

7 to 12 months
- walkers

One Year to 18 Months
- blocks: just a few soft, brightly colored ones to start off with, preferably with interesting designs or letters
- dolls: plain and huggable, easily washed
- simple puzzles and sorting/stacking toys will help baby learn

colors, sizes, increase manual dexterity and will satisfy urge to stack, organize and nest objects
- toys that appear and disappear, such as boxes that fit into larger boxes or hammer boards (babies love to pound)
- fill-and-dump toys, such as shovels and pails or dump trucks
- push and pull toys such as Popcorn Poppers give some support to a baby who's still wobbly on his or her feet; pull toys such as Oscar the Grouch, who pops in and out of a trash can as baby walks, should be given to a baby once he or she is steady and can walk looking over the shoulder as the toy is being pulled

Motion Makers

Automatic swings, jumpers and walkers all offer your baby a kind of autonomy he or she would not ordinarily enjoy at this age. Not only do they amuse your baby, but they give you a breather during those busy waking hours. Their value in terms of aiding physical development is questionable, and they all demand extra safety precautions.

Swings. These gadgets wind up and give your baby about five to ten minutes of soothing motion. The rhythmic sound calms and pleases a fussy baby. They should not be used much before your baby is 6 weeks old or after 6 months, when your baby can crawl out.

Possible Hazards:
- falling or slipping too far forward (not a problem if seat belts are properly used)
- bumping head if not careful in lifting baby out of the swing
- shattering springs

Jumpers. These fabric or plastic seats are suspended from doorjambs by an elastic or metal cord. A baby's feet barely touch the floor, so that he or she can push up and bounce. Jumpers should hold the weight of your baby and secure the body well without being too tight. The coils of the spring should stretch no more than an eighth or an inch apart, to avoid pinching tiny fingers. Some babies absolutely love jumpers; some may prefer other motion toys, such as walkers.

Possible Hazards:
- clamp may release
- strap may fray
- baby may bounce into sharp corner of door or wall
- some seat designs put too much pressure on baby's inner thighs
- baby may get "seasick" after continual or prolonged use
- may force development of leg muscles before physically ready

Walkers. Wheeled support seats give babies an opportunity to move about alone. Some believe a walker helps train a child to walk early, much as training wheels on bicycles do, though there is no proof to support this claim. The great advantage of walkers is that they allow crawling/cruising babies to have a taste of "walking" while being protected from falls by the bumperlike tray that surrounds baby. The flip side is that this same protection can hinder the development of your baby's fall reflex.

Possible Hazards:
- tipping over rugs, etc.
- falling down stairs
- finger entrapment

To avoid mishaps, the U.S. Consumer Product Safety Commission makes the following recommendations for selection and use of baby walkers:

- If you are buying an X-frame baby walker, look for one with protective covers over accessible coil springs, spacers between scissoring components and locking devices to prevent the X-frame from collapsing.
- Purchase a baby walker with a wheel base that is both wider and longer than the frame of the walker itself, so that it will be as stable as possible.
- Keep your infant and the walker on flat, smooth surfaces—away from carpets, door thresholds and other obstructions.
- Place guards at the tops of all stairways to prevent accidents.
- Keep doors closed, so that babies cannot slide their walkers toward the stairs.
- Watch your child, to help avoid falls or accidents.

Toy Safety

Manufacturers are not required to meet safety standards before putting a toy on the market. If they do submit a toy to be tested by the U.S. Consumer Product Safety Commission (CPSC), it is on a purely *voluntary* basis, so it is up to you to inspect toys for potential safety hazards, particularly if the manufacturer is not a mainstream company (manufacturing toys such as homemade dolls, wooden trucks or rattles) or the toys are imported. The CPSC offers the following suggestions for parents of infants and toddlers:

(1) Toys should not contain small parts that could become lodged in the windpipe, ears or nose or that have long cords that could possibly entangle or strangle.

(2) Be sure rattles are too large to go down baby's throat (to date, the largest rattle known to have lodged in a baby's throat had an end 1⅜ inches in diameter). The CPSC issued regulations requiring rattles to be a certain size, and constructed so that they will not separate into small pieces, but check any rattles you suspect may have been made before August 1978, the date these regulations went into effect.

(3) Labels should be checked for safety warnings such as "not recommended for children under 3 years" (not all toy-makers offer this warning when they ought to).

(4) Examine toys periodically; look for sharp edges and points; sand splintered wood surfaces; repair broken toys and discard those that cannot be fixed.

Although a toy can be sold without meeting safety standards the CPSC may order it recalled if shown to be hazardous. If you suspect a toy is potentially dangerous call the CPSC toll-free hot line (listed at the end of this section). Be sure to take a hard look at any second-hand toys you receive as gifts or buy as there are still some older unsafe toys which have never been recalled.

Picture Books

Like toys, books are tools you and your child can use not only for amusement but also for teaching and learning. Infants and toddlers enjoy the bright colors and shapes of picture books, have fun listening and helping turn the pages—usually before you're ready—and there is increasing evidence that suggests reading aloud at an early age speeds up your child's cognitive development. In *The Read-Aloud Handbook*, author Jim Trelease writes that, in infancy, "we are not concerned with 'understanding' as much as we are with 'conditioning' the child to your voice and to books," stimulating him or her to be drawn naturally to the activity of reading. Trelease tells an astonishing story of a handicapped little girl whose parents began reading to her at age 4 months. "By nine months the child was able to respond to the sight of certain books and convey to her parents that these were her favorites. By age five, she had taught herself to read."

In choosing books for your child, vary your selection to include some small, thick-paged ones that your baby can handle and "read" alone, along with others such as *Pat the Bunny*, which invite still more child involvement.

Information Sources

ADDITIONAL READING

The Complete Baby Book, by the editors of *Consumer Guide* (New York: Simon & Schuster, 1979). Guide to buying products and toys.

Good Things for Babies, by Sandy Jones. (Boston: Houghton Mifflin, 1976). Catalog of items for babies chosen for safety, usefulness and high quality.

The Read-Aloud Handbook, by Jim Trelease (New York: Penguin, 1982). Includes approximately 300 book suggestions according to age group.

ORGANIZATIONS

U.S. Consumer Product Safety Commission
Washington, DC 20207
Toll-free safety hot line for information or to report a product hazard or a product-related injury is (800) 638-CPSC.

Also see "Stimulating Your Baby's Senses" (p. 419) for more about toys, games and reading.

(11)

Health Questions

EMERGENCIES AND FIRST AID*

In case your child is vomiting blood, has sustained a crushing injury to the chest, severe or extensive burns or poisonous bites: Don't stop for anything except life-saving first aid. Rush directly to a hospital or other medical center.

*These emergency and first-aid instructions are based on the recommendations of the American Academy of Pediatrics, the American Heart Association and the Poison Control Center.

INFANT CPR (CARDIOPULMONARY RESUSCITATION)
Mouth-to-mouth resuscitation if breathing stops

(1) Listen carefully to be sure breathing has stopped completely.

(2) Wipe out any fluid or vomitus. If foreign object is in the throat, refer to "Choking" on facing page.

(3) Place your mouth over baby's mouth and nose.

(4) Give gentle breaths every 3 seconds (20 breaths per minute), using the air in your cheeks, not your lungs, and using only enough air to move baby's chest up and down.

Cardiac support if there is no pulse or heartbeat

(1) Check to make sure there is no heartbeat by feeling for pulse in baby's upper arm (neck is too chubby and short).

(2) Place baby on firm surface.

(3) Compress baby's breastbone one-half to one inch, using three fingers at level of nipples. Depress breastbone five times and then give another gentle breath, using the air in your cheeks, not your lungs. Repeat set of compressions followed by a breath in a 5:1 ratio.

Bleeding and Shock

Severe or heavy bleeding; baby is very pale, cold, breathing irregularly or in stupor (signs of shock):

- stop blood flow by covering wound with clean cloth and applying pressure for at least seven minutes
- do *not* use a tourniquet
- if baby is in shock, lay infant down flat and raise legs about eight to twelve inches above heart unless causes pain
- if head injured, elevate head and shoulders
- cover with light blanket to keep warm but not too hot
- take baby to hospital immediately

Choking

If infant is gasping for breath:

- turn upside down so gravity can dislodge object
- do *not* try to get it out yourself—you may push it farther down

If infant is unable to breathe:

- place baby's face down over the inside of your arm, with head lower than trunk
- rest your forearm on your thigh
- rapidly deliver four measured blows, with heel of hand, between infant's shoulder blades

If infant is still unable to breathe:

- roll baby over and place three fingers at level of nipples and depress breastbone one-half to one inch four times. Repeat if necessary
- then try to remove foreign object obstructing airway if you see it
- last resort is take to hospital immediately

Convulsions or "Fits"

Baby's lips and face may turn blue; eyes roll upward; limbs stiffen, then tremble; breathing is heavy. Convulsions will last two to ten minutes, and are usually the result of a head injury, high fever or, rarely, DPT vaccination.

(1) Place baby on bed or soft rug and clear the area of dangerous or hard objects.
(2) Try to loosen tight clothing, especially around the neck.
(3) Do *not* restrain baby during convulsion.
(4) Do *not* put anything in the mouth—baby will not swallow tongue.
(5) Once convulsion is over, lay baby on its side, with head lower than hips. Don't give anything by mouth.
(6) As soon as baby is calm, call physician or hospital emergency room for further advice (if you haven't already phoned).

Drowning

If infant is breathing and coughing:

- this will clear lungs
- do *not* resort to resuscitation

If baby is not breathing:

- do *not* leave even to get help
- turn on stomach for a second to let any water drain out of lungs
- perform mouth-to-mouth resuscitation (see box, p. 362)

Electrical Shock

If baby is part of the circuit, *do not touch with bare hands.*

- pull infant away from source, using wood or cloth
- if child is not breathing, perform mouth-to-mouth resuscitation (see box, p. 362)
- all electrical burns must be medically evaluated

Smoke Inhalation

If baby is not breathing, perform mouth-to-mouth resuscitation (see box, p. 362)

Poisoning

Caution: Antidote labels on products that suggest how to counteract the effects of poison may be out-of-date or incorrect.

Follow these instructions and *then* call 911 or "0" for operator if you don't have the number of your local poison control center.

TYPE OF POISON	WHAT TO DO
Swallowed Poison (any nonfood substance is a potential poison)	**(1)** if infant is awake and able to swallow, give milk or water only **(2)** call poison control center or M.D.
Inhaled Poison (fumes or gases)	**(1)** carry baby to fresh air **(2)** if not breathing, give mouth-to-mouth resuscitation (see box, p. 362) **(3)** air out the room(s) affected **(4)** call poison control center
Poisons in the Eye	**(1)** flood eye with lukewarm (never hot) water poured from a pitcher held 3 to 4 inches from eye for 15 minutes **(2)** call poison control center or M.D.
Poisons on the Skin	**(1)** remove any affected clothing **(2)** throw water on arms, hands, whatever is exposed **(3)** wash with soap and water, then rinse **(4)** call poison control center or M.D.

Always keep on hand Ipecac Syrup, which induces vomiting, and Epsom salts, which act as a laxative. They help get the poison out or dilute it. Do *not* use either one unless instructed to do so by your local poison control center or your doctor.

If you are unable to reach poison control or a doctor, make your baby vomit by giving two teaspoons of Ipecac Syrup if under 12 months and one tablespoon if over 1 year old: however, *do not use Ipecac Syrup if:*

- child is unconscious or having a convulsion
- substance swallowed was acid or strong alkali such as oven cleaner, drain cleaner, ammonia, lye
- substance swallowed was a petroleum product such as gasoline, turpentine, kerosene, lighter fluid, insecticide, furniture polish

In any of these three circumstances, if unable to contact either poison control center or a doctor, go to nearest hospital. *Take the container or jar with you to the emergency room.*

OTHER FIRST-AID INSTRUCTIONS

Bites or Stings

If infant is bitten by an animal:

- stop bleeding by pressing wound firmly with clean cloth
- wash wound with soap and water; hold wound under running water while soaping for 5 minutes
- cover with sterile, gauze-type dressing
- call the doctor

If infant is stung by an insect:

- call doctor promptly if there is any reaction such as hives, severe rash, pallor, weakness, nausea, vomiting, irregular breathing, collapse
- remove stinger, if present, with scraping motion of fingernail
- apply cold compresses to reduce swelling; meat tenderizer or a baking soda/water paste may also be used
- use calamine lotion for itching

Bruises

- rest injured part
- apply cold compresses for half an hour (but don't put ice next to the skin)
- if skin is broken, treat as a cut (see "Cuts and Scrapes" on facing page)

Burns and Scalds

For electrical burns, see "Electrical Shock," p. 364.
If baby suffers *minor burns* on small areas:

- on arm or leg, immerse in cold water
- on face or trunk, apply ice bag or cold wet packs intermittently
- call doctor
- nonadhesive dressing such as "Telfapad" should be used if available

If baby is burned on *large area*:

- apply cold, wet compresses or if leg or arm, soak in cold water
- call doctor or hospital
- cover burns with plastic wrap or clean sheet or towel
- use *no* ointment, grease or jelly
- keep child warm and go to hospital

Cuts and Scrapes

If child is bleeding from a large cut:

- stop bleeding by pressing wound firmly with clean cloth
- do *not* use iodine, Mercurochrome or first-aid ointment
- wash cut(s) with soap and running water; scrapes with dirt, gravel and/or cinders in them need to be thoroughly cleaned out immediately; may want to take baby to see doctor if procedure is too painful
- if cut is about one-quarter-inch deep, you may want to go to hospital or clinic for stitches to promote healing and prevent scarring

Head Injury or Severe Fall

- baby should rest
- call doctor before giving anything by mouth
- call doctor again if baby vomits more than once, is unusually weak, has personality changes (displays excessive irritability, confusion, stupor), vision problems or unequal pupils
- wake baby every one to two hours during the day or two to three times at night to make sure he or she can be easily awakened

Puncture Wounds

- press gently to encourage "cleansing" bleeding
- soak in warm water for 10 to 15 minutes
- cover with bandage
- consult physician if it gets more sore or red

Sunstroke

If baby becomes flushed, does not sweat, and you notice shallow breathing:

- act quickly to lower temperature, either by placing baby in shallow tub of cool water or sponging body with quick, light strokes until temperature drops; another approach is to wrap child in wet, cold sheets or towels until temperature goes down.

Remember, always get your baby to drink lots of fluids if exposed to the hot sun, and use lotion to guard against sunburn.

WHEN TO CALL THE DOCTOR: DAY OR NIGHT?

If you are like most new parents, you waver between wanting reassurance that your baby is okay and "bothering" the doctor unnecessarily. Any physician specializing in children knows that 2:00 A.M. phone calls come with the territory and prefers that you feel free to call even for something that turns out to be minor rather than hesitate with a problem that warrants immediate medical attention. An ideal time to get basic calling guidelines is the first well-baby checkup. Throw out some "What if . . . ?" situations; for instance, ask "What if my baby has a fever? Should I call right away or not until the temperature reaches a certain point?" "Is a relentless cough in the middle of the night reason to phone, or should I wait until morning?"

Below is a list of circumstances that are considered "midnight emergencies"—times when you should not wait until normal office hours. You may want to have your baby's doctor look over this checklist to help the discussion along. Regardless of what scenarios you work through, remember to trust your instincts. Every mother has at least one anecdote of how she knew her baby was ill despite the doctor's initial skepticism. If you have a gut feeling that something is wrong, even in the absence of obvious signs of sickness, persevere about having your child examined. In newborns, especially, any strange change in attitude or behavior, even without a fever, can be significant.

Call Immediately Regardless of the Hour

Besides obvious emergencies such as electric shock or poisoning, the American Academy of Pediatrics recommends calling baby's doctor promptly under the following circumstances:

- convulsions or "fits" (see p. 364)
- bleeding that cannot be stopped after applying pressure to the wound for seven minutes
- severe breathing difficulties; specifically, blue lips, nostrils enlarged with each breath, struggling for air
- cough that is loud, deep and dry, accompanied by a fever, or one that cannot be relieved after steaming up the bathroom or using a vaporizer or humidifier for half an hour
- blood-tinged bowel movement
- severe diarrhea in an infant

Many doctors would expand this midnight emergencies list to include:

- fever, specifically if rectal temperature is 104°F or higher after fever-reducing medication has been given or if feverish infant is hard to wake
- wheezing in infant less than 3 months old for over one hour
- vomiting in newborn under 2 months who throws up repeatedly or if baby vomits more than once after a head injury or bad fall
- diarrhea in baby who is hard to rouse, and eyes appear sunken; also in infant under 2 months if accompanied by listlessness, dry mouth, unusual thirst and baby has not wet a diaper within past six hours (less than six if infant is younger than 8 weeks)
- earache if baby has stiff neck, rectal temperature over 103°F or is hard to wake

If you remain uncertain about whether to call right away, refer to "The Top Three Illnesses: Fever, Diarrhea, Ear Infection" (p. 385) and "Common Problems from Allergies to Rashes" (p. 391).

Before getting the doctor on the line, spend a moment collecting your thoughts if possible. Jot down pertinent information, which may save time in the long run and ensures that you've covered all the bases:

(1) check for fever with rectal thermometer (see "How to Take Your Baby's Temperature," p. 386)
(2) note baby's skin color; general attitude and behavior (listless, irritable, no appetite); other symptoms, including cough, runny nose, pulling ear, abnormal bowel movements, along with how long they have lasted
(3) jot down any medications given, including baby aspirin or acetaminophen, decongestants, cough syrup, along with how much and when
(4) have phone number of nearby drugstore handy for the doctor
(5) get paper and pencil ready to take down M.D.'s directions

If your child's physician or the nurse makes you feel foolish for calling, either ignore it or think about switching doctors. After all, you are the client who is paying for medical care as well as for peace of mind. Remember, you will rely less on health professionals as you learn to "read" your baby, and the experience of conquering a cold or curing an ear infection will provide you with confidence, should similar problems occur again.

Tips on Measuring and Giving Medicine

Some liquids come with their own measuring cup or droppers, or your pharmacist may slip one in the prescription bag. If not, do *not* rely on a kitchen teaspoon to measure—its capacity can vary from as much as half a teaspoon to one and a half teaspoons—but buy your own calibrated medicine dropper or oral syringe. Not only is it perfectly accurate, but it also reduces spilling and wasting. The cardinal rule in giving your baby or small child medicine is to be nonchalant, don't let on that you know he or she probably won't like the taste; resist the temptation to call it candy.

Here are a few more suggestions including what to do if your baby puts up a fuss:

- coax baby's mouth open by putting your thumb on one cheek and your index finger on the other
- slip dropper or oral syringe between cheek and upper gum line to make spitting out more difficult and swallowing easier
- avoid mixing with baby's favorite juice or milk, since the funny taste may make him or her suspicious of the liquid for weeks afterward.

Even after your child looks healthy, it is important to use all the medicine for whatever length of time agreed on with the physician, since some bacteria are stubborn and difficult to wipe out completely. Don't make the mistake, either, of using a drug prescribed for a previous ailment even if the symptoms seem similar.

Information Sources

ADDITIONAL READING

Baby and Child Care, by Dr. Benjamin Spock (New York: Wallaby, 1977).
This old standby provides readable and comprehensive baby-care guidelines.

Baby Check-up Book, by R. Hillman (New York: Bantam, 1983). Especially good for the care of young children.

The Parents' Guide to Baby and Child Medical Care, ed. by Terril H. Hart, M.D. (Wayzata, MN: Meadowbrook Press, 1982).

Should I Call the Doctor?: Caring for Your Sick or Injured Child, by Christine A. Nelson, M.D. and Susan C. Pescar (New York: McGraw-Hill, 1983). Ranges from simple first-aid principles to emergency medical intervention.

Reference books available at both public libraries and medical libraries, specifically the annual editions of *Physicians' Desk Reference* and U.S. Pharmacopoeia's *USP DI: Advice for the Patient.* The journal *Pediatrics* may be useful if you want to do your own research on a particular illness. Also refer to periodicals listed in the appendix.

Also refer to "The Top Three Illnesses: Fever, Diarrhea, Ear Infection," p. 385, and "Common Problems from Allergies to Rashes," p. 391.

INFANT VITAMINS AND FLUORIDE DROPS: NECESSARY OR NOT?

Vitamin and Iron Supplements

Everyone agrees that your baby needs daily doses of certain vitamins and minerals, particularly vitamins A, C, D, E and iron. There is broad disagreement, however, on just how much is necessary and from what sources. Of particular importance is the iron question. In the first three months of life your baby dips into the iron stores that were built up in the final trimester in utero. These savings are gradually spent, and as the six-month mark approaches, your infant's supply of this blood-building mineral is getting low.

The following are various points of view regarding vitamin and iron supplements for both breast-fed and bottle-fed babies.

If your baby is breast-fed and was full-term	The American Academy of Pediatrics advises that no additional vitamins are needed if you have normal exposure to sunlight and are well nourished (except in some cases, such as strict vegetarians) but recommends that more iron be added to baby's diet beginning at about 4 to 6 months of age, through iron-fortified cereals or iron

drops; additional iron at this age will counterbalance normal depletion.

La Leche League advises that no additional vitamins or minerals are necessary for the infant, but strongly recommends that you take prenatal vitamins and iron pills until you stop nursing.

Other medical experts argue that infant vitamin and iron drops should be given from day one as insurance against vitamin and iron deficiency regardless of the mother's diet or use of iron-rich foods or formula.

If your baby is bottle-fed   The American Academy of Pediatrics suggests that if your baby is drinking iron-fortified formula, no supplements are necessary. When solid foods are started, at 4–6 months, they should include iron-fortified cereal.

In the case of formulas without iron or whole cow's milk, some iron supplement should be started by 4 months of age, either through iron-rich cereals or infant drops. Additional vitamins C and D may also be advised.

Iron is an essential blood-building ingredient, and all the vitamins are important for your baby's skin, bones and general development. As a form of extra insurance, then, there are those—parents and physicians alike—who opt for giving extra vitamins A, C and D and iron even to normal, full-term babies from birth on. However, many view these supplements as a waste of money and a hassle. Others, like the La Leche League, point to the color and sugar additives found in most drops and claim that artificial iron interferes with your baby's absorption of natural iron and the passing on of immunities from your milk. The Clinical Nutrition Branch of the government's National Institutes of Health, however, states that no scientific evidence exists to back up this claim.

Fluoride Supplements

The mineral fluoride, when absorbed in tooth enamel, provides an important line of defense by strengthening the surface against cavity-causing bacteria in the mouth and corrosive substances in the saliva. Fluoride is as important for baby teeth as for permanent ones, since decay often means losing a baby tooth early and removing support for neighboring teeth.

Although fluoride is found naturally in water, soil and some foods, the amounts vary, and higher levels are often needed in order to shield teeth well. Most communities add fluoride to central water supplies, but if yours does not, you can compensate by giving your child fluoride drops. Thanks to fluoride use, the incidence of tooth decay has dropped markedly in the U.S. However, overdoses of the mineral in children have been known to stain permanent teeth yellow (fluorosis).

Opponents of fluoride argue that because of higher levels of the mineral in the food we eat, supplements are not only unnecessary but could be harmful as well. Those in favor of some sort of supplement, whether it be in drinking water or some other form, still question how early infants should be given extra fluoride and, in the case of breast-fed babies, whether it is necessary at all. Below is a comparison of the main arguments on both sides.

Arguments Against Fluoride	Arguments For Fluoride
mineral is difficult for baby to metabolize in first weeks of life	no evidence exists that supplements are unsafe for baby's system in first weeks of life
fluoride unnecessary before 6 months, since teeth have not yet erupted; and in formula-fed infants under 6 months, proper dosage is complicated by a wide variety in feeding schedules	fluoride needed before 6 months of age to help in mineralization of baby teeth developing under gums as well as in partial development of permanent teeth
breast milk never contains more than trace amounts of fluoride, whether mother is in fluoridated or nonfluoridated community; consequently, this filtering out is nature's way of protecting the baby from too much	fluoride levels in blood and tissues are always low, because the body's bones and teeth are the first to sponge up the mineral; therefore, scant amount in human milk is not an example of nature's safeguarding the infant
easy to take in too much fluoride, causing fluorosis (yellow staining of permanent teeth)	dosage schedule has been lowered in children under 2 years to prevent fluorosis

Cavity prevention thanks to fluoride supplementation is undeniable; however, some believe that the margin of error between enough fluoride to strengthen teeth against decay and the staining of teeth from too much is dangerously narrow, particularly in children under 24 months. In studying this question, the American Academy of

Pediatrics drew up a revised fluoride dosage schedule that carefully regulates the daily amount of additional fluoride a child needs according to age and level of fluoride present in drinking water:

- if your drinking water contains less than 0.3 parts fluoride per million (ppm), your baby needs 0.25 milligrams extra fluoride (from drops or tablets) each day from the age of 2 weeks to 2 years
- if your drinking water contains over 0.3 ppm, it already supplies enough of the daily fluoride requirement, and no supplements are needed or advisable.

Both the American Academy of Pediatrics (AAP) and the government's National Institute for Dental Research (NIDR) agree that fluoride supplements should be begun soon after birth for both breast-fed and bottle-fed infants, though the AAP "recognizes the basis for the view that satisfactory reduction in prevalence of caries [cavities] can be accomplished by initiating fluoride supplementation as late as six months of age." For breast-fed babies, the NIDR adds the caution that if the mother drinks an optimally fluoridated water supply (over 0.3 ppm) the pediatrician should prescribe supplements only if 100 percent sure the baby's sole source of liquid is breast milk; in other words, that it takes no water or juices. Others take this even further, by recommending that breast-fed babies be given no supplements at all until they are in mid-infancy. Although the levels of fluoride found in human milk are very low—even in fluoridated areas—La Leche League maintains that the small amount is sufficient for a baby's needs, citing studies that show the number of cavities for unsupplemented breast-fed babies and supplemented bottle-fed to be roughly the same. NIDR and AAP would argue that more fluoride could not hurt and could, in fact, provide an even stronger shield against cavities.

Factors to Weigh

There are two schools of thought about fluoride drops as well as about vitamin and iron supplements. Knowing the arguments for and against should help you to arrive at an informed decision, with help from your baby's doctor. As Dr. Jean Lockhart of the American Academy of Pediatrics says, "There is probably more variance among pediatricians on the advice they give pertaining to nutrition—including vitamins, minerals, fluoride and feeding patterns—than on other pediatric topics. This reflects geographic and cultural differences as well as the lag in available data on implications of changes in childhood diet for later adult years." Regardless of what you decide, it is wise to reevaluate supplements periodically, given your baby's constantly changing eating habits, and particularly if your family moves to a new area, where the level of fluoride in the water may be different.

Information Sources

ORGANIZATION

National Caries Program
National Institute of Dental Research
5333 Westbard Ave., Room 594
Bethesda, MD 20205
Free pamphlets on fluoride supplements and dental care.

IMMUNIZATIONS: RISKS VERSUS BENEFITS

Trips to the doctor will generally coincide with your baby's immunization timetable. Beginning at 2 months, as newborn immunities start to wear off, and stretching until entrance into kindergarten, your child needs periodic vaccinations to safeguard against the "Big Seven" childhood diseases: diphtheria, pertussis (whooping cough), tetanus (lockjaw), polio, measles, mumps and rubella. Within the next decade this list may grow longer, to include protection from other infectious diseases. And perhaps one day there will be antiparasitic and antitumor vaccines.

In addition to whether to circumcise and breast-feed or bottle-feed, your consent to vaccinate your child represents a major decision concerning his or her health. The legality of refusing immunization has become a hot issue in the past few years, as the incidence of certain diseases has dropped, throwing the spotlight instead on adverse reactions to the vaccines themselves. Because vaccinating a child means exposure to small amounts of diseaselike substances that stimulate production of special antibodies in defense, the possibility of side effects always exists. Some parents question whether the benefits of certain vaccines are worth these potential risks. Public-health experts point out that the lowered incidence of some childhood infections has lulled us into a dangerously false sense of security. Unlike smallpox, these seven diseases have not been wiped off the face of the earth. In parts of the world, such as Great Britain and Sweden, where well-publicized adverse reactions to vaccines led to reduced immunization for some diseases, widespread outbreaks soon followed. Though the more lethal infections—diphtheria, whooping cough, tetanus, polio—

have been squelched substantially, the government's Centers for Disease Control and the American Academy of Pediatrics urge continued immunization to prevent their revival. Ardent opponents believe that a proper diet and careful hygiene are equally effective in controlling the Big Seven.

Outlined below are descriptions of these diseases and their dangers.

Diphtheria (means skin or leather)
- as bacteria take hold, gray membrane begins to form in throat
- interferes with breathing
- produces poison that damages heart, kidneys and nerves
- 10 percent of cases are fatal

Tetanus (means muscle spasms, also called lockjaw)
- caused by contaminated dirt getting into wounds
- causes painful muscular contractions, striking first muscles in neck and jaw
- 50 percent of cases are fatal

Pertussis (means intense cough, also called whooping cough)
- characterized by coughing fits and eventual tightening of the throat; whooping sound comes from gasping for air between coughs
- most severe in young infants
- can cause ear infections, pneumonia and convulsions; rare but most serious is brain damage

Polio (poliomyelitis means gray, pale marrow)
- virus inflames and destroys nerve tissue in spinal cord or brain
- causes paralysis, usually of arms or legs but also of the breathing muscles
- 10 percent of cases are fatal

Measles (means spots)
- most serious common childhood disease
- always causes high fever (103°F – 105°F) and rash; usually lasts 10 days
- may cause pneumonia or ear infection
- causes deafness, blindness, convulsions and/or inflammation of the brain in 1 of every 1000 children who get the disease
- of children who develop a brain disorder from measles, 1 in 10 dies

Rubella (means reddish) or **German Measles**
- when contracted by pregnant women, can cause miscarriage,

stillbirth or multiple birth defects including deafness and heart disease
- usually a mild disease with mild fever, rash and swollen glands, generally lasting only a few days

Mumps
- usually causes fever and swelling of salivary glands (chipmunklike appearance)
- may cause inflammation of pancreas
- may cause a temporary brain disorder
- can result in permanent deafness

What to Expect

Vaccines contain specific germs that have been either killed, chemically disarmed (toxoids) or kept alive but weakened (attenuated). Before they are used, each batch is double-tested, first by the manufacturer, then by the U.S. Food and Drug Administration. These vaccines stimulate your child's immune system to form a specialized army of antibodies to fight each disease. If exposed to the same bacterium or virus in the future, your child's army of antibodies is already in place and standing guard.

The following is the inoculation timetable recommended by the American Academy of Pediatrics.

	DPT	Polio	Measles	TB Test	Rubella	Mumps	Tetanus-Diphtheria
2 months	x	x					
4 months	x	x					
6 months	x						
1 year				x			
15 months			x		x	x	
1.5 years	x	x					
4–6 years	x	x					
14–16 years							x

No vaccine is perfect, and because it must be powerful enough to immunize your child, some side effects are normal and usually predictable. Any serious reactions including a fever of 103°F or higher should be reported immediately to your child's doctor or clinic (see "Ways to Avoid Problems" on facing page).

Possible Side Effects of Vaccines

REACTIONS TO MOST VACCINES

Local: Mild swelling, redness and tenderness at injection site.
Systemic: Crankiness, fever, chills, rash and/or headache may occur after a killed vaccine; live viruses such as measles and rubella may cause fever and rash one to several weeks after inoculation; most reactions subside within 24 hours and can be controlled with Infant Tylenol or similar products.

REACTIONS TO SPECIFIC VACCINES

Polio: Reactions are uncommon.
Measles: A few children may get a low fever (under 101°F) or faint rash within one to two weeks after shot.
Mumps: Same as measles, but without a rash and with some swelling of the glands.
Rubella: Possible low fever (under 101°F), rash or swollen glands in the neck or behind ears one to two weeks after the shot.
Diphtheria, Pertussis, Tetanus: Slight fever, possibly headaches, chills, vomiting; prolonged screaming or unusual crying and sometimes effects on the central nervous system such as involuntary muscle contractions or convulsions.

Risks Versus Benefits

Controversy surrounding the safety of vaccines is due partly to conflicting statistics. According to official figures from the U.S. Public Health Service, the incidence of serious side effects is as follows:

POLIO

1 in 8.1 million who receive *oral* polio vaccine develops permanent paralysis; there is virtually no risk with *injectable* (killed) polio vaccine.

MEASLES, MUMPS AND RUBELLA

No statistics, but "very rarely" will children have a serious reaction, such as inflammation of the brain (encephalitis), convulsions with fever or nerve deafness.

DIPHTHERIA, PERTUSSIS AND TETANUS (DPT)

1 in 1,750 will experience convulsion(s) or episodes of limpness; 5 percent may develop a temperature greater than 102°F and unusual crying may occur in 1 in 1,000; rarely, about once in every 110,000 shots, inflammation of the brain (encephalitis) may occur, and permanent brain damage about once in every 310,000 shots.

At the core of the immunization debate lies the safety of the DPT vaccine, where the P—pertussis—is the villain. Of all vaccines, pertussis is considered the most reactive, but it is the only one to date able to keep the disease itself at bay. People scared about the P challenge the Public Health Service figures and cite a preliminary 1979 study at UCLA involving 7000 children, which found the incidence of "serious reactions" such as high fever, collapse and convulsions as high as 1 in 875. The study notes, however, that all cases "returned to their normal baseline state within 48 hours of immunization and all were judged to have normal neurological examinations when seen by the author within 2 weeks of their reaction." Presented with the discrepancy between these and the government's figures, vaccine proponents point out the questionable validity of a single study.

Parents still wonder if it would not be wiser to risk their child's catching whooping cough than take the chance, however slight, that he or she might suffer permanent side effects from the vaccine. "Whooping cough in itself," answers Dr. Alan Hinman, chief of immunization at the government's Centers for Disease Control, "poses the risk of brain damage—a ten times greater risk than the vaccine— even with antibiotics. Medication can prevent pneumonia in this case, but may not shorten the course of the illness, which often spans a few months. My advice continues to be that the benefits far outweigh the risks."

In the 1970s, the pertussis vaccine became very controversial in England, and immunization levels fell from approximately 80 percent of all children in England to about 30 percent. From 1976 to 1981, following the decline in the number of youngsters protected against whooping cough, there was a 2.3-fold increase in the rate of whooping cough for children under 1 year; a 4.4-fold increase in the rate of disease among the ages 1 to 4 years; and a 1.8-fold increase in the rate of disease for children 5 to 9 years of age.

Ways to Avoid Problems

(1) *Before your baby gets his or her first shots,* be sure you have gone through the following list, taken from the American Academy of Pediatrics' *Red Book,* outlining when shots should be withheld.

Volunteer any pertinent information including allergies or "bugs" going around your household to the doctor or nurse beforehand—don't wait to be asked. The vaccine should *not* be given if the child:

- is sick with a high fever (minor infections not associated with fever such as common cold are not reason to defer immunization)
- is under medical treatment that lowers resistance or immunity such as radiation therapy, chemotherapy, steroids (true only for live vaccines)
- had plasma or blood transfusion given within past eight weeks (true only for live vaccines)
- had a reaction to a prior vaccine.

The pertussis component of the DPT vaccine should not be given if a child has a progressive neurological disorder, and some pediatricians would go beyond the recommendations of the American Academy of Pediatrics to include a child whose sibling(s) had a seizure or other serious reaction or who comes from a family with a history of convulsions or neurological disorders.

(2) Understand fully the possible side effects before your child is inoculated. Ask to see information sheets or vaccine package inserts. Although many immunizations are required by law, you have the right to refuse them until all your questions regarding risks and benefits have been satisfactorily answered.

(3) Watch for reactions to the shot(s). Don't hesitate to call your doctor's office in the event of fever over 101°F or any unusual behavior. A cool, wet washcloth usually eases the discomfort of local painful swelling. Ask the doctor about acetaminophen such as Infant Tylenol, to reduce the fever.

(4) *Before subsequent shots,* review any reactions from the previous one. A child should never receive another DPT vaccine if he or she experienced any one of the following, states the American Academy of Pediatrics' *Red Book*:

- screaming episodes, usually a prolonged period of peculiar crying during which your baby cannot be comforted
- fever of 103°F or higher (some put the limit at 105°F)
- extreme sleepiness or limpness
- involuntary muscle spasms/convulsions
- collapse, turning pale and going into shock.

(5) If there has been a significant reaction, discuss leaving out the P component entirely the next time.

(6) Be sure the shots are given on time; in some cases spacing is important to ensure effectiveness (but interruption of the schedule with a delay between doses does not usually interfere with the final immunity achieved). It is not necessary to start the series over again even if a long time has elapsed.

(7) Ask for a form from your physician to record the dates and types of vaccines. You may have to insist that it be filled out. It is important to keep vaccination records in a safe place, as you will need the record when enrolling your child in day care or school.

(8) If you're concerned about the fee for each vaccination at the doctor's office, check with your local county health department, because you may be able to get them free or for just a few dollars.

(9) All states require children to be immunized, but state laws vary regarding just which vaccines are necessary. Some exemptions are allowed on medical or religious grounds. To find out more about your legal rights in the event that you refuse immunization, see the organization listed below in "Information Sources".

Factors to Weigh

Until these bacteria and viruses are totally snuffed out, anyone not safeguarded by immunization is an open target for the disease. Clearly, a low fever or rash is a small price to pay for protection against a potentially harmful form of the illness. Don't be paranoid about the side effects, but by keeping a watchful eye out for reactions and reporting them promptly you can usually head off more serious complications. It is easy to be railroaded into vaccinating your child, particularly since that is the law, but be sure you feel you know enough before giving the green light. The American Academy of Pediatrics emphasizes that "parents should be informed of the possible side effects of all vaccines and of the risk of the diseases by their physicians."

Though no vaccine "brew" is perfect, the threat of severe disability and death from the Big Seven childhood diseases has been dramatically controlled. Since development of the polio vaccine in 1955, for example, annual cases of the crippling disease have dropped from 22,000 to 2 (in 1982). Intensive immunization research continues in the U.S. and other countries, focusing particular attention on developing a less reactive pertussis vaccine, which, according to the Centers for Disease Control, is on the horizon.

Information Sources

ORGANIZATIONS

American Natural Hygiene Society
698 Brooklawn Ave.
Bridgeport, CT 06604

Letters for requesting exemption by school authorities are available for a fee from this parents' organization.

Immunization Division
Centers for Disease Control (CDC)
1600 Clifton Rd., NE
Atlanta, GA 30333
"Make Measles a Memory—Immunize!" and other pamphlets that discuss benefits of inoculations; single copies are available free from the CDC.

CRIB DEATH: WHAT YOU SHOULD KNOW

Telling you not to worry about crib death—sudden infant death syndrome (SIDS)—won't do much good, since its possibility is bound to cross your mind more than once during the first year of your baby's life. By definition, SIDS is the sudden death of an infant or young child that is unexpected and unexplained even after an extensive autopsy. Though it is a relatively rare phenomenon, striking 2 in 1000 babies, still it figures as the leading cause of death in babies aged 1 month to 12 months. Researchers generally agree that while most SIDS victims appear normal, they probably have subtle differences that cannot yet be perceived by those studying this phenomenon. The incidence of SIDS is higher among males than females. Although SIDS does not strike children in specific social or economic strata or geographical areas, sudden death tends to occur more frequently during cool-weather months when respiratory infection is greater.

The exact causes of this syndrome remain a mystery, but, according to the government-sponsored National SIDS Clearinghouse, researchers have at least ruled out several factors that do *not* cause crib death in the majority of cases:

- SIDS is not considered hereditary
- SIDS is not contagious
- SIDS is not caused by suffocation by an external source such as bedding
- SIDS is not caused by vomiting
- SIDS is not caused by choking
- SIDS is not caused by neglect.

In addition, babies less at risk appear to be firstborns, those whose mothers are nonsmokers and those born to mothers over 20 years old.

Scientists continue to search for all the conditions responsible for sudden infant death in order to identify babies prone to SIDS and develop preventive safeguards. Although some progress has been made, so far all researchers really know is that SIDS is the result of not one but a combination of factors. Areas of study include developmental changes during life in utero and during the newborn period, sleep physiology, nervous-system abnormalities, heart and respiratory patterns, metabolic and biochemical defects as well as numerous environmental factors. One element that confuses the picture is that the period in which most SIDS babies die—between 2 and 6 months—coincides with a time of first exposure to many new things, such as foods, germs from nonfamily members and vaccines. The number of potential contributing factors tends to generate a new SIDS theory each week, often creating the illusion that the cause of crib death has been uncovered. It is important to remember that no single theory has yet been proven, so even with the growing body of scientific data, the typical SIDS victim cannot be identified beforehand.

Can SIDS Be Prevented?

Without definitive answers, crib death remains unpredictable and therefore unpreventable, except perhaps for a small number of babies at risk for SIDS due to a condition called apnea, meaning prolonged lapses in breathing. All infants occasionally take pauses between breaths, but for a few these lapses are dangerously long, and respiration may stop altogether. Infantile apnea is considered serious only when breathing stops for as long as 20 seconds or when breathing stops for shorter periods of time and is associated with symptoms of a bluish tint around the mouth and nostrils or pale skin color or a slow heartbeat or pulse. Sometimes an underlying cause of infantile apnea can be detected and corrected; in other cases there is no cure. Preliminary research, however, suggests that babies tend to outgrow apnea by about 6 or 8 months of age.

Children who experience such breathing irregularities and blue spells are considered at high risk for SIDS. One option for their treatment is to attach the infant to a home apnea monitor that sounds an alarm any time respiration or the heart rate slows down. When the monitor signals, this alarm alone may sometimes reactivate breathing. Most of the time, however, further stimulation such as a gentle shake, or mouth-to-mouth resuscitation, may be necessary.

The decision to monitor a baby should be made in consultation with a qualified physician. It's important to remember that monitors are not a cure for apnea. Definitely steer away from advertisements for monitors, special pillows and other gadgets that promise to protect your child from crib death. Opinions are mixed on the benefits of apnea monitors, as they can be costly not only in dollars but in emotional strain for the family. Local chapters of the National SIDS

Foundation offer guidance and support for those parents with children diagnosed as being at high risk for SIDS.

The relationship between infantile apnea and sudden infant death remains unclear; certainly most victims of SIDS have not exhibited previous breathing problems. Since preventive measures are not known at this time, the one thing that parents can do is visit their pediatrician or family physician if they observe or sense changes in their infant's development or behavior. Dr. Howard Hoffman, Chief of the Biometry Branch at the government's National Institute for Child Health and Human Development, suggests, "Personally, I would advise parents to pay extra attention to their baby during the second and third months regarding any change in behavior, listlessness or infection, particularly respiratory problems."

It is not only useless to worry, but probably unnecessary, since SIDS is not a common occurrence; as the National SIDS Clearinghouse emphasizes, out of 1000 babies born, 998 do *not* fall victim to crib death.

Information Sources

ADDITIONAL READING

Coping with Sudden Infant Death Syndrome, by John De Frain (Lexington, MA: Lexington Books, 1983).

ORGANIZATIONS

National SIDS Clearinghouse
1555 Wilson Blvd., #600
Rosslyn, VA 22209
SIDS Hotline (703) 528-8480 (they will call you back if you are calling long distance).
Provides fact sheets, information and educational materials free of charge.
Referral service to parent support groups, SIDS counseling.

National SIDS Foundation
2 Metro Plaza, #204
8240 Professional Pl.
Landover, MD 20785
Nationwide network of volunteer chapters to help families with high-risk infants, those diagnosed with respiratory irregularities, and also provides support and counseling to families of SIDS victims.
Publishes booklets and a newsletter, including "At Home with a Monitor: A Guide For Parents."

Promotes and supports medical research into the cause and prevention of SIDS and SIDS-related concerns.

National Institute for Child Health and Human Development
Center for Research for Mothers and Children
7910 Woodmont Ave.
Bethesda, MD 20205
This government agency is in the forefront of SIDS research.
Single copies of the reprint "An Evaluation and Assessment of the State of the Science: SIDS" (NIH Pub No. 82-2304) is available free from NICHD, Office of Research Reporting, NIH, Bldg. 31, Room 2A-32, Bethesda, MD 20205.

Also, your local county health department can refer you to local SIDS programs and support organizations.

THE TOP THREE ILLNESSES: FEVER, DIARRHEA, EAR INFECTION

Most babies are pretty healthy for the first three months. They give you a chance to "read" them, to become familiar with their eating, sleeping and activity patterns. When they first get sick—and all infants do—initially it's a guessing game, but after enough episodes of runny noses and flushed faces you will learn to recognize when to seek medical advice. At the beginning, your biggest concerns are likely to be fever, diarrhea and ear infection. Here is a rundown on each, with some general guidelines about what to do if and when they develop. The rule of thumb is, when in doubt, call your doctor (for more details, see "When to Call the Doctor: Day or Night?" p. 368).

Fever

Major Symptoms: Temperature, Irritability, "Fits." A fever signals that your child's body is fighting some illness—usually an infection—though the degree of fever generally has surprisingly little to do with the seriousness of the infection.

The pattern of "behavior" of a fever, however, often provides helpful clues in diagnosing the illness. Fever is actually a good sign, because it means your baby's white cells are fighting off the invading germs and sending messengers (termed "pyrogens," a fever-producing substance) to the brain to turn up the body heat to assist your baby's antibody system, sometimes halting germ growth, often inhibiting growth of some viruses.

How to Take Your Baby's Temperature

Fever is considered any temperature of one degree or more above normal. Measured on a *rectal* thermometer normal is 99.6°F—one degree higher than oral. But "normal" varies from child to child and is influenced by the amount of activity and the time of day. Lowest readings are seen in the early morning, while late afternoon shows the highest of the day. Use of a fever-detector tape across the forehead or registering the temperature under the armpit are fine methods, but a rectal thermometer is preferred because it provides a more accurate reading.

(1) Be sure to shake the rectal thermometer so it is well below the normal 98.6°F mark, and grease the stubby, rounded mercury bulb with petroleum jelly or baby oil.

(2) Place your baby on his or her stomach across your lap. Insert the thermometer about one inch or a bit farther into the rectum. Don't worry—you won't hurt the baby. Hold the thermometer loosely with one hand to keep it in place, while holding the buttocks firmly together with the other. Another position is to put the baby on its back so he or she can see you and see what's going on. Hold feet up with one hand and hold the thermometer comfortably against the bottom with the other, so if the baby moves, your hand and the thermometer will move with it.

(3) Hold the thermometer in the rectum for three minutes—yes, it seems like forever. Gently lay it aside while you rediaper your baby; the thermometer reading won't change until you shake it down.

(4) To read the thermometer, hold it horizontally in one hand at eye level and slowly roll it back and forth between your thumb and finger until the column of silver or colored mercury comes into focus. Write down the reading and the time of day.

(5) After cleaning it, put the thermometer in a safe place, out of reach of the baby, since mercury is poisonous and broken glass is dangerous.

If your baby has a fairly high fever but remains playful and cheerful, the sickness is not likely to be serious and you need not worry. However, any fever should warn you to watch carefully and seek medical attention if it persists for several days or if your child appears to be sick and weak.

When to call the doctor

- a rectal temperature above normal 99.6°F in an infant less than 4 weeks old
- a rectal temperature 103°F or more
- a rectal temperature 101°F or more that continues for 72 hours

- persistent vomiting
- persistent diarrhea
- crying as if in pain
- difficult breathing
- excessive sleepiness and baby is hard to rouse
- rubbing ear or rolling head

Harmful effects of running a temperature are rare because of the body's built-in mechanism designed to keep temperatures from rising above the 106°F danger level. For about 3 to 4 babies in 100, however, a fever will irritate the brain enough to set off twitching, stiffening of the limbs and violent shaking. The temperature threshold of such convulsions or seizures varies from child to child, but once a child has had one, chances are that the same temperature reached again will trigger a similar seizure. These are not epileptic, but febrile, convulsions, and your child will return to normal with no permanent damage. Follow the procedures outlined under "Convulsions or 'Fits,'" p. 364.

Fevers usually do not need to be treated unless your child is really uncomfortable or the temperature risks spiking sharply to 105°F or more, posing the threat of convulsions. On the other hand, all this newly generated heat needs to be released eventually. The key in caring for your feverish baby is to allow his or her own body stabilizing mechanisms to work:

- keep the child cool and dress lightly; also keep room on the cool side
- use no blankets, just a sheet
- give plenty of cool, clear liquids, which work to release heat much the way a water-cooled car engine does
- take clothes off if temperature is 103°F or more, sponge baby in tub with lukewarm water or use damp washcloth while baby lies on the bed. This brings "warmed" blood to skin's surface, where evaporation of the water cools it in turn. Don't use ice-cold water, because it will bring on chills, which only raise the temperature again
- use fever-reducing drugs only if your child is really uncomfortable or if suggested by the doctor. Aspirin, which reduces fever, is suspected of contributing to the rare but life-threatening illness called Reye's Syndrome when given to children with a viral infection, particularly the flu or chicken pox (most cases occur between the ages of 5 and 15). Acetaminophen such as Tempra or Tylenol is preferred to aspirin by many pediatricians for reducing fever, although an acetaminophen overdose is potentially life-threatening and much more difficult to reverse than an aspirin overdose.

- be aware that convulsions are a possibility if temperature hits 105°F. If they occur, try to stay calm and see the step-by-step directions on p. 364.

Diarrhea

Major Symptom: Frequent, Loose Watery Stools. For the first two years of life, your baby's intestines are highly sensitive to infection. During this time, diarrhea can result even from a nonintestinal bug caught from your sore throat or your husband's cold. The infection makes for greenish-yellow, foul-smelling and very watery stools, often expelled with some force. Because your infant is so tiny, water loss through diarrhea can endanger its supply of necessary fluids and minerals and possibly lead to dehydration. Most cases, though, are mild, lasting only a day or so, and you can correct the slight fluid imbalance quite easily. For a baby of under 3 months, however, even a single large, watery bowel movement can be serious, and any time diarrhea is accompanied by other signs of illness, such as vomiting, seek medical advice.

When to call the doctor

- one or more large, watery bowel movements, especially in infants under 8 weeks
- frequent, watery, definitely green stools
- blood or pus in stools (but try to recall whether your baby ate beets recently)
- unusual vomiting
- diarrhea along with a fever of 101°F or higher (taken rectally) in an infant under 3 months

If diarrhea is mild, the goal in treating your baby is to be sure to replace the fluid and minerals he or she is losing, until the infection subsides. Your doctor will have specific suggestions, but common remedies include:

- offering liquids frequently, especially clear fluids (water, very weak tea, but don't use honey in tea if baby is under 12 months to avoid infant botulism)
- continuing to breast-feed
- diluting infant formula
- cutting back on solids for a day except perhaps for a little yogurt, rice, applesauce or banana (all easily digestible)
- using an over-the-counter prepared oral solution to replace essential minerals (electrolytes) and water lost, along with enough sugar to speed intake and provide calories.

If your baby is listless and has parched lips and scanty urine over a six-hour period, keep him or her on clear fluids until you contact the doctor, since this may be a sign of a dangerous level of dehydration. If the doctor is unavailable, go to the hospital emergency room.

Remember that diarrhea often defies easy diagnosis, so if you are worried, get in touch with your baby's physician.

Ear Infection

Major Symptoms: Unexplained Crying, Pulling Ear. With all the colds your baby is likely to get, some of the germ-filled mucus from the nose is bound to travel occasionally to the connecting ear canal (which is one reason to use a bulb syringe on your child's nose if the cold is severe). Sometimes a viral or bacterial infection—termed "otitis media," meaning inflammation of the middle ear—takes hold, usually several days after the cold has been around. Besides nasal congestion, this common illness during infancy is linked to exposure to household cigarette smoke and a predisposition to certain allergies.

The problem area is the Eustachian tube, which leads from the middle ear to the back of the throat. This canal permits air to enter the middle ear and equalize the pressure on both sides of the eardrum. When germs from the nose and throat start growing in the Eustachian tube, the air supply is blocked, and inflammation may occur. In some cases this can provide an ideal warm, moist home in which bacteria can flourish. Pain is caused by fluid pressing against the sensitive nerves of both the middle ear and the drum.

In secretory otitis media, the fluid or secretion in the middle-ear cavity is not thick and does not produce much pressure on the drum, so there may be few symptoms. However, acute purulent otitis media (pronounced pur'rou-lent, which means containing or forming pus) usually will cause your baby to wake during the night crying or moaning because of pain. Other symptoms include pulling at one or both ears, loss of appetite, fever, weakness and perhaps nausea or vomiting.

When to call the doctor

- if baby has rectal temperature above 103°F and you have trouble waking him or her or if you notice a stiff neck, phone immediately
- if you notice pus or any discharge, the baby's eardrums may have burst, so call right away
- if you suspect an ear problem even if your baby's temperature is normal, make a doctor's appointment

Diagnosis is accomplished simply by inspecting the eardrum with an otoscope, so that the doctor can judge from its appearance if the middle ear, which lies behind, is infected. If its usual pearly whiteness has turned deep red or if the drum is bulging, the middle ear is inflamed. But a shade anywhere in between makes the decision judgmental. Whether an infection is viral or bacterial cannot be determined just by looking, so, though some ear infections are viral and therefore untreatable with drugs, antibiotics are commonly prescribed just in case. If left untreated, a bacterial infection can spread and cause mastoid infection, brain disease and meningitis. There are those doctors, though, who routinely puncture the eardrum to draw out a sample of fluid to test before prescribing a baby antibiotics.

An ampicillinlike antibiotic is normally prescribed for a ten-day period, followed by another look at the ears. If the middle ear still is not pearly white, another antibiotic may be suggested. Decongestants and antihistamines are sometimes recommended to shrink mucus in nasal passages and the Eustachian tube, but use of such medications remains controversial; they do cause side effects ranging from hyperactivity to mild sedation.

RECURRENT FLARE-UPS

Next to regular checkups, ear infections are the most common reason for doctor visits, the highest incidence being among babies age 6 months to 2 years, then declining, but picking up again between 5 and 6 years, when children start school. An ear, nose and throat specialist, called an otolaryngologist, may be worth consulting if your child has recurrent ear infections or is not hearing well. An estimated one million operations are performed annually to insert a tiny ventilation tube into the eardrum. This surgical procedure, termed tympanostomy, is rarely done in infants under 24 months, partly because at about 2 years, chronic infections often stop, possibly due to the Eustachian tube's growing straighter and wider as well as a child's increasing immunity to viruses and bacteria. While many pediatricians are not keen on using these tubes, child-development specialists frequently rave about the progress in language and learning skills after a youngster has had a tympanostomy.

There is not much you can do to prevent middle ear infection, particularly when colds are prevalent. Once your baby is old enough, teach him or her to blow the nose slowly and gently, so mucus is not driven up into the Eustachian tube. Also try to eliminate exposure to suspected allergens (food and airborne substances) and keep your child away from cigarette smoke. Another suggestion you may want to discuss with your doctor is elevating your child's head and shoulders slightly while sleeping. Something else to consider is buying an Earscope for about $20, which may save you trips to the doctor's when you suspect a problem (for more information about this device, write Nash & Associates, PO Box 300, 504 Shaw Ave., Ferndale, CA

95536). But there is no substitute for prompt professional diagnosis and treatment to avoid hearing loss or other long-term effects.

COMMON PROBLEMS FROM ALLERGIES TO RASHES

Colds, coughs and other maladies are to be expected, particularly once your baby starts playing with other children. And if you are rarely sick, get ready for a change. Soon after your sore throat disappears, your son or daughter may come down with a runny nose and then you may catch a cold. Germs get passed back and forth, especially during the winter months, and it may be rare for everyone in the family to be healthy at the same time. Luckily, most childhood illnesses require only a watchful eye, plenty of rest and such old-fashioned medicine as chicken soup. This also applies in some cases to the three most common illnesses during infancy, described in the preceding section. If you are just plain worried and it's the middle of the night, refer to "When to Call the Doctor: Day or Night?" (p. 368).

Allergies and Asthma

Major Symptoms: Rashes, Diarrhea, Wheezing. In the first year or so of life, your baby's system is still adjusting to its new environment, and along the way may develop an unusual sensitivity to what he or she eats, inhales or touches. For some reason, an ordinarily harmless substance like milk or dust is treated as a threat by the body's defense system, causing it to release histamines—chemicals that expand blood vessels and allow serum to ooze into tissues—which is called an antibody attack. These allergic reactions, which tend to run in families, often mimic childhood illnesses such as colds and intestinal infections or turn up in a variety of skin rashes. In infancy the most likely triggers, called allergens, are foods and airborne substances such as household dust.

Some tip-offs to allergies include frequent intestinal upsets or spitting up large amounts of formula, chronic stuffy nose or chest cold, recurring middle ear infections and skin rashes, especially on the cheeks, inside arms, or diaper area. In determining whether your baby's condition is an illness or an allergy, you are the best observer, so keep track of possible cause-and-effect relationships to review with the doctor. Consult your doctor about use of antihistamines and decongestants such as Actifed and Dimetane which relieve nasal congestion and symptoms of hay fever and other allergies but do not affect the overall course of an illness. More immediate medical attention is advised, however, if your child is losing fluids through diarrhea or has real difficulty breathing.

Wheezing, specifically when your baby exhales, may well mean asthma, loosely translated from the Greek word for "a panting." Symptoms of this common illness tend to mimic bronchitis: first a swelling of the tiny tubes running from breathing passages into the lungs; then a thick mucus buildup. This swelling sets off dry coughing spasms or wheezing, which eventually loosens the mucus, narrowing and restricting the airways. In infants, asthma is usually set off by an infection. When it accompanies a chest infection, it is termed asthmatic bronchitis.

If you notice your child is wheezing and fighting to breathe, sit him or her upright and try to do something calming—perhaps read a book together. Then start a vaporizer or steam up the bathroom and sit there with your child to see if that helps. Wait to call the doctor until morning if it settles down, but don't hesitate to pick up the phone if you are just plain worried. The doctor may order theophylline preparations, which come in liquid form, rectal solutions or small pellets to be mixed with soft foods such as applesauce. If asthmatic bronchitis is suspected, seek medical attention promptly, since both the infection and cough must be treated.

Below are some of the more common allergens that bother allergic children, the reactions they generally trigger and a few suggestions for how to take care of them. Fortunately, allergies that begin when a child is very young are frequently outgrown.

Potential Allergens	Reaction	Care
Foods: including cow's milk, citrus fruits, nuts, tomatoes, wheat, corn, eggs, peanut butter, strawberries, chocolate, fish, shellfish	diarrhea, cramps, rashes, specifically hives (large red welts), eczema (dry, scaly patches in skin folds of elbows and behind knees), itching, scratching	keep notes of which food or foods together seem to cause the reaction; investigate food substitutes including soy-based formulas
Airborne Substances: pet dander, household dust, down or feather pillows; sprays such as for insects	stuffy or runny nose, sneezing or wheezing	keep pets and down and feather pillows out of baby's room; sprays are available to reduce amount of pet hair in air; dust and vacuum daily
Skin Irritants: some plastics, synthetic fabrics, wool, detergents	rash will break out on part of skin touching irritant	use common sense and keep irritants away or find substitutes; dress

Potential Allergens	Reaction	Care
not thoroughly rinsed from clothes, claytype play materials, perfumed substances such as lotions		in cotton instead of synthetics; put clothes through second clear-rinse cycle in washing machine

Unless you can pinpoint the troublemaker, a visit to an allergist may be a wise investment, particularly in cases of severe asthma attacks.

Colds

Major Symptom: Runny Nose. A succession of runny noses is likely to begin about the time your baby has started to play with other children. Colds are viral infections of the nose and throat that usually stubbornly run their full course anywhere from four or five days to a week or so. Expect two or three the first year, though three times that number is not unusual. The first sign of a cold is often fussiness, followed by clear, watery mucus streaming from your baby's nose. In two to three days the bubbly mucus will thicken and turn cloudy, plugging or stuffing up the nasal passages. Other symptoms may include sneezing, coughing, loss of appetite, red eyes or fever.

Since antibiotics are powerless against viruses, the only cure for a cold is time and tissues. While you wait, the most important thing is to try to confine the virus to the nose and stop it from spreading into ear and lung passages. You can help by drawing mucus out of the baby's nose periodically with a bulb syringe (described in the following checklist) and making sure your child gets enough rest and fluids to help the body heal itself.

- *Easing congestion/stuffy nose.* Plug in a vaporizer or humidifier in the nursery or entertain yourselves in a steamy bathroom while hot water pours from faucets or shower head; do not give decongestants, antihistamines or nose drops unless you've discussed it first with the doctor.
- *Flushing out germs.* Lots of clear liquids are best, such as chicken noddle soup, warm tea with a bit of sugar (no honey if your baby is not yet 1 year old, since there is potential for botulism poisoning) or vitamin C–rich fruit juices such as Cranapple (watch out for orange juice, as it may trigger diarrhea in young infants).
- *Relieving discomfort and fever:* See "The Top Three Illnesses: Fever, Diarrhea, Ear Infection" (p. 385) for a discussion on how to take care of a temperature above 99.6°F.
- *Clearing out nose.* Use a soft rubber bulb syringe to draw mucus

gently out of the nasal passages so it won't travel up through ear canals; once breathing is easier, the baby may nurse more and its appetite may pick up.

As with most infant ailments, colds can piggyback other illnesses, such as croup or a middle ear infection, that warrant prompt medical attention.

When to call the doctor

- if cold lasts longer than ten days
- if baby is very weak with not even energy to cry loudly
- if baby nurses poorly or won't drink more than half of usual bottle even when nose is clear
- if there is a frequent or deep wheezing cough even without fever
- if breathing is labored, not just noisy, so baby actually has difficulty drawing in air
- if baby cries or moans as if in pain for an hour or more
- if stuffy or runny nose lasts over three days in baby under 12 months

Colic

Major Symptoms: Crying, Screaming, Cramps. Not every baby with periodic, inexplicable howling is suffering from colic (from the Greek word for colon). Crying from colic differs from most other types of crying because it is maddeningly regular and the baby is usually inconsolable. The condition usually sets in about the second week after birth and fades away by the end of the third month. Generally crying episodes occur six days out of seven, starting up somewhere between 6:00 P.M. and midnight each evening and lasting anywhere from 45 minutes to four hours. Though colic itself poses no medical threat to your child's health, the baby does experience considerable discomfort, probably from a combination of tension and stomach or intestinal pain. Often babies either draw their legs up to their abdomens and scream or stick their legs out straight, many times passing gas. The cause of colic is probably something they are trying to digest or the digestive system itself, but no one knows for sure. Most medical experts predict the colic puzzle will ultimately be solved by pieces borrowed from two or more of the following theories:

(1) Food allergies: cow's milk, either from formula or from the mother's milk if she consumes dairy products (there's a large body of evidence supporting this as a contributing factor)
(2) Faulty feeding habits: the mother's diet contains too many food

additives such as diet soft drinks; fluoride and other vitamin and mineral supplements cause stomach cramps; baby swallows too much air while eating; baby sucks hard to satisfy sucking needs and gets too much food; baby cannot tolerate carbohydrates; or baby has tendency toward allergies in general (usually both parents are allergic)

(3) Kink in the intestines: after six months curled up in utero, baby's bowels may take time to straighten enough to let waste pass smoothly

(4) Underdeveloped nervous system: babies are tense and high-strung (hypertonic) until their nervous systems mature

(5) Progesterone withdrawal: your baby's body was used to this relaxant, borrowed from you while in utero, and the smooth muscle tends to tense as baby readjusts

(6) Nervous, uptight parents: you unwittingly communicate your anxiety to your baby, causing him or her to respond in kind; this can be a chicken-or-egg situation—in other words, which came first, your tension or your baby's caterwauling?

Don't expect to get understanding and sympathy from parents and grandparents who have never lived with a colicky baby. Above all, remember it's only a matter of time before your son or daughter will outgrow colic. Here are some ways to try to relieve and relax you and your child:

- take a warm bath together
- lay baby across your knees or place baby stomach down on hot water bottle wrapped in towel
- move baby's legs gently in bicycle motion to help expel gas
- put baby in the car seat and go for a ride
- play soft music or cassette tape, such as "Suite Baby Dreams," with familiar, womblike sounds
- hold your baby through naps or try a hammock with a battery-operated device designed to lull baby with heartbeat sounds
- let baby sleep with you (skin-to-skin contact)
- put a loudly ticking clock in the nursery
- minimize outside stimulation; for instance, dim lights and don't turn on the vacuum cleaner
- try more frequent nursing but limit the amount each time and make sure baby doesn't gulp or suck too fast
- carry baby around in front carrier such as a Snugli, to satisfy need for physical contact
- consult with your baby's doctor about switching to soybean-based formula or eliminating dairy products from your diet if you're nursing

- discuss use of antispasmodic drugs that are prescribed for severe cases to relax baby's digestive tract

Constipation

Unusual Bowel Movements. Your baby is not truly constipated unless his or her stools are hard, dry or difficult to pass. Regularity and frequency of bowel movements are unimportant so long as it's not been more than three or four days since the last one. A baby's intestines can get stopped up if stools are hard, which may happen in bottle-fed infants or when an infant's diet lacks sufficient fluids. It's possible, too, that the answer is lack of enough fibrous food to move things along, a problem particularly if an illness has dulled your baby's appetite.

In toddlers, constipation is occasionally psychological. After a painful or difficult bowel movement your child may hold back for fear of being hurt again, or a refusal to "go" could be an effort at proving some independence.

For ordinary constipation, you may want to try one or a combination of the following:

- increase baby's fluid intake
- add about one tablespoon of prune juice or brown sugar or molasses to eight ounces of milk once a day
- try fruits and vegetables if your baby has been on solid foods for a while; especially effective are strained, stewed prunes
- no laxative, mineral oil or enema unless you've discussed it first with the doctor.

Constipation is not, in itself, an illness. Seek medical advice only if it lasts over a week, if "prune-juice therapy" doesn't do the trick or if it is paired with any of the following symptoms:

When to call the doctor

- blood in the stool
- frequent and unexplained projectile vomiting
- tummy is bloated; but remember, all babies' stomachs stick out because of the lack of tone in stomach muscles
- pale, listless, weak, very irritable
- baby seems to have tremendous difficulty passing a stool. Keep in mind that babies naturally grimace and grunt and turn pink during a bowel movement

Coughs

Major Symptoms: Dry and Raspy, Wet with Phlegm, Barking. A cough, like a fever, signals that your baby's body is defending itself against some foreign invader. The coughing reflex is designed to blow out whatever material is irritating your baby's throat or breathing passages, a sort of barking dog guarding the lungs from invasion or clearing them of germ-filled mucus. The reflex is triggered by any irritant such as a speck of dust entering the nose or throat (particularly if the bedroom air is dry), by a ticklish sore throat, excess mucus due to an allergic reaction or mucus/phlegm produced by a viral or bacterial infection.

Because a cough is one mechanism your child has of self-protective healing, the cough should not be suppressed unless it is wearing your baby out, preventing sleep or sorely scraping the throat. But since comfort measures may mask important clues, try to identify the underlying cause before doing anything to make your child more comfortable.

Symptoms	Possible Cause
dry frequent cough but no mucus brought up	arid room air; sore throat
wet cough, bringing up lots of phlegm/mucus	a cold (especially if coughing is heaviest at night or first thing in the morning); postnasal drip
crackling sounds at end of each breath from chest, with lots of mucus brought up; irritable, not playful and has poor appetite	viral or bacterial infection (temperature higher if bacterial)
wheezing, particularly when exhaling	asthma or bronchitis (see p. 391)
raspy, foghorn sound when inhaling that strikes suddenly and may seem as though baby is choking	croup (see p. 398)

If you are sure that your baby's cough is caused only by a cold, then you can treat it like a viral infection, with lots of fluids, plenty of rest and by moistening the room air with a vaporizer. Decongestants may help dry up a loose, wet cough. Watch for other symptoms such as fever; labored or difficult breathing; irritability; listlessness. The danger with a cough is that it might also be a symptom of bacterial infection—for instance, pneumonia—which could become serious if left untreated.

When to call the doctor

- if there are severe breathing problems; trouble exhaling; raspy or violent, barking cough; blue lips or nostrils are enlarging with each breath
- if baby is running a fever and loud, deep, dry cough cannot be relieved by half an hour with the vaporizer or steaming up the bathroom
- if a cough lasts longer than ten days without signs of improvement even if you think it is only caused by a cold; antibiotics may be prescribed in event of bacterial respiratory infection

Croup

Major Symptoms: Violent Cough During the Night. Croup nearly always comes on suddenly in the middle of the night and is usually caused by a virus that attacks the larynx (voice box) and the trachea (windpipe). Named for the hoarse, barking noise that produces laryngitis in older children and adults, croup swells the larynx, making it difficult for an infant to get air. When your child wakes up struggling to breathe, he or she will panic, and that causes the muscles of the airway to go into more spasms. You may notice the rib cage and area above the breastbone sink deeply each time your child struggles to inhale.

Try to stay calm. Immediately steam up the bathroom by turning on all the hot-water faucets. After about 15 to 30 minutes the moist air should reduce the swelling of the larynx to let more air past. Once the coughing fit is over, a lollipop or Popsicle may also soothe the throat. Croup tends to improve by morning but may recur for two to three nights.

When to call the doctor

- if baby has a fever and you suspect croup, call immediately
- if barking cough continues despite half an hour of vaporizing; an expectorant cough medicine may be suggested

Rashes

Major Symptoms: Pimples; Red, Raw Skin; Blisters. Small eruptions in your baby's skin or changes in its color or texture could come from wet diapers, allergies, bacterial or fungal infections, or normal adjustment to summer heat.

Type	Symptoms	Care
CRADLE CAP	greasy, dirty-looking crust on scalp	soften crust with baby oil or a bit of petroleum jelly before bed; shampoo with mild soap and comb off in the morning; usually it will clear up in a few days
DIAPER RASH	bright pink or red, usually caused by damp diaper, but sometimes temporary rash is due to food allergy	discussed below in detail
ECZEMA	dry, scaly patches in tiny babies; starts on cheeks or forehead in older infants; usually found in skin folds behind knees or in elbows; usually allergic reaction to certain foods, sometimes caused by teething	hypoallergenic lotion or ointment may help; (see "Allergies and Asthma," p. 391)
HEAT RASH	tiny pink pimples surrounded by patches of pink skin, usually on neck and shoulders; may blister, dry up and turn tan	sponge rash, pat dry, dust with cornstarch or baby powder and dress baby lightly with loose clothing; no ointments, as these block pores all the more
IMPETIGO	open, blisterlike pustules seen first in any moist area of body (armpit, groin, etc.) that spread easily; usually symptom of bacterial infection	sores should be looked at by a doctor; boil anything that comes in contact with baby, such as diapers, shirts, sheets, washcloths, eating utensils; scrub tub thoroughly after bathing baby (see "When to Call the Doctor," next page)

All babies at some point develop a skin rash on the diaper area but some are more prone to it than others. When something wet lies against the skin for a long period of time, it softens the top layer, which can peel away, get raw and occasionally become infected. If you notice a pungent, ammonia smell in the diaper, this comes from the increasing number of ammonia-producing germs in the urine as your baby gets older, and it is a further irritant to already raw skin.

The best way to treat diaper rash is to keep the area clean and dry, so as to limit as much as possible the growth of ammonia bacteria, either by disinfecting cloth diapers or using the disposable type. Techniques that may also help include:

- *change baby frequently*—at the least sign of dampness
- wash bottom thoroughly but very gently with mild soap and soft washcloth that doesn't contain perfumes or other potential irritants; rinse and dry well
- expose rash to air as much as possible by avoiding plastic pants, which trap moisture; try letting baby sleep without a diaper
- slip in diaper liners
- smooth on water-proofing cream such as petroleum jelly or special diaper-rash ointments; more expensive prescription ointment is another alternative
- wash diapers in laundry bleach (or use disposable type if ammonia is a problem); if possible, hang outdoors to dry

Most rashes—except for impetigo, which usually means the presence of bacterial infection—come and go, requiring no more treatment than keeping skin clean and dry. Some problems do warrant a check by your baby's doctor, though.

When to call the doctor

- if any rash or pimple dramatically changes color or shape; for instance, turns bright red and enlarges
- if rash looks like bleeding or bruising under the skin, unless you know for sure what caused it
- if diaper rash is caused by frequent loose, watery stools (first refer to "Diarrhea," p. 388)
- if rash worsens and continues for more than five days or so

A good description of the skin problem over the phone may preclude an office visit, so before calling your doctor, make a note of the following: where the rash started; if it has spread and if so, where; if it looks different on different parts of the body; if it's wet and weepy or dry and flaky; and its color (red, crimson, pink).

Spitting Up and Vomiting

Spitting up or vomiting either can be perfectly normal or can signal some underlying illness. In rare instances, persistent forceful vomiting could mean an obstruction or abnormality in your baby's digestive tract. Most of the time, though, spitting up is limited to the table- spoon or two of milk your infant burps out soon after feeding. During the first few months of life, the ringed muscle valve that closes off the food pipe from the stomach is still unskilled in keeping food down. Consequently, any excess fluids or solids are frequently sent back up, especially if your baby is squeezed or moved about soon after finishing a meal. What comes up is likely to appear to be much more than it actually is, and if your child continues to put on weight, the loss of a little food is unimportant.

Spitting up with force or vomiting is not unusual either, and is probably due to indigestion or some other common illness. If you suspect an upset stomach, take your child's temperature first, then try:

- waiting an hour before feeding again unless the baby seems hungry
- staying away from solids; restart feeding with half an ounce of cold, sweet fruit juice or tea with a little sugar (not honey) every 10 to 15 minutes for one hour, then increase to one ounce at 10–15 minute intervals for the next hour, followed by 2 ounces the third hour at the same time intervals.

Projectile vomiting, which jets out sometimes up to two feet, especial- ly in newborns, should not be ignored.

When you should call the doctor

- if baby spits up/vomits at every feeding (not just once or twice daily)
- if baby seems to throw up as much as he or she takes in (only eats a little and brings up all of it)
- if baby has to be coaxed to eat and lacks appetite
- if baby seems pale, listless, very irritable and stools are not their usual color or consistency
- if baby has projectile vomiting as frequently as once or twice daily.

Thrush

Major Symptom: White Spots in the Mouth. If nursing becomes uncomfortable for your baby and if your nipples become mysteriously sore, look inside your child's mouth for signs of thrush. This is a common fungal (yeast) infection a baby easily picks up and one quickly recognizable by the white scumlike spots it makes on the tongue and the insides of cheeks and gums. Except for mild discomfort for your baby and perhaps tender nipples for you, thrush isn't serious. But, as with any infection, it warrants prompt care and possibly a visit to the doctor. Antibiotics may be prescribed, but if you prefer to try home remedies first, La Leche League offers a few suggestions.

- *Relieve your baby's symptoms.* Dissolve a level teaspoon of baking soda or salt in a cup of boiled water and then swab baby's mouth firmly, especially the tongue, insides of cheeks and gums, after each nursing. Use fresh, sterilized cotton swabs each time you dip into the solution, which you mix fresh daily.
- *Relieve your sore nipples.* Bathe nipples in vinegar solution (1 tablespoon to 1 cup of water) after breast-feeding and then apply a soothing coat of petroleum jelly or lanolin to prevent dryness and cracking; another approach is to ask your doctor about a special ointment for treating a yeast infection.

To help avoid thrush in the first place, don't breast-feed another baby or let another woman nurse your baby. Keep toys clean, and don't share them with other young infants.

Information Sources

ADDITIONAL READING

The Child's Health Encyclopedia, by Boston Children's Medical Center (New York: Dell, 1975).

Healing at Home: A Guide to Health Care for Children, by Mary Howell, M.D. (Boston: Beacon, 1978).

A Parents' Guide to Telephone Medicine, by Jeffrey Brown, M.D. (New York: Perigee Books, 1980).

The Well Child Book, by Mike Samuels, M.D., and Nancy Samuels (New York: Summit Books, 1982).

CHILD-PROOFING: FROM POISONOUS PLANTS TO POPCORN

Don't underestimate your son's or daughter's insatiable curiosity. Accidents tend to occur more often as the ability to roll over, crawl and grasp increases. From about the age of 6 months on, your baby's mobility plus the desire to explore and put everything imaginable into the mouth will demand a watchful eye. While you don't want to be overprotective and confine this inquisitive mind too much, it's necessary to comb your home systematically—on your hands and knees—for potential hazards. Think of anything that could burn, bruise, cut or poison a curious, fearless and uncoordinated baby.

Here are a few basic safeguards for every room in the house:

- *Remove* to an out-of-reach shelf anything that could be swallowed or secure it with cabinet locks or drawer latches; all potentially poisonous substances such as medications and cleaning fluids should be sealed with child-proof caps and stored only in the original containers; put on green Mr. Yuk stickers, available from your local poison control center.
- *Hunt* for hot spots and put guards up to keep baby from radiators, registers, floor furnaces; be very careful if you use free-standing heaters; to prevent scalding, turn water-heater temperature to no hotter than 120°F.
- *Inspect* furniture for sharp edges and pad or tape them heavily or purchase specially made rounded plastic stick-ons for corners; consider moving your chrome-and-glass coffee table to another, unused room for a while.
- *Tape* over or plug guards into all unused electrical outlets to avoid shocks to curious fingers; plastic cover plates are available for those outlets in constant use; tape long electrical cords to the floor or against the wall or buy cord shorteners at a hardware store.
- *Ensure* against accidental drowning by keeping all toilet seats closed.

Keep in mind that as your baby grows, accident possibilities will change. Be sure to stay ahead of them and reevaluate every room in your home often, since spurts in development happen overnight.

Inside and Out

- Keep stairs free of objects, remove any slippery rug at the bottom and replace with a thick, secure one; ideally, gates should be set up at the top and the bottom. Plastic mesh ones are preferred to the accordion-style ones (for more about safety gates, see "Car Seats, Cribs and Other Essential Equipment," p. 341).
- Lock all trunks, cedar chests, hope chests.
- Put away those objects easily turned over, such as lightweight floor lamps, vases, fireplace tools.
- Secure scatter rugs with rubber mats.

- Watch out for flaking paint, which could contain lead, or loose insulation made of asbestos.
- Check out all your houseplants and those around the yard, since many are harmful when chewed, swallowed or rubbed on the skin. If necessary, take a sample leaf with you to a plant store or nursery for positive identification and find out if it is poisonous. It might also be wise to double-check with your local poison control center. Some *common poisonous* varieties include azalea, Christmas pepper, daffodil, English ivy, hydrangea, iris, mistletoe, philodendron, rhododendron, tomato leaves and wisteria. Several popular houseplants that you don't have to put out of reach, because they are not poisonous, include African violet, begonia, coleus, jade, poinsettia, schefflera, spider and wandering Jew.

POISONOUS PLANTS

Angel's-Trumpet (*Satura suaveolens*)
Azalea (*Rhododendron simsii*)
Bird of Paradise Flower (*Strelitzia reginae*)
Black Nightshade (*Solanum nigrum*)
Buttercup (*Ranunculus*)
Caladium (*Caladium*)
Castorbean (*Ricinus communis*)
Choke Cherry (*Prunus virginiana*)
Christmas Pepper (*Capsicum annum*)
Climbing Nightshade (*Solanum dulcamara*)
Daffodil (*Narcissus pseudonarcissus*)
Daphne (*Daphne mezereum*)
Deadly Nightshade (*Atropa belladonna*)
Delphinium (*Delphinium*)
Dumbcane (*Dieffenbachia*)
Elephant Ear (*Colocasia esculenta*)
English Ivy (*Hedera helix*)
Foxglove (*Digitalis purpurea*)
Fruit pits: apple, peach, apricot, wild cherry, pear, plum
Hens-and-Chicks (*Lantana*)
Holly (*Ilex aquifolium*)
Hyacinth (*Hyacinthus orientalis*)
Hydrangea (*Hydrangea macrophylla*)
Iris (*Iris*)
Jack-in-the-Pulpit (*Arisaema triphyllum*)
Jerusalem Cherry (*Solanum pseudocapsicum*)
Jimson Weed (*Satura stramomium*)
Jonquil (*Narcissus*)
Lily of the Valley (*Convallaria majalis*)

Mayapple *(Podophyllum peltatum)*
Mistletoe *(Viscum album)*
Morning Glory *(Ipomoea learii)*
Mountain Laurel *(Kalmia latifolia)*
Narcissus *(Narcissus)*
Nephthytis *(Nephthytis)*
Oleander *(Nerium oleander)*
Philodendron *(Philodendron)*
Pokewood *(Phytolacca americana)*
Pothos *(Scindapsus aureus, Rhaphidophora aurea)*
Privet *(Ligustrum vulgare)*
Rhododendron *(Rhododendron ponticum)*
Rhubarb leaves *(Rheum officinale)*
Sweet Pea *(Lathyrus odoratus)*
Swiss Cheese Plant *(Monstera deliciosa)*
Tomato leaves *(Lycopersicon esculentum)*
Yew *(Taxus)*
Virginia Creeper *(Parthenocissus quinque folia)*
Wisteria *(Wisteria)*

NONPOISONOUS PLANTS

African Violet *(Saintpaulia ionantha)*
Begonia *(Begonia)*
Christmas Cactus *(Schlumbergera bridgesii)*
Coleus *(Coleus blumei)*
Dandelion *(Taraxacum officinale)*
Dracaena *(Dracaena)*
Firethorn *(Pyracantha coccinea)*
Impatiens *(Impatiens)*
Jade *(Crassula argentea)*
Marigold *(Tagetes)*
Peperomia *(Peperomia caperata)*
Poinsettia *(Euphorbia pulcherrima)*
Purple Passion *(Cynura aurantiaca)*
Rose *(Rosa)*
Schefflera *(Brassaia actinophylla)*
Snake Plant *(Sansevieria trifasciata)*
Spider *(Chlorophytum comosum)*
Swedish Ivy *(Plectranthus australia)*
Wandering Jew *(Tradescantia fluminensis)*
Wax Plant *(Hoya carnosa)*
Wild Strawberry *(Fragaria)*
Zebra Plant *(Aphelandra squarrosa)*

Nursery

Precautions regarding cribs, mattresses and so on are discussed in detail in "Car Seats, Cribs and Other Essential Equipment" (p. 341). Some general safety guidelines for your baby's bedroom include:

- keep crib away from window, venetian-blind cords and radiators
- block access to window, even before your baby can climb
- position changing table so you don't need to turn your back, yet keep powders and creams out of baby's reach
- remove large toys from crib once baby can assume a standing position, so they won't be used as stepping-stools
- dress baby in flame-resistant sleepwear
- keep crib sides up.

Bathroom

Toddlers between 12 months and 2 years love to climb, open doors and drawers, take things apart and play in water. This makes any bathroom in the house potentially dangerous for a toddler on the prowl. You may want to get in the habit of keeping the bathroom doors shut. An added safety measure is to cover the doorknobs with special plastic slip-away covers. Additional safeguards include:

- lock medicine cabinets even if they seem out of reach
- prevent falls in the bathtub by using suction-lined rubber mat
- cover bathtub faucet with a soft rubber protector (available commercially; see "Information Sources," p. 408).

Of course, never leave your child alone for a second when he or she is in the bathtub.

Storage Areas

Once your child begins to roam, consider taking some precautions. In the garage, for instance, be sure insect sprays, car wax and the like are out of reach. Yard equipment such as lawnmowers and bicycles should be tucked away from curious toddlers, in a safe corner. Also:

- take doors off unused refrigerators or block the door latch from catching
- lock large picnic coolers
- check for safety latches on front-opening washers and dryers
- set up gate to guard basement stairs.

Kitchen

This is potentially one of the most dangerous rooms in the home. Store all detergents, household cleaners, plastic wrap, chewable vitamins and pet medication out of reach. If necessary, install latches, although storage in high cabinets is preferred. Other safeguards include:

- turning pot handles toward the wall, so they cannot be pulled off the stove
- storing knives and other sharp utensils high on the wall, perhaps in an enclosed rack
- watching baby's utensils for any chipping or peeling; metal flaking may contain poisonous substances (it's best to buy stainless steel).

If you are buying new kitchen appliances, consider a cooking range with rear controls and a wall-mounted oven. For a discussion about high-chair safety, see "High Chair Versus Portable Seat" (p. 350).

Other Precautions: Q-Tips, Popcorn and Nuts

Babies are little vacuum cleaners—everything imaginable goes into the mouth. After all, it's the most effective way of discovering what's what. The danger here is not so much swallowing, say, a nickel or a button, but of getting it stuck in the windpipe, which, in a 12-month-old, is no larger than your little finger. Be on the lookout for any object within your baby's reach that measures an inch or less in diameter or is sharp and risks damaging the body—tacks, pins, screws, jewelry, pens, pencils. Some safety precautions you might consider include the following:

- Cut off any buttons or decorations on toys, stuffed animals, dolls, cars (some toys, too, contain tiny batteries); also see "Pounding Toys, Puzzles, Picture Books" (p. 357).
- Keep balloons—inflated or not—away from the baby, who could choke on them.
- Wait to give baby popcorn, nuts, raw carrot sticks and celery stalks until he or she is able to chew them up; these are easily inhaled and can get stuck in the breathing passage.
- Don't allow your baby to play with any plastic bags, particularly dry-cleaning garment bags, for fear of suffocation.
- *Never feed honey* until after your baby's first birthday; it may contain bacteria that in a baby's intestines become lethal and may produce infant botulism (these spores are not killed by cooking).
- Dust talcum powder sparingly and carefully over your baby (cornstarch is preferred by many pediatricians); overgenerous sprinkling, especially around the face, mouth and nose, can be inhaled, clog airways and lead to serious respiratory problems; baby-powder containers are unsafe toys unless empty and washed out.

- Cleaning with cotton-tipped sticks such as Q-Tips is unnecessary and possibly hazardous; any part of the body you need to keep clean can be washed with a washcloth.
- Baby rattles that are quite small pose a real risk; regulations are in effect to control the size and shape, but check any older ones you think might have been made prior to 1978.

It cannot hurt to familiarize yourself with the various emergency services close to home. Keep handy the phone number of your baby's doctor, poison control center, hospital and ambulance service. Figure out possible escape routes in the event of fire. And, finally, review "Emergencies and First Aid," (p. 362).

Information Sources

ORGANIZATIONS

American Red Cross
Your local chapter probably offers courses on child safety.

Consumer Product Safety Commission
Washington, DC 20207
Toll-free hot line (800) 638-CPSC.

National Home Safety Council
Home Safety Department
P.O. Box 11933
Chicago, IL 60611
Toll-free hot line is (800) 621-7619 (in Illinois, (312) 527-4800). Publishes safety bulletins, brochures, fact sheets.

Poison Control Center (PCC)
Your local PCC can give you on-the-spot advice on handling emergencies; inquire about Mr. Yuk stickers and other PCC information; TTY (teletypewriter) lines for the deaf.

ADDITIONAL RESOURCES

F&H Child Safety Co.
Box 2228
Evansville, IN 47714
Brochure of various safety products such as corner guards.

True Love Care Products
Box 541
Dennis, MA 20638
Brochure of Safety Bear bathtub spout safety cover, soft rubber protectors and other products.

Growing Up

LANDMARKS IN DEVELOPMENT: THE FIRST EIGHTEEN MONTHS

Changes during the first 18 months will seem to happen overnight. The pace is, of course, highly individual. You may notice your baby's forging ahead of peers in one area while lagging behind in another. If development is markedly slow in any area—responding to voices, finding enough balance for walking, imitating sounds, mastering body control—reassure yourself by breezing through the next section, "Early Detection: Catching Problems in Time" (p. 415). Here is a rundown of what you are likely to see your baby doing as he or she progresses through the first year and a half. Suggestions geared to month-by-month development are described in "Stimulating Your Baby's Senses" (p. 419). For a more comprehensive picture of growth spurts and plateaus there are dozens of excellent books on the subject (see "Information Sources," p. 415).

Birth Through Three Months

The first six weeks are a sort of waking-up period, when your baby makes the transition from womb to the outside world, so there's a great deal of sleeping now and little interest in learning. Toward the end of the second month, however, innate curiosity takes hold and more waking hours are used to absorb the surroundings. By far the greatest treat for you at this juncture is seeing your baby crack that first smile. By the age of two or three months, your baby may be sleeping through the night.

Body Development	Approximate Age Range
Holds head off of bed for a few moments while lying on stomach	Birth and 1 month
Holds head upright lying on stomach	5 weeks and 3 months
Holds head steady when you hold baby in sitting position	6 weeks and 4 months
Rolls over from front to back, or from back to front	8 weeks and 5 months
Takes part of weight on own legs when held steady	12 weeks and 8 months

Eye/Hand Coordination	
Follows an object with eyes for a short distance	Birth and 1½ months
Follows with eyes from one side all the way to the other side of head	6 weeks and 4 months
Brings hands together in front of body	6 weeks and 3½ months
Grasps toy placed in fingers	10 weeks and 4½ months

Speech Development	
Pays attention to sounds	Birth and 1½ months
Makes vocal sounds other than crying	Birth and 1½ months
Laughs	6 weeks and 3½ months
Squeals	6 weeks and 4½ months
Turns eyes and head in direction of sounds	12 weeks and 6 months

Social Behavior	
Looks at your face	Birth and 1 month
Smiles when you smile or play with baby	Birth and 2 months
Smiles on his or her own	6 weeks and 5 months

Four to Six Months

As your baby gains better head, neck and shoulder control, he or she is able to view the world from a sitting position. Now, too, these strengthened muscles can be put to work and for the first time can coordinate more than one skill to perform a single task. Your son or daughter may shake a rattle, for example, listen to the sound and study it all at the same time. Because of this suddenly expanding world and the onslaught of new unknowns, the need for your reassuring presence grows proportionately and marks the first phase of attachment or dependence.

Body Development	Approximate Age Range
Sits without support when placed in a sitting position	5 months and 8 months
Develops strength and better coordination	4 months and 6 months
Gets self into sitting position in crib or on the floor	6 months and 11 months
Stands holding on	6 months and 12 months

Eye/Hand Coordination	
Passes a toy from one hand to the other	4 months and 7½ months
Grasps a small object from a flat surface	4 months and 8 months

Speech Development	
Turns toward your voice	4 months and 8 months
Says "Dada" or "Mama"	6 months and 10 months
Imitates the speech sounds you make	6 months and 11 months

Social Behavior	
Pulls back when you tug on a toy in baby's hand	4 months and 10 months
Tries to get a toy that's out of reach	5 months and 9 months
Feeds self crackers, cookies and so on	5 months and 8 months
Plays peek-a-boo	6 months and 10 months
Starts to discriminate, may prefer one toy to another	4 months and 6 months

Expresses negative feelings such as making
a face at a food not liked   4 months and 6 months

Seven to Nine Months

These are months of constant practice as your baby tests out motor
skills, first by crawling; then, much later, by experiments in standing.
Your son or daughter is just beginning to sense, too, that his or her
actions have some consequence, and loves to see the cause and effect
of grasping an object with the whole hand, letting it go, watching it
drop, then hearing the "clunk." All sounds are interesting now, and
imitations of them will come out as coos and squeals sprinkled with a
few vowels or even a "Dada" or "Mama" if you haven't heard it yet.
Along with a growing awareness of cause and effect inevitably comes
the sense of "baby power" and, with increased mobility, the second
phase of dependence.

Body Development	Approximate Age Range
Begins to crawl	7 months and 12 months
Stands for a moment alone	8 months and 13 months
Walks holding on to furniture	7½ months and 13 months

Eye/Hand Coordination	
Picks up a small object using thumb and finger	7 months and 10 months
Brings together two toys held in hands	7 months and 12 months

Speech Development	
Turns head and shoulders toward familiar sounds, even when baby cannot see what's happening	7 months and 10 months
Responds selectively to emotional tones of parents' voices	7 months and 10 months

Social Behavior	
Smiles at familar faces	7 months and 10 months
Plays pat-a-cake	7 months and 13 months
Forms attachment to stuffed animal or blanket	7½ months and 14 months

| Increasing level of curiosity | 9 months and 14 months |
| Cries and gets upset with strangers, termed "separation anxiety" | 7 months or earlier |

Ten Months to First Birthday

Babies are now starting to relate more to others, by playing simple games, understanding and obeying words and commands, and showing some sensitivity to the moods of those around them. Along with a finer interest in the world comes a greater mastery of self: finger and thumb feeding, dressing and undressing, and standing alone well— even some skill in identifying parts of the body.

Body Development	Approximate Age Range
Stands unassisted	10 months and 14 months
Continues to crawl and cruise	10 months and 14 months
Walks alone across a room	10½ months and 15 months

Eye/Hand Coordination	
Points to body parts such as toes	10 months and 14 months
Feeds self entire meal with hands	10 months and 14 months
Scribbles with a pencil or crayon	11 months and 24 months
Steers cup to mouth	10 months and 18 months
Drinks from cup without assistance	10 months and 16 months
Shows preference in use of one hand	11 months and 14 months

Speech Development	
Uses "Dada" or "Mama" to mean one specific person	10 months and 14 months
Imitates sounds—showing that baby can hear and match them with own sound production	11 months and 15 months
Shows understanding of some words by appropriate behavior (points or looks at familiar objects, people)	11 months and 15 months
Jabbers in response to human voices, cries when there is thunder or may frown when scolded	11 months and 16 months

Social Behavior	Approximate Age Range
Learns what "no" means	10 months to 13 months
Displays moods	10 months to 13 months
Plays alongside yet not "with" other children	12 months to 14 months
Stares with interest at strangers, especially other babies	10 months and 14 months

Twelve to Eighteen Months

Personality begins to shine through as your baby learns better to express emotions—jealousy, affection, sympathy—displays a sense of humor and throws an occasional temper tantrum. A tottering walk steadies, and locomotion speeds up once again, bringing a counter-reaction of dependence and special attachment to familiar people and places. There is usually a blossoming of new forms of expression such as scribbling, listening or turning about to music, and looking at picture books with you. More independent behavior, though, also leads to testing just how much he or she can get away with. In the next few months, expect to be working through your own disciplinary techniques (for more, see "Discipline: Different Approaches," p. 442).

Body Development	Approximate Age Range
Starts to walk more smoothly	15 months and 18 months
Tries to run	15 months and 18 months
Likes to climb into your lap	12 months and 18 months
Uses whole arm to play ball	18 months and 2 years

Eye/Hand Coordination	
Eats with spoon and fork	18 months and 2 years
Loves to throw objects	15 months and 18 months
Puts things into containers	15 months and 18 months
Scribbles with pencil or crayon	12 months and 2 years

Speech Development	
Begins to identify different parts of body	12 months and 16 months
Uses a few single words—not complete or pronounced perfectly, but clearly meaningful	12 months and 18 months

Recognizes and responds to name	12 months and 14 months
Drops consonants at end of words, such as "boo" for book and "ca" for cat	18 months onward

Social Behavior

Loves an audience	12 months and 18 months
Teasing and sense of humor evident	12 months onward
Personality development most dramatic	14 months to 2 years
Tests parents	15 months onward

Information Sources

ADDITIONAL READING

The First Twelve Months of Life, by Frank Caplan (New York: Grosset and Dunlap, 1979). Provides monthly growth charts divided into motor, language, mental and social skills, which are designed to give you a yardstick by which to measure your child's progress.

Growing Child. This monthly newsletter, written by child-development specialists at Purdue University, tracks child's development every month during the first 6 years. For subscription information, write to 22 N. Second St., PO Box 620, Lafayette, IN 47902.

Infants and Mothers: Difference in Development, by Dr. T. Berry Brazelton (New York: Delta, 1979). This book traces the growth and development of three children and illustrates that the range of normalcy is very wide.

EARLY DETECTION: CATCHING PROBLEMS IN TIME

During the first two years your child's health is closely monitored, beginning with newborn evaluations and blood tests and on through periodic examinations. Few physicians include developmental screening as part of their routine infant checkups; however, your input, based on day-to-day observations, can fill in the blanks. If developmental problems are picked up early, chances are that they will be easier to correct. A wait-and-see approach may be suggested by one pediatrician if your toddler seems to be lagging in fine-motor coordination, for example, while a child-development specialist might advise specific infant-stimulation exercises.

This section singles out some of the areas where your observations are particularly valuable and where prompt detection of problems is especially important: vision, hearing, speech, foot and leg formation.

Vision

That first smile directed at you should give you a special glow for more than one reason—it's proof your baby can see and is able to coordinate the appropriate muscles. Failure to smile in response to your smile by 8 weeks, and 3 months at the latest, may indicate an eye problem. If the vision centers in your baby's brain are continually receiving mixed signals—as would happen if one eye were much weaker than the other or if the eyes did not move in unison—these "image-catchers" would begin to deteriorate and ultimately shut down altogether. That is why it's so important to spot any trouble right away. Signs of possible eye problems include:

- failure to make eye contact with you
- holding things very close to see them
- squinting or closing one eye frequently
- constantly favoring one eye when looking at an object
- inability to pick up small objects with accuracy
- turning one or both eyes in or out for a noticeable period of time.

Recent research suggests that if one eye is weaker or fails to function, it is likely to occur around the fourth or fifth month after birth. If you suspect vision difficulty, first ask your baby's doctor to take a look, and see if it is suggested that you go to an eye doctor. Cross-eye (strabismus) can be surgically realigned with excellent results, and a very weak or "lazy" eye may be corrected with glasses or an eye patch worn over the good eye to force the weaker one to work harder and strengthen itself.

Hearing

Hearing loss deprives your child of a crucial dimension of stimulation and dramatically inhibits speech development. Babies particularly vulnerable are those who have a history of upper-respiratory infections, chronic ear infections or a family history of deafness. If your baby falls into one of these categories or if you notice any of the first signs of hearing loss listed below, you may want to consider taking your baby to see an ear specialist (audiologist/otologist).

- newborn not startled when someone claps sharply within 3–6 feet and not soothed by mother's voice

- at 3 months baby does not turn eyes toward sound
- between 3 and 6 months baby doesn't react to mother's voice, does not imitate own noises such as "oooh" and does not enjoy sound-making toys
- between 6 and 10 months baby doesn't respond to own name, and fails to understand "no" and "bye-bye"
- at 8 months baby does not turn toward a whispered voice or sound of a rattle or spoon stirring in a cup when the sound originates three feet away
- between 10 and 15 months toddler cannot point to or look at familiar objects or people when asked
- between 15 and 18 months child is unable to follow simple spoken directions and does not seem able to expand his or her understanding of words
- between 18 and 24 months child uses gestures—pantomime— instead of verbal clues to establish needs and watches parents' faces intently

Your baby can be fitted with a hearing aid in the first few months of life. Even with a hearing loss of 70 to 75 percent this will enable your child to hear speech. Ear surgery is another option, depending on the reason for the hearing loss.

Speech

The quality of your baby's hearing is intimately linked with the ability to reproduce sounds and, ultimately, learn a language. Other ingredients basic to speech are cognitive skill—knowing how to put sounds together in a meaningful way—and social interaction—your baby needs a "receiver" for the message he or she wants to try out. The steps involved in language-building are discussed further in "Talking: From First Sounds to Sentences" (p. 440), and suggestions about the role you can play in this development can be found in "Stimulating Your Baby's Senses" (p. 419).

Generally, delays in speech are the result of a lack of either the necessary small-motor skills, motivation or stimulation. Problems with articulation—true speech defects—cannot be detected with real accuracy until about 24 months. Here is a general idea of how your baby's speech should be progressing. Remember that omission of sounds and difficulty with certain combinations of letters and particular vowels are all normal.

2 months	vocalizes a little
3 months	chuckles and coos
4 months	laughs out loud
6 months	babbles (about half of all babies babble, making two or more sounds at this age)

8–9 months	says "Dada," then "Mama," the easiest consonant/vowel combinations, as first words
11–15 months	enjoys listening to some sounds and imitating
12 months	speaks two or three words
18 months	uses a few simple words though not complete or perfectly pronounced
24 months	strings several words together to make a sentence (vocabulary increases 30 percent)

If your baby has not uttered a single intelligible word by the first birthday, this may flag a hearing problem.

Foot and Leg Formation

Your baby's doctor will be on the lookout for any serious structural abnormalities such as hip dislocation, so don't worry. Bow legs, toeing in and flat feet are all normal in babies and young children. Your baby was, after all, curled up for nine months in the womb, so straightening out is bound to take a little time. And feet appear flat because muscle and fat have filled in for what will, in a couple of years, become the arch. True flat feet resulting from an unusual bone structure in the instep won't show up until then. If pigeon toes or bow legs are very pronounced or lopsided (with one leg or foot much worse than the other), call it to the attention of your baby's physician.

Usually your baby's sleeping position gradually corrects any odd foot formations formed in utero, but there are a few simple things you can do to help it along:

- each time you change diaper, simple gentle stretching of limbs and feet opposite the direction they "naturally" take
- turn feet outward while your baby sleeps on stomach

If these aren't effective, ask your doctor about tying the heels of your baby's stretch suit or sleeper together at night to ensure that the feet will stay pointed duck-fashion. Stubborn cases may require temporary splints or corrective shoes.

Information Sources

ORGANIZATIONS

Alexander Graham Bell Society
3417 Volta Place, NW
Washington, DC 20007
Write for more details on possible hearing loss.

American Optometric Association
243 N. Lindberg Blvd.
St. Louis, MO 63141
Send stamped, self-addressed envelope for information on children's vision care and the importance of eye exams.

National Society to Prevent Blindness
79 Madison Ave.
New York, NY 10016
Send stamped, self-addressed envelope for pamphlets including "Home Eye Test for Preschoolers" and "Signs of Possible Eye Trouble in Children."

STIMULATING YOUR BABY'S SENSES

Though much of your baby's physical and mental development is already programmed to unfold in a specific sequence and within a predetermined time frame, other skills also require cultivation and nurturing from you, especially in the areas of language acquisition and sensorimotor skills. Experts disagree, however, on the amount of stimulation that is necessary or wise, particularly in the area of intelligence, where too much pressure from parents to develop can make a baby anxious and nervous. Overdoing it is clearly a serious danger in large-motor skills, since encouraging sitting or standing before a baby's bones and muscles are strong enough can cause permanent bodily damage.

Here are some suggested approaches and activities to help you encourage your child to grow and learn. Remember, each child develops at a different rate, and if your baby was born prematurely, he or she may need more time to "catch up."

Curiosity and Motivation

While your baby is born with a natural desire to explore and discover, you can enhance this instinct by providing a wide variety of stimuli. It also helps to tailor your "teaching" to what is capturing the baby's interest at the time. Motivating your baby early to learn and to be curious about the world will encourage development now and pay dividends in future intellectual growth. Child development specialists share these suggestions:

- hang mobiles over crib; consider putting one on the right and another on the left to encourage your newborn to use both sides of the body and to discourage forming a side preference

- place a good, unbreakable mirror toy in the crib (at about 3 months)
- allow baby to roam through child-proofed home rather than confining him or her to one room or a playpen (at about 6 to 8 months)
- let child turn on lights, the radio or television, flush toilet (expect these activities around 8 to 14 months)
- talk to your baby about what you are doing or what he or she is doing; about the shapes and textures of objects (starting at about 7 months—particularly effective between 14 and 24 months, when your child begins showing signs of imagination and originality)
- take baby on excursions to interesting places, such as the zoo or a museum; even the grocery store provides lots of stimulus
- fill bathtub or wading pool with an inch or two of water and toss in toys that are ideal for filling and spilling (from about 10 months onward).

If you choose activities that you enjoy, your baby will sense your interest. The theory is that the more your child notices your involvement, the greater his or her own enthusiasm to learn.

Sensorimotor Development

Good sensorimotor performance helps your baby explore and solve problems, since these skills bridge the gap between what your baby senses—sees, smells, hears, tastes—and the physical reaction—reaching, grabbing, turning, smiling. Your child's brain and entire central nervous system receive and interpret the signals arriving from sense organs and organize and produce the appropriate responses.

- Offer objects that provide a variety of stimuli for the senses and involve some small-motor coordination: sponges to squeeze, pots and pans to bang, even food to touch and play with at mealtime (at about 6 or 7 months)
- Help your baby practice grasp-release movement—opening and shutting fist, throwing—by fastening simple toys to both sides of the high chair with a short cord or elastic so you needn't stoop to pick them up each time—throwing practice will go on tirelessly as your baby learns this important movement (at about 7 months).
- Set out a shoe box filled with toys; dump them out, then drop them, one by one, back into the box, asking your baby to help (at about 8 months).

Intelligence

Intellectual growth cannot be rushed, as it must wait for memory banks and sensorimotor skills to mature. Yet, while intense training sessions to force your baby's budding intellect are likely to do more harm than good, you can safely lay the groundwork for future problem-solving, logical thinking and imagination by stimulating your baby's natural need to know and by offering opportunities to apply emerging concepts. Until your baby's memory banks begin to develop (between about 8 and 14 months), his or her view of reality focuses on the concrete rather than the abstract or unseen. The stepping-stone to taking in more sophisticated abstract concepts, such as means-end relationship, cause and effect, and language, is the grasp of object permanence; that is, understanding that even when an object or person is not seen, it continues to exist. Though your baby won't be able to demonstrate this fully until about 9 months of age, you can start the wheels moving months sooner by exposing your child to objects that disappear, then reappear without long time lags in between.

- Play peek-a-boo or cover your head or the baby's head with a light scarf or lift a sheet up between the two of you, then remove or lower it.
- Let your baby hear your voice before you come into view when nap time is over.
- Provide open-ended containers with small objects to "hide" inside.

Once object permanence is established, you can sharpen an 11-month-old's intellect a bit by presenting the challenge of a cause-and-effect problem. For example, attach a string to a toy and show your baby how the string can be used to bring the object closer; then let him or her try to do it alone.

Language

More than any other area of development, your baby's language acquisition interfaces with the growth of other skills: hearing and imitating sounds (sensorimotor), seeing words as labels for objects, people and ideas (cognitive) and recognizing them as a form of communication (social). The quality and pace of learning to talk depend largely on outside stimulation, since most babies speak only if actively encouraged to or in the face of a real need. Use the following checklist and games as the framework for helping, and refer to "Talking: From First Sounds to Sentences" (p. 440) for an idea of when your baby can understand and participate in these language activities.

- Talk in ordinary, full sentences, using simple vocabulary.
- Make easy sounds such as "oooh" and encourage your baby to repeat them, or imitate what he or she says each time (and offer praise when your child repeats it, as this has been shown to stimulate even more "talking" or dialogue).
- Make connections between what your child is doing and another idea or object.
- Listen intently to your child's messages, guess at meanings and interpret.
- Use lots of gestures—in other words, be a ham—so your baby learns to associate the action with the words you're using to describe them (for instance, reach out as you command, "Give it to me," or ask, "Where's baby?" look around and then say, "There's baby!").
- Give directions to see if your baby understands (this can begin at about 11 months).

By all means nurture curiosity, since interest is a prime motivator in developing language skills. For more on speech development, see "Landmarks in Development: The First Eighteen Months" (p. 409) and "Early Detection: Catching Problems in time" (p. 415).

Information Sources

ADDITIONAL READING

The Baby Exercise Book for the First 15 Months, by Ganine Levy (New York: Pantheon, 1980).

Baby Learning Through Play: A Parents' Guide for the First Two Years, by Ira Gordon (New York: St. Martin's, 1978).

Infant Massage, by Vimala Schneider (New York: Bantam, 1982).

Learning Games for the First Three Years, by Joseph Sparling and Isabelle Lewis (New York: Berkley, 1980).

Learning While Growing: Cognitive Development, by the National Institute of Mental Health. Available for $2.25 from the Government Printing Office, stock number 017-024-01719-7. G.P.O., Superintendent of Documents, Washington, D.C. 20402.

CRYING AND SLEEPING

Coping with Crying

It takes a few months to learn the language of your baby's crying. Soon you'll discover your infant's skill at expressing different needs and feelings just by varying the pitch, duration and intensity of each cry. Unlike other languages, however, there will always be some untranslatable howls and whimpers. Once you have eliminated hunger, fatigue and pain from the list of possible causes, figuring out what's wrong becomes a matter of trial and error. Generally, a very young infant is comforted by a womblike environment such as warmth, rocking motions, physical contact and rhythmic sounds; while an older baby, more fascinated with his or her new world, is cheered up by simple distractions such as toys, picture books or even the switching on and off of a lamp. Researchers are increasingly interested in the role tension and stress play in babies' crying.

Do what you can to stop tears, trust your instincts and experiment, but realize, too, that it's not humanly possible to interpret each cry. To help you with some guesswork, a few possible causes of crying are outlined next, according to age. Some suggestions and remedies follow, along with a few words about spoiling.

Like the first 50 miles on a new car, your newborn has to "break in" the digestive tract and central nervous system. In addition to this physical development, the baby must adjust emotionally to an environment that lacks all the familiar sounds and feelings of the womb. Crying is the only way an infant has to express such stress. Some observers suggest that the "tension theory" solves the mystery behind much of the unexplained crying during the first 12 weeks, particularly since it occurs mainly in the evening, after a stress-filled day.

You'll soon find the best ways to comfort your own baby, but to get you started, here's a shopping list of some you might try:

- Pick up and hold your baby. If he or she stops bawling then hunger probably is not the problem; perhaps it is loneliness or the need to feel close to your body.
- Rock your baby or use any rhythmic motion; the advantage of a rocking chair is that it can calm both of you (one study, though, indicated that rocking only encouraged babies to cry more, whereas rocking when calm encouraged more quiet periods).
- Offer a pacifier. This satisfies an infant's tremendous urge to suck and is relaxing, too, for an overtired baby (for further discussion, see "Pacifiers," p. 354).

- Spin some records that have a soft, steady beat; special cassette tapes full of womb sounds may work; humming sounds also seem to please babies; some mothers swear by the sound of their vacuum cleaners.
- Lay the baby on his or her stomach in the bassinet or crib if you suspect the reason is sheer fatigue, and gently rub or pat the back for a minute or so. Some parents and pediatricians suggest that if this fails, the baby simply isn't ready to rest, while others advise leaving the room so the baby can cry itself to sleep (suggested waiting-it-out times vary from 5 to 30 minutes).
- Strap the baby in the stroller and take a walk.
- Put the baby in a car seat and go for a drive, preferably taking a route that is not stop-and-go.
- Swaddle your newborn: warm and hold snugly in a blanket (until the nervous system has fully matured, a newborn lacks a sense of where the body parts are, and wrapping helps identify or define what's where and, as a result, gives more security).

If screaming persists and you're still stymied, check your baby from head to toe. Some possible reasons for provoking tears could be:

- a wet or soiled diaper, particularly if there's a rash
- baby is too warm or is thirsty
- air bubble, which burping will ease
- tight clothing, including disposable diapers.

The other possibility is colic. Usually during a colic attack, a baby's stomach bloats and hardens. Often the knees are drawn up, gas may be passed and crying will be loud and long. This is discussed more fully in "Colic" (p. 394).

As your baby grows, the repertoire of communication skills broadens. Though crying fits will occasionally be sparked by a need to blow off steam or frustration at limited communication skills, they are likely to be expressions of loneliness, boredom, fear of strange people and a sense of loss because of separation from you. The misery of teething enters the picture now, too, from about 5 or 6 months onward. Simply understanding what sets off the crying and responding instinctively and appropriately is all that's needed. Some of the remedies listed for babies under 3 months still apply, along with several other techniques:

- take baby's mind off the problem—sometimes babies continue howling simply because they don't think to stop; by distracting child with a toy or making a funny face, you focus attention away from it and break the crying chain
- arrange for your baby to keep you company—if space allows,

put child in the kitchen while you're working or at least in view of you, near the door, or try a windup swing or other motion-maker (see "Pounding Toys, Puzzles, Picture Books," p. 357)

- relieve teething discomfort (see "Pearly Whites: Teething and Dental Care," p. 435).

Spoiling

If you rush to the rescue at every whimper, will your baby gradually begin to demand even more—eventually unwarranted—attention? For the first three months, most early-childhood-development specialists not only agree that the chance of this is very small, but point out that answering your infant's distress provides a sense of security that actually enables him or her to become less dependent in the months to come. Small babies who receive consistent positive feedback seem to cry less and slip more easily into regular sleeping and eating patterns.

Views on spoiling infants over 3 months old, however, vary considerably. Since babies become more aware of cause-and-effect relationships as they grow, and of their power to command your attention simply by crying, some experts believe this naturally leads to manipulative behavior. Others maintain that a cry for your attention should always be answered. In the end, you have to do what you feel comfortable with and what you sense is best for your baby and your family.

Sickness and Crying

Parents have a sixth sense about when their children are sick. You'll notice subtle changes in behavior and general appearance, and crying usually increases in frequency and length when a baby isn't well. This "pain" cry could come from an ear infection (particularly if it's during the night), a stomachache or a respiratory infection. Phone the doctor if the baby also coughs a great deal, develops diarrhea or vomits, or runs a temperature that doesn't drop (see "When to Call the Doctor: Day or Night?" p. 368 and "The Top Three Illnesses: Fever, Diarrhea, Ear Infections," p. 385).

Keep in mind that, thanks to the fast pace of your child's development, almost any effective crying cure has a limited "shelf life." What worked like magic last night may not work this afternoon. On the positive side, developmental psychologists tell us that infants' cries are often responses to change, and change means learning and growth.

Solid Night's Sleep

Sleep patterns during the first year of life are for the most part shaped by your baby's gradual adjustment to his or her new world. The first few weeks are spent in deep, nourishing sleep to ease the transition from fetus to newborn and to support all the changes in body function, waking only to take in food for fuel. As the baby pulls out of the newborn stage and takes a greater interest in the world, waking hours will lengthen. Toward the end of 12 months, in fact, growing attraction to, and curiosity about, the new world and attachment to you may keep your baby awake even when he or she is dead-tired.

Of all your concerns about sleeping—your baby's and yours—putting your child to bed will be second only to middle-of-the-night wakings. Approaches to both these problems vary greatly even among baby-care specialists, so you will have to rely largely on your own instincts, personal style and child-rearing philosophy in choosing which is best. First, though, to get an idea of how you can expect sleeping patterns to evolve the first year, keep in mind that sleep requirements for babies are as individual as for adults. Your baby's nap could, for instance, last anywhere from 20 minutes to four hours once or twice daily.

Age	Typical Sleeping Patterns
Birth–3 months	3–4 weeks: wakes to eat, falls back to sleep after being fed (at intervals of 3–4 hours)
	6 weeks: wakes up before feeling hungry; longest single waking period lasts 2 hours, usually in late afternoon
3–6 months	12 weeks: sleeps 6 hours at a stretch, with two 2-hour naps morning and afternoon
	sleeps better and more predictably
	outgrows middle-of-the-night feeding but may continue to wake up
	longest single sleeping period about 6 hours, waking for 3½ hours at a stretch
6–12 months	likely to sleep 12 hours at night, with 2 daytime naps
	as awareness of people and surroundings grows, may develop "separation anxiety" and wake in night screaming (night terrors)
	able to force self to stay awake and reluctant to leave "all the fun" (9 months)
	excited over new discoveries, now that he or she

Age	Typical Sleeping Patterns
	is so mobile, and thus, more reluctant to go to bed or even nap
12–36 months	naps cut in half; best time to put baby down is after early lunch, to ensure an uninterrupted 10-to-12 hour night.

Problem #1: Waking in the Middle of the Night

Neither one of you is going to sleep through the night if a night feeding is still expected or if you and the baby both formed the habit of waking up at a time when your baby was colicky or sick. Some suggestions for eliminating middle-of-the-night feedings include:

- trying to wait four hours or more between feedings during the day, so baby's stomach adjusts to being less full for that extended period of time
- gradually reducing amount of night feeding, say from 6 ounces one week to 4 ounces the next, then to 2 ounces, followed by none
- feeding just before you go to bed even if you must wake baby to do so, but keep the amount fairly low, since urination tends to wake up babies
- introducing solids such as cereal prior to four months is discouraged for many reasons (see "Nutrition: Introducing Solids and Giving up the Bottle," p. 429).

Some experts advise that you break the waking habit in two to three days by gritting your teeth and letting your baby cry it out, probably for 20 to 30 minutes the first night and less time the second and third nights. Others argue that these waking patterns should be altered gradually and that allowing your child to howl that long could damage both your psyches. They advocate five-minute crying intervals, with half-minute checks in between when you look in on your baby, pat and softly reassure that everything is all right. Most experts do agree, however, that a baby should never be removed from the crib under these circumstances and definitely not moved into the parents' room to relieve nighttime loneliness. Your baby needs to feel secure but at the same time should be encouraged to develop his or her own resources for comfort—cuddling a toy, sucking a fist or blanket and so on. The five-minute time limit should be ignored, though, if crying is caused by night terrors.

Problem #2: Getting Baby to Go to Bed Without a Fuss

It's natural that your toddler would rather stay up and be with you than leave the family to go to bed, but you can make it easier by easing your child gradually into bedtime and sleep. Spend the last hour or so together in happy but quiet activity, then go through a read-for-sleep routine every night; for instance, look at a picture book, kiss stuffed animals, play a music box, say good night. Both the security of those peaceful pre-bed moments and the every-night ritual will help condition your child to accepting the idea of going to bed.

Family Bed: Good or Bad Habit?

One mother cannot imagine a restful night without her baby tucked in bed close beside her, while another parent feels the kicking, snoring and flailing arms rob her of a hard-earned, solid eight hours of sleep. Is an open-bed policy good or bad for you and your baby? There is no proof either way, and advocates of the family bed and advocates of separate rooms claim their approaches promote happier, healthier and better-adjusted children.

Those in favor of family-bedding believe unlimited access to parents during a child's dependent years instills the security necessary for true independence later on. Those opposed to the idea feel that the sooner a baby learns to depend on its own emotional resources and recognize the parents' rights to privacy, the better. Your own position depends on your child-rearing philosophy, your child's temperament and the life-style you and your mate desire. Many couples, for instance, value those night hours alone not simply for the freedom to have sex but for getting back in touch with each other after a day of being shared with their baby. Lack of privacy at night, however, is unimportant to others and simply means an extension of daytime communication and closeness with their child. The following are some of the arguments for and against making your bed the "family bed."

AGAINST	IN FAVOR
Forms a bad habit that will be difficult to break	Child will separate self naturally as he or she feels emotionally more secure
Restricts your sexual relationship with mate	Children in other cultures bundle with parents, with no reported emotional handicaps formed
Encourages excessive dependence	Cultivates independence later by

AGAINST	IN FAVOR
	supplying as much security as possible in early years
Deprives parents of needed sleep by restless babies and toddlers whose size cramps everybody in anything but a queen- or king-size bed	Gives parents more rest because they know children are safe and sleeping soundly; eliminates trip to another room because of night terrors or feedings

No one knows what long-term developmental effects, if any, are related to making your bed the property of the entire family, but welcoming your youngster occasionally into bed with you after a nightmare or just because he or she is feeling particularly lonely that night seems unlikely to cause permanent emotional scars or develop into a habit as some pediatricians claim. At one end of the spectrum are those who believe that 6 months is the cutoff age for bed-sharing, and even for a few hours' of middle-of-the-night consolation. At the other extreme, strong advocates of the family bed would like not only to see small children sleep in their parents' bed but suggest installing another mattress in the master bedroom as babies grow and the family expands.

Information Sources

ADDITIONAL READING

Baby and Child Care, by Penelope Leach (New York: Knopf, 1981). In-depth explanations about crying and sleeping patterns in babies.

Crying Baby, Sleepless Nights, by Sandra Jones (New York: Warner, 1983). Helpful advice for parents with especially miserable babies.

The Family Bed: An Age-Old Concept in Child-Rearing, by Tine Thevenin (Self-published, 1976). This "classic" is available by writing the author at PO Box 16004, Minneapolis, MN 55416.

NUTRITION: INTRODUCING SOLIDS AND GIVING UP THE BOTTLE

Once solid foods are introduced, the weaning process begins. The question of when to start offering baby cereal and other nonliquid delicacies has come full circle. Before the availability of commercially prepared baby foods, in the 1930s, babies went right from breast milk to table food, often around 12 months of age. Then, in the 1940s and 1950s, when store-bought baby food became popular and parents were eager to see their babies gain weight rapidly, spoonfuls of cereal were given as early as one month. Now the pendulum rests between these two extremes, coinciding with the resurgence in breast-feeding and the widespread belief that both mother's milk and commercial formula meet all known nutritional requirements for the first half year. The iron stored in the baby's liver during life in utero dwindles, usually between 5 and 6 months, which is one reason why an iron supplement and/or iron-fortified cereal is recommended by the second half of the first year.

The American Academy of Pediatrics advises starting solids between 4 and 6 months, with the caveat that it depends on an individual infant's stage of development, rate of growth and level of activity. Prior to 4 months, a baby's intestinal tract and kidneys may not be ready to handle certain solids. Furthermore, the extrusion reflex, meaning the tongue-thrusting action used for sucking, which would interfere with swallowing nonliquid foods, does not disappear until about 4 or 5 months. Another reason to delay starting solids is to wait until the neck muscles are strong enough to allow the head to turn, so babies can signal if they've had enough to eat. Many pediatricians worry about overfeeding, citing numerous studies that show that obesity is more of a problem when it has occurred early in life.

The desire for eight hours of uninterrupted sleep, or at least for fewer nighttime feedings, is one motive for feeding solids early. There is no proof that semisolids make a difference; in fact, many strained baby foods have about the same caloric density as milk. Even many of those pediatricians who still think cereal before bedtime may help parents get more rest concur with the stance of the American Academy of Pediatrics that "no nutritional advantage results from the introduction of supplemental foods prior to 4 to 6 months of age. This conclusion is essentially the same as in the Committee [of Nutrition] statement of 1958, but it deserves reemphasis because of the continuing widespread and possibly harmful effects of introducing supplemental foods at 1 or 2 months of age, or earlier."

The sequence of foods is not critical, but iron-fortified single-grain infant cereal is usually the first choice and goes down well, although it might take several days before a full teaspoon stays in the mouth. Not only is your baby learning how to swallow semisolid foods, but don't underestimate how strange the taste and texture of both the cereal and spoon may seem. As one nutritionist describes it, "The amount of food your baby consumes at first is unimportant; it's the quality of experience." Offer next mild-tasting pureed vegetables such as carrots and squash, although frequently applesauce, mashed bananas and other fruits are suggested instead because many babies are less inclined

to reject them than vegetables. Only one new food should be introduced at a time, starting with a couple of tablespoons of it each day.
Wait about five days before another food is added, to allow for any
allergy or sensitivity to show up, so that that particular food can be
temporarily eliminated. The signs of an allergy are nasal congestion,
rash, vomiting, diarrhea or a change in personality such as increased
irritability. Some of the foods that are known to be least allergenic
and most easily digestible include rice cereal, bananas, carrots, lamb,
barley cereal, applesauce, yellow squash, veal, oatmeal, pears, sweet
potatoes and chicken.

TYPICAL FOOD PROGRESSION

Age	Daily Fare
Birth to 4 or 6 months	Breast milk or iron-fortified formula
4 to 6 months	Iron-fortified dry infant cereal mixed with milk or water, and perhaps mashed fruit, such as banana
7 to 8 months	Carrots, squash and other vegetables and/or pears and other fruits
9 to 10 months	Yogurt, cottage cheese, lean meat, fish or poultry pureed and strained
11 to 12 months	Finger foods including rice, mashed vegetables, spaghetti, slices of soft fruit, tiny pieces of meat, bread
12 months and older	adult foods (unsalted); perhaps weaned from bottle or breast, and cow's milk is introduced

Don't mistake thirst for hunger, particularly in hot weather. Babies
need lots of water because of their large body surface area as
compared to their body weight.

If you buy commercially prepared baby food, read the labels carefully.
Most prepared baby food is salt-free and contains no monosodium
glutamate (MSG). Sweeteners are used in many extratart fruits as well
as in custards, puddings and other desserts, which is reason most
nutritionists are not keen on such foods. The Society of Nutrition
Education advises parents to purchase plain, rather than mixed,
vegetables, meats and cereals "for the best value nutritionally and
economically."

Homemade baby foods, of course, have the advantage of being much cheaper than commercially prepared products, but there are pediatricians who worry about excessive calories and salt. Here are some other suggestions to keep in mind when preparing baby foods:

- wash your hands and utensils
- peel fruits and vegetables to reduce amount of dirt, microorganisms or pesticide residues and tough fiber for baby to digest
- steam carrots and other fruits and vegetables until barely tender, so as to lose as few nutrients as possible
- don't add salt, sugar or fats, and go easy with other seasoning
- cooked foods should not be left to stand at room temperature but should be eaten or refrigerated promptly after cooking
- store covered in refrigerator for no longer than two days
- freeze pureed food in ice-cube trays; once frozen, pack cubes in labeled, dated, airtight freezer bags. Use within one month.

Storage suggestions for commercial baby foods should also be heeded. Of course, check the expiration date on the lid before buying it.

- wash food jar and lid thoroughly before opening
- be sure you hear the pop when you open jar; in the center of each cap is a safety button, which should be concave (sunken), guaranteeing that the vacuum seal is intact so look and listen
- avoid feeding directly from the jar if the remainder of the food is to be used for another meal, because the digestive enzymes from the baby's saliva can contaminate the leftover food
- keep an opened jar of fruits covered in the refrigerator for no more than three days, and save meats and vegetables for no more than two days
- smell food and discard if it has any odd odor whatsoever; also, don't use if the food is no longer liquified and just doesn't look right
- don't refrigerate ordinary canned foods because of the lead content or the soldered seams; instead remove the contents from the can and store in another container

POTPOURRI OF PRECAUTIONS

Honey, nuts, even popcorn all have something in common ... they are dangerous. Other foods, such as wheat, eggs and strawberries, are troublemakers, possibly causing allergic reactions. Here is a checklist of foods to think first about, and it may be a good idea to leave this list with any babysitter who might give your child snacks or meals.

No popcorn, nuts, seeds, carrots, mini-hotdogs until your baby is able to chew them; these are easily inhaled and can get lodged in the throat.

No honey until your baby is 1 year old; it may contain bacteria that in an infant's intestines become lethal and produce botulism; these spores are *not* destroyed by cooking.

Salt has been cited as a possible factor contributing to high blood pressure; researchers speculate that high salt intake might predispose children to hypertension later in life. The sodium found naturally in foods is fine— necessary, in fact— but don't add salt to either commercial or homemade baby food.

Spinach, beets, turnips or collard greens should not be given to young infants, cautions the American Academy of Pediatrics. These vegetables are high in nitrates, which, if converted to nitrites by bacteria while the food is being stored, can be absorbed into the bloodstream and reduce the amount of oxygen circulating in the blood. In serious cases, this may lead to methemoglobinemia, a condition marked by blue skin and breathing difficulty.

No cow's milk until baby is one year old. Whole, 2 percent or skim milk contains much more protein than mother's milk or infant formula and may overload baby's kidneys. The high level of salt is another concern. Even an overweight baby should not be given skim or 2 percent until 12 months, because it lacks essential fatty acids vital for growth.

Eating Habits

During the first 12 months an infant faces tremendous challenges, only one of which is learning about new foods and new ways to eat. Perhaps in no other area of the development of young children is progress more individual. Nowadays patience is encouraged and parents are warned about the consequences of pressuring their child to eat. The emphasis on providing a casual, positive setting even with finicky eaters, however, does not rule out insisting on reasonable mealtime behavior. Certainly a 7-month-old's playing with pureed peas in the hair is all part of mastering new feeding techniques, but standing up in a high chair and throwing food across the room is best not ignored. Some specific suggestions for instilling good habits and avoiding bad ones include the following:

- Be patient with the baby's first efforts, and don't offer heaping portions, which might be intimidating.
- Introduce new textures and flavors gradually, yet enlarge the baby's experience with a variety of foods prepared in different ways.
- Allow your baby to fumble with forks and spoons designed for tiny hands, which, after all, is the only way to learn how to use them.
- Avoid laughing at your child's clumsiness, since this reaction may cause the baby to spill or splatter food deliberately to get your attention; don't become disturbed by unintentional mistakes; one way to prevent anger is to put newspapers or a plastic drop cloth on the floor to catch whatever lands or splashes.
- Expect a baby's appetite to vary from day to day—it's normal for squash to be a favorite one week yet refused the next.
- Anticipate new stages, particularly the 18-month refusal-to-eat phase, and keep reminding yourself that your child will not starve.
- Consider a Sassy Seat or other gadget that rests right on the table, so the baby can eat with the rest of the family.

Rarely do children—or adults, for that matter—like the "right" foods. Remember that diets should be balanced over a week or two—not every meal or every day—although a baby needs certain foods regularly, such as milk. You have no reason to worry even with a picky eater, so long as your baby has energy to spare and continues to put on weight.

Giving Up the Bottle

Graduating to the cup represents another milestone in your baby's development. Like learning how to use a spoon, it requires patience and parental involvement. The independence a baby feels when drinking from a bottle, along with the no-spills advantage, are reasons parents are reluctant to offer a cup. Some experts think it's best to get infants started on a cup sometime around 8 months, before they get too attached to bottles, and many parents introduce the cup in addition to breast- or bottle-feedings at about 5 months, knowing it will take several more months before their child is taking in the necessary 16 ounces of milk a day by cup. Most dentists advise that babies stop sucking on bottles by their first birthday, to ensure proper development of teeth and jaws. There are other child-care professionals, however, who say there's no harm in waiting till your child is two before giving up the bottle. If your baby is too dependent on the bottle, especially if it rarely leaves the hand all day, filling up on liquids is bound to interfere with his or her interest in trying solid foods and probably keeps a child from learning to sit at the table and eat.

Once you decide when you want to get your child off the bottle and onto the cup, here are a few different approaches you might consider trying:

- Wean from the bottle gradually, spreading it over about two weeks, dropping one bottle at a time.
- Go cold turkey, and don't offer the bottle at all.
- Try an abrupt switch by filling bottle with water so the baby loses interest in the taste (if you meet with too much resistance, dilute the juice or milk gradually).

Information Sources

ADDITIONAL READING

No-Nonsense Nutrition for Your Baby's First Year, by JoAnn Hesline, Annette Natow and Barbara Raven (Boston: CBI Publishing, 1978).

ORGANIZATIONS

For questions about infant nutrition, call the Beech-Nut Nutrition Hotline. Its toll-free hot-line service operates Monday through Friday from 9:00 A.M. to 4:00 P.M. E.S.T.: (800) 523-6633 (in PA, call [800] 492-2384).

National Child Nutrition Project
46 Bayard St.
New Brunswick, NJ 08901
Clearinghouse on nutrition.

PEARLY WHITES: TEETHING AND DENTAL CARE

Similar to nearly every other aspect of child development, there is no strict timetable for the appearance of baby teeth. The "typical" baby will cut the first tooth at about 6 months, but many get their first as early as 3 months or as late as 1 year. While the timing varies considerably from baby to baby, the sequence of appearance of each pearly white generally does not. There are exceptions, but usually they erupt in this order:

Central incisor, 7½ months ————————————————————————

Lateral incisor, 9 months ——————————————————————

Cuspid (pointed, also called eye or canine), 16 months————

First (primary) molar, 14 months ———————————————

Second molar, 24 months ——————————————————

First permanent molar, 6 years ——————————————

UPPER

First permanent molar, 6 years ————————————————

Second molar, 20 months ————————————————

First (primary) molar, 12 months ————————————

LOWER

Cuspid (pointed, also called eye or canine), 16 months ——

Lateral incisor, 7 months——————————————————

Central incisor, 6 months——————————————————

If eruption of your baby's first teeth deviates widely from this progression, it may mean he or she is missing a tooth, and dental X rays may be advisable later on.

Cutting teeth is a more or less continuous process until about 2⅓ to 3 years, when all 20 baby teeth are in place. This can be uncomfortable and may be responsible for many of your baby's complaints. Some signs of teething are straightforward, while others may mimic real illness, such as an ear infection or colic, and call for some close evaluation on your part. It's possible, too, that teeth breaking through gum tissues allow introduction of bacteria into your child's bloodstream and thus the child is actually sick at the same time. Whatever the reason, most pediatricians advise calling the office any time there are symptoms of illness even if you suspect it is "only teething." The following is a checklist of the classic signs of this rite of passage:

- fussiness and fretfulness
- gnawing on everything, including the coffee table
- red, swollen and tender gums (cheeks may even be warm)
- loss of appetite and refusal to nurse or suck bottle for more than a few minutes even when hungry, often followed by angry crying
- fever that comes and goes
- stuffy nose, wheezing and watery eyes
- eczema (often skin rash on cheeks)
- waking at night.

A surplus of saliva produced while teething can also cause your baby to drool, spit up or vomit and have a mild case of diarrhea.

Remedies for Teething

Discomfort generally lasts only a few days with any one tooth and can be relieved by offering your baby something hard and cold to chew on, though at times gums may be too sore even for gnawing. Should teething seriously interfere with sleeping and eating, it's time to call the doctor and probably try a pain reliever such as Infants' Tylenol. But for day-to-day relief, try some of these remedies:

- simple massage or pressure on baby's gums with your finger
- liquid-filled teething rings cooled in the refrigerator (if frozen, may damage gum tissue; be sure rings are marked "non-toxic"), pacifiers or other rubber-edged objects (the smaller, the better, since they can reach back teeth), or an ordinary large wooden kitchen spoon may do the trick
- refrigerated wet washcloth to gnaw on, homemade water popsicles or ice cubes (but stay alert to make sure they don't get caught in the throat)
- numbing ointment such as Nuk or Orajel, available at drug and grocery stores
- teething biscuits, but check with doctor first, as baby may be allergic to wheat or grains found in these biscuits or may be too young to swallow the chunks bitten off
- waterproof cheeks and chin with cream such as Vaseline, to protect against excess saliva
- liquid baby medication such as Infants' Tylenol is best given before bedtime or at mealtime and has an immediate, almost suspiciously quieting effect, so don't give it too often.

Dental Care

Your child won't be seeing a dentist or pedodontist (specialist in pediatric dentistry) until about age 2½ or 3, but you should begin preventive dental care early on—even before that first tooth appears— by wiping gums after each feeding and later by keeping the new teeth clean by swabbing with moistened gauze or a soft, child-size toothbrush. Babies are very oral, or mouth conscious, so they usually enjoy this attention. Be careful, though, not to hurt the gums by using too much pressure. Decay of baby teeth can start as soon as a tooth appears, so be particularly careful not to let your child suck on a bottle containing anything but water when in bed or at nap time. The natural sugars in milk and juices left around the teeth mix with bacteria in the mouth to form enamel-eating acid. Some experts even go so far as to recommend that milk and juice be offered only at mealtimes, not around the clock, followed by mouth-cleaning, as described earlier. Even mother's milk has been known to cause cavities if proper feeding habits and oral cleanliness are not maintained. It is healthier for the teeth to have regularly scheduled feedings than "on-demand" feedings, which tend to keep food in the baby's mouth more hours per day. Dr. Michael Roberts at the government's National Institute of Dental Research cautions against giving apple juice except in very diluted form when a baby is sick and needs extra fluids, since its high sugar content and relatively low nutritional value contribute to cavities, especially in the upper front teeth.

If you move to a community with a different water supply or to a home that draws from well water, call a dentist in the area for information on the recommended amount of fluoride supplementation, and double-check this with your baby's new doctor. (See "Infant Vitamins and Fluoride Drops: Necessary or Not?" p. 371).

Information Sources

ADDITIONAL READING

Bureau of Health Education and Audiovisual Services
American Dental Association
211 E. Chicago Ave.
Chicago, IL 60611
Pamphlet titled "Your Child's Teeth," which describes development, diet, proper care and orthodontics, is available for $0.25.

CRAWLING, CRUISING AND WALKING

As a newborn, your baby's movements are simple reflexes—involuntary muscle movements—that ensure enough nourishment (rooting or sucking reflex) and help protect from harm (startle, or "Moro," reflex). While reflexes involve simple, short-distance messages from nerves to muscle fibers, more sophisticated voluntary movement involves the brain circuitry, so that your baby can slowly begin to command its own actions. Just how well nerves transmit messages and muscles respond marks the level of neuromuscular growth. Only as bones and muscles strengthen, however, can your baby put these skills to use in sitting, creeping, crawling, standing and walking.

Here's an idea of how and when your baby is likely to progress to each major physical milestone:

AGE	MOBILITY
1 month	extends legs when stood on hard surface; automatic striding movements; turns head to side; limbs are bent and fists clenched; by end of first month baby should hold head up for about 3 seconds
2 months	holds head up for 10 seconds; kicks
4 months	supports self securely even with arms stretched far out in front
5 months	baby "swims"; rocking on belly while lifting head, chest, arms; when held in standing position, braces self against surface and stretches legs; stands when supported on tip-toes; arms bent and hands semi-flexed
6–7 months	should be able to sit unsupported for a few moments (if unable by 9 months, seek medical advice)
7 months	reaches for toy with one hand while supporting self with other; turns from back to stomach
6–12 months	half of all babies start to creep or crawl
9 months	stands on soles of feet; when held up by hands, can stand for at least a minute and can support weight
10 months	creeping: moving backward and forward propelled by arms only; begins to crawl and rock on hands and feet
12 months	should be able to pull self erect with a pair of helping hands, and can "cruise" along sofa or coffee table; if held by hand, will take steps forward, but little more than half of all babies actually walk before first birthday
18 months	should be able to walk independently

A word of caution about encouraging your baby to walk before his or her body is ready: Permanent damage can be done to bone and muscle structures, if your baby takes too much weight and pressure on them before they're strong enough. Jumpers and walkers are discussed separately in "Pounding Toys, Puzzles, Picture Books" (p. 357).

TALKING: FROM FIRST
SOUNDS TO SENTENCES

Your baby begins communicating moments after birth with newborn murmurs and squeals, but that communication won't become language until the child is able to capture and articulate a wealth of sounds (develop sensorimotor skills) and understand, store and recall their meanings (cognitive skills). For speech to take place, these skills must also meet with a certain level of curiosity and desire for self-expression. This is where your encouragement and interaction can play such a significant role. The broad steps your baby takes toward learning language in these first two years will start with hearing, then imitating, sounds, repeating them, seeing connections between them and actions of other people—a cry will bring you running, a chuckle will make you smile—associating a sound or word with an object or idea—seeing the car means "bye-bye" or "Dada"—and finally combining different sounds and words for more sophisticated communication. The "typical" baby will progress through the stages outlined below, but keep in mind that the timing of language acquisition is most unpredictable. Babies with otherwise perfectly normal development may be inexplicably slow to speak—Einstein was 4 years old before he spoke. Girls generally are quicker to learn than boys. If your household is bilingual, proficiency in one or both languages may be delayed but will catch up by the time your child enters kindergarten.

AGE	SPEECH DEVELOPMENT
4 months	makes sounds; coos and babbles
	connects the way they feel in the throat and on the tongue with their sound (storing auditory and motor patterns)
	notes your response to baby's different noises
6 months	laughs, chuckles, squeals, expresses emotions via sounds
	babbles, trying out vowel sounds punctuated with a few easy consonants (p, b, m, t, d), forming "Mama" and/or "Dada" (incidentally, these are the first words uttered by babies around the world)
	copies your intonation and modulation by varying volume, pitch and tone

AGE	SPEECH DEVELOPMENT
	pays more attention to other nonvoice noises such as music, associating the sound with its source
8 months	continues cooing and babbling; begins imitating your mouth and jaw movements
9–15 months	first word
9 months	strings nonsense syllables together
	mimics other throat and mouth sounds such as tongue clicks, hisses, coughs
	may use "Dada" and "Mama" as specific names
11 months	expands passive vocabulary (for example, understands more words such as "no" and recognizes own name)
	may utter 2 or 3 words but will substitute or omit difficult consonants, saying "ca" instead of cat
	recognizes words as symbols for objects or ideas
12 months	babbles in short "sentences," mimicking your tone and intonation
14–24 months	forms single-word sentences such as "Eat," meaning, "I want to eat" or "I'm eating"
	speech flourishes during this period, but some children hold back until they are 3 years old; if hearing is good, don't be overly concerned, so long as your baby has a good passive vocabulary; in other words, understands speech and your commands
24 months	puts 2 words together for sentences and begins to learn proper word order and rules of grammar (generally needs about a 50-word vocabulary to do so)
	continues to have trouble with certain consonants and letter combinations such as cracker = cwacker or three = tree or free
	has active vocabulary of about 300 words, but these may be unintelligible to strangers

DISCIPLINE: DIFFERENT APPROACHES

The word "discipline" too often conjures up only the idea of punishment, but in its fullest sense it also means teaching, explaining and rewarding. Everyone agrees that a child needs to learn what is acceptable behavior and what is not in order to get along with others, to develop self-control and to form a strong sense of self-esteem. Where there is wide disagreement, however, is on how and when to correct unacceptable behavior and whether the behavior of any baby under the age of 12 months can actually be called "bad."

Approaches in discipline where the ultimate goal is to help a child feel secure and act responsibly range from responding to all cries and protests to ignoring a great many of them. Some early-child-development experts reassure parents that it is only after the third month of life that babies can be spoiled, since it is only then that they are aware of their power to manipulate through fussing or whining. Others, like British child psychologist Penelope Leach, believe that "babies are not grown up or clever enough to be spoiled" and that instead of a baby's demanding more as he or she is given more, "parents who always meet their baby's demands fully and without unnecessary delay have less work, less drudgery and less stress." At the other extreme, setting limits very early on is the best way to cultivate a child's sense of security, according to Dr. William John Turtle, author of *Dr. Turtle's Babies.* Ignoring "unnecessary fussing" as soon as your baby is 8 weeks old will lay the foundation for respecting your authority and others' rights later on. Taking the opportunity to establish ground rules when an infant is young, argues Dr. Turtle, will pay off later, when the baby is mobile and needs—particularly for safety's sake—to respond obediently to commands of "no" and "don't."

Though there is no agreement on the timing, guidelines on how to discipline young babies are less controversial:

- keep emotion out of your response, because baby will focus on your reactions rather than on what you are teaching; furthermore, showing annoyance, exasperation or anger at protests or squirming usually only heats up the situation and is counterproductive
- be careful not to let your baby feel its behavior will affect your level of affection; in others words, you can show disapproval or disappointment while giving assurance of your unconditional love
- reward good behavior with smiles, hugs and praise; withdraw attention to show displeasure for bad behavior
- set firm limits, and above all be consistent about sticking to

them; if not, baby may become confused and unsure about what is expected, thereby creating possible anxiety and more fussiness

- present a united front with your husband; the two of you should agree on all the rules, since it takes only one parent to lose the other's hard-won ground quickly
- keep expectations realistic regarding how fast your baby can learn; resign yourself to much repetition

The specific ways you will want to correct, teach, explain and reward will depend on your temperament and your baby's. They will also need to be greatly modified as your child grows and begins to understand more sophisticated forms of communication. For infants and toddlers, Dr. Turtle advises simply ignoring unpleasant behavior unless it is truly disruptive or the bid for attention that it indicates is warranted. If that fails, "isolation," or withdrawing your attention by putting the baby in the playpen or crib for a few minutes until he or she calms down, is an approach that usually works without resorting to physical punishment or injuring the child's self-esteem. This restriction of movement for an active 1-year-old, however, may serve only to intensify the child's frustration.

No one has yet come up with a foolproof child-rearing method, so go with your own instincts, expect to make mistakes and try not to worry too much—children are remarkably resilient creatures. If you find, however, that all your effort seems ineffective and you come to dislike your baby, talk to other parents and to your baby's doctor about your feelings (and seek advice about sources of help). Parents Anonymous has a toll-free 24-hour hot line to help parents deal with anger, frustrations and other conflicted feelings about their children. Little has been written on training infants and young toddlers, but for older children, books such as *Parent Effectiveness Training* offer various approaches.

Information Sources

ADDITIONAL READING

Discipline: Preparing for Parenthood, by Dr. Lee Salk (New York: Bantam, 1980).

Dr. Turtle's Babies, by Dr. William John Turtle (New York: Popular Library, 1973).

How to Influence Children, by Charles Schaefer (New York: Van Nostrand Reinhold, 1983).

How to Parent, by Dr. Fitzhugh Dodson (New York: Signet, 1980).

Love and Discipline, by Barbara Brenner (New York: Ballantine, 1983).

P.E.T.—Parent Effectiveness Training, by Dr. Thomas Gordon (New York: Plume, 1975).

ORGANIZATIONS

Parents Anonymous
22330 Hawthorne Blvd., #208
Torrance, CA 90505
Toll-free 24-hour hot line is 800-421-0350 (in California 800-352-0386).

National Committee for Prevention of Child Abuse
332 S. Michigan Ave., #1250
Chicago, IL 60604
The booklet "You Can Prevent Child Abuse" and a sample copy of "Caring," its national newsletter, are available free.

PREDICTING YOUR BABY'S FUTURE SIZE

The first year of life sees a 50 percent increase in your baby's body length, a four-inch growth in head circumference and the doubling of brain weight. Total body weight doubles by five months of age and triples by your child's first birthday. The chart below shows ranges of small, average and large babies' weights and heights as checkpoints throughout the first 12 months.

BABY'S AGE	SMALL		AVERAGE		LARGE	
	Height	Weight	Height	Weight	Height	Weight
3 mos.	less than 22 in.	less than 10 lbs.	22–24.5 in.	10–13 lbs.	24.5–25 in.	13–16 lbs.
6 mos.	less than 24.5 in.	less than 14 lbs.	24.25–26 in.	14–17 lbs.	26–27.25 in.	17–20 lbs.
9 mos.	less than 26 in.	less than 16 lbs.	26–28 in.	16–20 lbs.	28–30 in.	20–24 lbs.
12 mos.	less than 28 in.	less than 17.25 lbs.	28–29 in.	17–22 lbs.	29–31 in.	22–27 lbs.

Adapted from *Infant Care,* published by the U.S. Dept. of Health and Human Services.

Birth weight is not a good indicator of your baby's size as an adult. A strapping nine-pound newborn boy will not necessarily grow up to be the size of a middle linebacker on the football team, and a dainty five-pound baby girl may very well outgrow the size of the standard ballerina. By age 2, however, you can get some rough idea of whether your child will grow to be small, average or large. If you have a boy, double his height in centimeters; if you have a daughter, double her height and then subtract 10 to 12 centimeters from that amount.

Abnormal growth that is not explained by heredity can indicate illness or an imbalance in your child's endocrine system. For this reason your baby's doctor will be recording weight and perhaps head measurements at each well-baby visit, to keep tabs on the steadiness of growth—this is more important than the amount or speed of physical development. By the time your child is 3, you should have some idea of whether the pace is normal. If you suspect a problem, you may want to consult a pediatric endocrinologist, who can run some simple tests to find out for sure.

BABY RECORDS

It is so easy to misplace important documents; for example, you may forget that your baby's birth certificate is in *Our Baby's First Seven Years* or in a drawer full of old car-insurance policies and other papers. Think about keeping *all* baby records in one file, somewhere in a safe place. Items you will probably want to include in the file are:

- copy of birth certificate
- blood type, Rh factor
- name of health-insurance company and policy number
- certificate of baptism
- immunization record (wallet-size card listing the date for each inoculation given by your baby's doctor; you may want to keep another record of shots and drops just in case you lose the card)
- child health-record booklet to keep track of illnesses or injuries along with any medical treatment
- canceled checks or other proof of child-care expenses if you qualify for the IRS tax credit

There are several other legal matters you may want to consider for your child during the first year.

Authorization for medical treatment. In the event that you are away and your baby needs prompt medical attention requiring a parent's or guardian's approval, you may want to leave a signed authorization form with whoever is caring for your child in your absence. Ask your baby's doctor about obtaining the necessary forms.

Social security number. If your baby receives U.S. savings bonds, stocks or other monetary gifts, you will want to put them in a separate savings account, since IRS taxes are less for children's dividend income than for adults'. In order to open an account, however, your baby needs a social security number, which can be obtained by applying to your local social security office. Be sure to take along with you a copy of your baby's birth certificate and two pieces of ID for you (such as driver's license or passport).

Fingerprinting. In order to trace missing or kidnapped children, police departments in several states have programs to fingerprint children of all ages. Check with your local police department if this interests you. The American Civil Liberties Union advises that you keep the fingerprint documents yourself rather than let them become police property.

Appendix

ORGANIZATIONS AND GOVERNMENT RESOURCES

These organizations complement the individual listings in the "Information Sources," found at the end of most sections.

Alcohol, Drug Abuse and Mental Health Administration
5600 Fishers La.
Rockville, MD 20857
This government agency publishes such pamphlets as "Importance of Play" and "Pre-Term Babies," and sponsors ongoing research on subjects including maternal/infant bonding.

Alliance for Perinatal Research and Services (APRS)
P.O. Box 6358
Alexandria, VA 22306
APRS is an interdisciplinary group with areas of expertise including childbirth preparation for men and women, fathers (issues related to pregnancy and postpartum), breastfeeding; books, tapes, publications.

American Academy of Pediatrics (AAP)
1801 Hinman Ave.
Evanston, IL 60204
AAP has a publications catalog available, with useful inexpensive pamphlets on topics such as first aid and child-restraint systems.

American College of Nurse-Midwives (ACNM)
1522 K St., NW, #110
Washington, DC 20005
ACNM establishes and maintains standards for the practice of nurse-midwifery and can refer you to certified nurse-midwives practicing where you live.

American College of Obstetricians and Gynecologists (ACOG)
Resource Center
600 Maryland Ave., SW
Washington, DC 20024
ACOG sets national standards in obstetrical education and practice; free copies of a number of patient-information booklets are available on such topics as alcohol during pregnancy.

American Foundation for Maternal and Child Health
30 Beekman Pl.
New York, NY 10022
This foundation, headed by Doris Haire, acts as a clearinghouse on birth practices and makes available such pamphlets as "How the FDA Determines The Safety of Drugs: Just How 'Safe' is Safe?" Send a self-addressed, stamped envelope for pamphlets.

American Red Cross National Headquarters
Health Services
17th and D Sts., NW
Washington, DC 20006
Local American Red Cross chapters sponsor such courses as Preparation for Parenthood and Parenting, Baby-sitting, as well as programs in safety and accident prevention.

ASPO-Lamaze
1840 Wilson Blvd., #204
Arlington, VA 22201
The American Society of Psycho-prophylaxis in Obstetrics promotes the Lamaze method of prepared childbirth and sponsors a nationally standardized teacher certification program. ASPO also publishes the magazine *Genesis* and makes other literature available to its members.

Association for Childhood Education International (ACEI)
3615 Wisconsin Ave., NW
Washington, DC 20016
ACEI focuses on children, from infancy through early adolescence, and has numerous publications available.

Cesarean/Support, Education, Concern
22 Forest Rd.
Farmington, MA 01701
C/SEC publishes booklets on a range of topics including father-attended cesarean birth.

Coalition for the Medical Rights of Women (CMRW)
1638-B Haight St.
San Francisco, CA 94117
CMRW is consumer-oriented and publishes several booklets on prenatal issues as well as the newsletter *Second Opinion*.

Consumer Product Safety Commission (CPSC)
Washington, DC 20207
CPSC sponsors toll-free hot line (800) 638-CPSC to handle requests for publications and questions on safety standards for cribs, toys and other accessories for infants and children. CPSC should be notified about any product-related injuries.

Cybele Society
Suite 414, Peyton Bldg.
Spokane, WA 99201
This national professional organization focuses on hospital family-centered maternity care. Many of their publications, such as "The Cybele Cluster: A Single Room Maternity Care System for High- and Low-Risk Families," are useful, par-

ticularly for those interested in implementing a family-centered approach.

Its Resource Center contains more than 2000 articles and books on family-oriented maternal and newborn care and is available to nonmembers for a fee.

The Farm
P.O. Box 156
Summertown, TN 38483
Lay midwives from The Farm serve as an informal clearinghouse on home childbirth and publish *Spiritual Midwifery* and other books.

Food and Drug Administration
5600 Fishers La.
Rockville, MD 20857
This government agency regulates such obstetrical devices as ultrasound scans (sonograms) and pharmaceuticals such as the morning-sickness drug Bendectin.

Healthy Mothers, Healthy Babies
  Coalition
Department of Public Affairs
Public Health Service
200 Independence Ave., SW, Rm.
  721-H
Washington, DC 20201
This coalition is an informal association of organizations including the American Academy of Pediatrics, American College of Obstetricians and Gynecologists, March of Dimes and U.S. Public Health Service. It publishes a quarterly newsletter and a directory (both of which are primarily distributed to coalition members and in turn to hospitals and clinics).

International Childbirth Education
  Association (ICEA)

PO Box 20048
Minneapolis, MN 55420
ICEA is an interdisciplinary organization that operates a mail-order bookstore and publishes a newsletter and numerous pamphlets on maternal and newborn health.

La Leche League International
  (LLLI)
9616 Minneapolis Ave.
Franklin Park, IL 60131
LLLI has local chapters throughout the U.S. and breast-feeding support groups for mothers; a newsletter and other literature are available to nonmembers.

Military Family Resource Center
% Joy Duva, 6501 Loisdale Court
Springfield, VA 22150
Member of Healthy Mothers, Healthy Babies Coalition which can provide information to military spouses.

National Association of
  Childbearing Centers
Box 1, Route 1
Perkiomenville, PA 18074
This organization serves as an information clearinghouse on out-of-hospital birth centers.

National Association of Parents and
  Professionals for Safe
  Alternatives in Childbirth
  (NAPSAC)
PO Box 428
Marble Hill, MO 63764
NAPSAC publishes such books as *Twenty-First Century Obstetrics Now!* and is concerned about obstetrical interventions and hospital practice.

National Center for Health
  Statistics (NCHS)

Natality Branch
U.S. Public Health Service
3700 East-West Hwy.
Hyattsville, MD 20782
NCHS can give you the latest statistics; for example, the cesarean rate in the Midwest among specific age groups.

National Committee for Prevention of Child Abuse
332 S. Michigan Ave., #1250
Chicago, IL 60604
A booklet, "You Can Prevent Child Abuse," and a sample copy of *Caring*, national newsletter, are available.

National Foundation—March of Dimes
Public Health Education Department
1275 Mamaroneck Ave.
White Plains, NY 10605
The March of Dimes distributes free pamphlets and fact sheets on such concerns as birth defects, prematurity, toxoplasmosis; catalog is available. Makes referrals to genetic specialists in your area.

National Health Information Clearinghouse (NHIC)
PO Box 1133
Washington, DC 20013
(800) 336-4797
NHIC can refer you to organizations that can best answer your questions. Has a data base of 1500 health-information resources and maintains a health-information library of 750 books, 200 periodicals and vertical files on 550 health subjects.

National Institutes of Health
National Institute of Child

Health and Human Development (NICHD)
Office of Research Reporting
Bldg. 31, Room 2A-32
Bethesda, MD 20205
NICHD is sponsoring research on hundreds of concerns ranging from sports during pregnancy to sudden infant death syndrome.
Reports, special publications, and conference proceedings such as *Antenatal Diagnosis* and *Cesarean Childbirth* are produced by NICHD.

National Poison Center Network
Children's Hospital of Pittsburgh
125 DeSoto St.
Pittsburgh, PA 15213
The national headquarters can direct you to one of its 55 poison control centers near you; for a small fee will provide Mr. Yuk stickers and aids in teaching your child about poisons.

National Poison Control Clearinghouse
5600 Fishers La.
Rockville, MD 20857
This clearinghouse can provide you with the phone number and address of the poison control center nearest you, at your written request.

National Self-Help Clearinghouse
184 Fifth Ave.
New York, NY 10010
This clearinghouse has the names of parent groups in your community. If you form a group, let them know so they can put others in touch with you.

National Women's Health Network
224 7th St., SE
Washington, DC 20003

This organization monitors legislative and regulatory developments in Washington and also publishes numerous publications on a variety of topics.

Nurse's Association of the American College of Obstetricians and Gynecologists (NAACOG)
600 Maryland Ave., SW
Washington, DC 20024
NAACOG may be able to help you locate local childbirth-preparation groups and other resources.

U.S. Department of Health and Human Services
Office of Human Development Services
Hubert Humphrey Bldg., Rm. 309F
200 Independence Ave., SW
Washington, DC 20201
Along with the National Institutes of Health, this government agency is concerned with maternal and infant care and publishes *Prenatal Care, Infant Care* and other government bestsellers that are sold by the Government Printing Office (see "Catalogs and Publication Lists, p. 455).

U.S. Pharmacopoeia (USP)
12601 Twinbrook Pkwy.
Rockville, MD 20852
USP, a nonprofit private agency that sets standards for all drugs marketed in the U.S., publishes a newsletter for consumers and several reference books, including *About Your Medicines During Pregnancy, Labor and Breast-feeding;* its data base is accessible.

RESEARCH ON YOUR OWN

The organizations and government agencies we have listed are a good starting point for doing your own research. The March of Dimes Foundation, for example, will send you its fact sheets and cite pertinent articles published in medical journals. Check into the availability of periodicals, textbooks and other literature.

(1) Your obstetrician, midwife, family practitioner or pediatrician probably subscribes to several medical journals.
(2) Most hospital libraries are open to the public.
(3) Most local chapters of ASPO-Lamaze, La Leche League, Red Cross and so forth have lending libraries.
(4) Most university medical libraries have an impressive number of titles.

If you want to read about the most recent findings, for instance, on the effects of sonograms on the unborn baby, consult *Index Medicus,* which is available at many public libraries, most hospital libraries and all medical libraries. *Index Medicus* is issued each month and indexes over 2500 journals, in addition to monographs and conference proceedings. The publisher of *Index Medicus,* the National Library of Medicine, provides the MEDLINE and MEDLARS search services through local medical libraries. For a small fee ($2.00 and up), the librarian can provide you with a print-out of all the articles published in journals indexed in *Index Medicus* on any subject. To obtain a current list of Literature Search titles (key words), send your name and address, typed on a gummed label, to: Literature Search Program, Reference Section, National Library of Medicine, 8600 Rockville Pike, Bethesda, MD 20209.

You may find some medical journals are weighty and technical, while others are more accessible to the lay person, such as the British journal *Lancet,* which has a reputation for accepting scientific work that is extremely promising but still tentative. Here is a sampling of journals that you might find helpful:

> *American Journal of Maternal Child Nursing*
> *American Journal of Nurse-Midwifery*
> *American Journal of Obstetrics and Gynecology*
> *American Journal of Public Health*
> *Birth: Issues in Perinatal Care and Education Briefs*
> *British Journal of Obstetrics and Gynaecology*
> *Child Development Abstracts and Bibliography*
> *Contemporary Ob/Gyn*
> *Journal of the American Medical Association*
> *Journal of Pediatrics*
> *Lancet*
> *New England Journal of Medicine*
> *Obstetrical and Gynecological Survey*
> *Obstetrics and Gynecology*
> *Pediatrics*
> *Science*
> *Women and Health*

Also remember to contact the National Health Information Clearinghouse for organizations and societies that focus on specific subjects of concern to you.

MAGAZINES AND NEWSLETTERS

The subscription prices quoted here probably have increased, so you may want to do some double-checking before sending any money. Free sample copies are often available.

Baby Talk

This monthly magazine contains primarily brief, general-interest articles for new parents. $6.75/yr. Subscription address: 185 Madison Ave., New York, NY 10016.

Birth

This magazine, sponsored by ICEA and ASPO-Lamaze, publishes new studies and abstracts and evaluates articles from medical journals on many issues of concern to expectant parents, including early hospital discharge and the adjustment to motherhood. $12.00/yr. Subscription address: 110 El Camino Real, Berkeley, CA 94705.

Briefs

This digest magazine carries several short abstracts from medical journals, such as on saunas during pregnancy, and discusses other issues concerning maternity and child care. It is published by the Maternity Center Association, the oldest out-of-hospital birth facility in the U.S. $8.00/yr. Subscription address: Charles B. Slack, Inc., 6900 Grove Rd., Thorofare, NJ 08086.

Childbirth Alternatives Quarterly

This newsletter is consumer-oriented, with articles on midwifery, home birth, birth stories and reprints of articles about mothers and children. $10.00/yr. Subscription address: CAQ, % Ashford, Bin 62—SLAC, Stanford, CA 94305.

Childbirth Educator

This quarterly magazine for childbirth instructors includes first-rate feature articles on subjects ranging from positions during labor to nursing bras. $10.00/year. Subscription address: Dept. ABM, 352 Evelyn St., Paramus, NJ 07652.

FDA Consumer

This newsletter covers current information on numerous health issues ranging from caffeine intake during pregnancy to electronic fetal monitors. $21.00/yr. Subscription address: Superintendent of Documents, Government Printing Office, Washington, DC 20402.

Genesis

Each issue of this magazine, published by ASPO-Lamaze, focuses primarily on one subject, such as vaginal birth after cesarean. $10.00/yr. for single parents and $15.00/yr. for couples. Subscription address: PO Box 33429, Farragut Station, Washington, DC 20033.

Growing Child

This personal monthly newsletter tracks a child's development from birth to 6 years of age. Subscribers also receive another newsletter, *Growing Parents*, and a catalog of toys and books. $11.95/yr. Send expected birth date or your child's birth date to PO Box 620, Lafayette, IN 47902.

ICEA News

This newsletter carries news about legislative and regulatory developments as well as articles on such topics as vaginal breech deliveries and is published by the International Childbirth Education Association. $5.00/yr. for nonmembers. Subscription address: P.O. Box 20048, Minneapolis, MN 55420.

Mothering
This quarterly magazine is oriented toward holistic childbirth and parenting, with an emphasis on midwifery and natural baby products. $8.00/yr. Subscription address: PO Box 2208, Albuquerque, NM 87103.

Mothers Today
This bimonthly magazine includes information of general interest to new parents, along with editorials. $6.00/yr. Subscription address: 212 Arbor Rd., Franklin Lakes, NJ 07417.

NAPSAC News
This newsletter reports on political and professional activities primarily with regard to home births and is published by the National Association of Parents and Professionals for Safe Alternatives in Childbirth. $10.00/yr. Subscription address: P.O. Box 428, Marble Hill, MO 63764.

New Parent Adviser
This magazine sponsored by Johnson & Johnson contains many useful articles primarily about concerns during the first few months postpartum. Available only from hospital maternity wards.

News From H.O.M.E.
This quarterly newsletter covers such topics as herbal remedies during pregnancy and other concerns of particular interest to those planning a home birth. $12.00/yr. Subscription address: HOME, 18515 Owl Run Way, Germantown, MD 20874.

Parent's Choice
This bimonthly tabloid contains advice to parents on selecting the best television programs, music, books,

toys and games. $10.00/yr. Subscription address: Box 185, Waban, MA 02168.

Parents Magazine
This monthly magazine has columns on topics ranging from travel during pregnancy to toilet training. $12.00/yr. Subscription address: PO Box 7000, Bergenfield, NJ 97621.

Pediatrics For Parents
This monthly newsletter reports on an array of child health and safety topics such as tips on how to give medicines to an infant. $12.00/yr. Subscription address: 176 Mt. Hope Ave., Bangor, ME 04401.

Practical Parenting Newsletter
This bimonthly newsletter, published by author Vicki Lansky, offers useful hints on everything from weaning to helping shy children. $6.50/yr. Subscription address: 18326B Minnetonka Blvd., Deephaven, MN 55391.

Pre-Parent Adviser
This newsletter sponsored by Johnson & Johnson contains a lot of information useful to expectant mothers and fathers. Available from many childbirth educators but not by subscription.

Salk Letter
This monthly newsletter, written by Dr. Lee Salk, includes regular features on new medical findings, treatment of health problems for children of all ages and interviews with child psychologists. $18.00/yr. Subscription address: 941 Park Ave., New York, NY 10028.

Working Mother
This monthly magazine offers advice on such topics as good-quality child care and preparing quick family din-

ners. $14.00/yr. Subscription address: PO Box 10609, Des Moines, IA 50336.

CATALOGS AND PUBLICATION LISTS

The information trail continues. These catalogs let you know about new books for expectant mothers and new parents.

American Academy of Pediatrics
1801 Hinman Ave.
Evanston, IL 60204
Free publications list available, which includes patient-education materials such as "Child Health Record" and "Human Milk Banking."

American College of Obstetricians
  and Gynecologists
Resource Center
600 Maryland Ave., SW
Washington, DC 20024
Free list of ACOG's patient information booklets.

Birth and Life Bookstore
PO Box 70625
Seattle, WA 98107
This is the oldest mail-order house. It carries hundreds of titles, many of which can no longer be purchased at your local bookstore. Write for a free copy of "Imprints."

Child Welfare League
67 Irving Pl.
New York, NY 10003
Free catalog of the League's publications, which include "The Essentials of Parenting in the First Years of Life."

Consumer Information Center
Pueblo, CO 81007
Government publications are available from this clearinghouse, as is a free catalog.

FDA Consumer Information
5700 Fishers La., Rm. 15B32
Rockville, MD 20857
Catalog available describing publications, slide shows and films produced by the U.S. Food and Drug Administration.

Government Printing Office (GPO)
Superintendent of Documents
Washington, DC 20402
GPO sells hundreds of titles, but to order you must know the GPO stock number and price; a free catalog is available.

Growing Child Store
PO Box 620
Lafayette, IN 47902
This catalog full of books and toys for infants and toddlers is free to subscribers of the monthly newsletter *Growing Child*; otherwise it costs $1.00.

Health Education Associates, Inc.
211 South Easton Rd.
Glenside, PA 19038
Free catalog is available, listing inexpensive pamphlets for new parents, including such titles as "Fathers Ask: Questions About Breast-feeding."

Healthy Mothers Coalition Directory of Education Materials
Office of Public Affairs
Public Health Service
200 Independence Ave., SW
Washington, DC 20201
This directory lists services and information available from coalition members; write for price and availability.

ICEA Bookcenter
PO Box 20048
Minneapolis, MN 55420
This mail-order bookstore is run by the International Childbirth Education Association; a free copy of *ICEA Bookmarks*, which reviews new books and ICEA's own publications about pregnancy, childbirth, breast-feeding and early child care, is available if you send a stamped, self-addressed #10 (business) envelope to receive a copy of the most recent booklist ($.20 postage) or *Bookmarks* ($.37 postage).

Informal Birth and Parenting Bookstore
501 Berkeley Ave.
Ann Arbor, MI 48103
This mail-order bookstore specializes in publications and manuals for those planning a home birth.

National Institute of Child Health and Human Development
Office of Research Reporting
NIH Bldg. 31, Rm. 2A-32
Bethesda, MD 20205
Free publications list of NICHD materials and reprints from various medical journals.

National Institutes of Health
Office of Communications, OD
Division of Public Information
Editorial Operations Branch
Bethesda, MD 20205
NIH publications list is a valuable resource, which includes research news and other information from all the Institutes.

Orange Cat
442 Church St.
Garverville, CA 95440
This mail-order bookstore carries titles on birth and parenting; for example, "Herbs, Helps and Pressure Points For Pregnancy and Childbirth" and the cassette tape "Suite Baby Dreams."

The Pennypress
1100 23rd Ave. E.
Seattle, WA 98112
Free list of books and pamphlets on childbirth and parenting, including such titles as "Obstetric Tests and Technology" and "When Your Baby Has Jaundice."

KEY TELEPHONE NUMBERS

Emergency Ambulance
_____

Fire
_____

Police
_____

Baby's Doctor Weekdays:
_____

Evenings and Weekends:
_____

Pharmacy
_____

Mother's Office
_____

Father's Office
_____

Neighbor(s)
_____
_____

Nearest Relative
_____

Babysitter or Day-Care Center
_____
_____

Poison Control Center (local toll-free number)
_____

National Sudden Infant Death Syndrome Foundation 301-459-3388
_____

Consumer Product Safety Commission 800-638-CPSC (in MD: 800-492-8363)
_____

National Health Clearinghouse 800-336-4797 (in VA, call collect: 703-522-2590)
_____

Parents Anonymous 800-421-0350 (in CA: 800-352-0386)
_____

Index